The PRACTICAL ENCYCLOPEDIA *of* SEX *and* HEALTH

The PRACTICAL ENCYCLOPEDIA *of* SEX *and* HEALTH

From Aphrodisiacs and Hormones to Potency,
Stress, Vasectomy and Yeast Infection

By STEFAN BECHTEL
AND THE EDITORS OF **Men's Health**
AND ***PREVENTION*** MAGAZINES

Rodale Press, Emmaus, Pennsylvania

Editor: Alice Feinstein
Cover and Book Designer: Acey Lee
Cover Photographer: James McLoughlin

The table on page 74 is reproduced and modified with the permission of the Population Council, from James Trussell et al, "Contraceptive Failure in the United States: An Update," *Studies in Family Planning* 21, no. 1 (January/February 1992).

Library of Congress Cataloging-in-Publication Data

Bechtel, Stefan.
    The practical encyclopedia of sex and health : from aphrodisiacs and hormones to potency, stress, vasectomy and yeast infection / by Stefan Bechtel and the editors of Men's health and Prevention magazines.
        p.   cm.
    Includes index.
    ISBN 0–87596–163–0   hardcover
    1. Hygiene, Sexual—Encyclopedias.   I. Men's health (Magazine)
II. Prevention (Emmaus, Pa.)   III. Title.
RA788.B43   1993
613.9′03 — dc20   92–35043
                                                                CIP

Distributed in the book trade by St. Martin's Press

              8   10   9   hardcover

NOTICE

This book is meant to increase your knowledge of human sexuality. Because everyone is different, a physician must diagnose conditions and supervise the treatment of individual health and sexuality problems. The information here is designed to help you make informed choices about your health. It is not intended as a substitute for any treatment prescribed by your doctor.

To the woman in the red dress

CONTENTS

x

FOREWORD

Sexual health is something of an enigma for many of us: It is taken for granted when we have it and sorely missed when we don't. Furthermore, sexual health is assumed by so many of us to be automatic that we pay little attention to how it can be maintained. Here, more than in most other areas of health, people are often unaware of fundamental preventive measures they can follow to ensure healthy sexual functioning. Regrettably, the medical profession has largely ignored this issue, with most primary care physicians doing little in terms of preventive counseling in their contacts with patients. In fact, even in situations where sexual problems are likely to occur—for example, in the aftermath of a heart attack, in association with alcoholism or other forms of drug abuse, in the medical management of people with high blood pressure—many physicians are themselves unaware of the requisite biomedical and psychological facts that would prevent a sizable percentage of the sexual difficulties that arise. Add to this the reality that many practicing physicians are personally uncomfortable discussing issues of sexuality with their patients, and it becomes obvious that there is a real vacuum of information related to sexual health even in contemporary American society.

At one level, many of the sexual problems that occur are still regarded as trivial in the sense that they are neither life-threatening nor even associated with major health consequences, in the ordinary way we think about our health. But this is a skewed assessment—and an assessment that can be tossed out the window when you or someone you love is affected. After all, these seemingly "trivial" sexual problems have a great deal to do with the quality of our lives. Just ask a woman who is dealing with a nonexistent sex drive during her menopausal years, or a man who can't control his ejaculations, or a 28-year-old who can't consummate his marriage if their problem is trivial or important.

Today more than at any time in the last 50 years, sexual behavior is also linked to a number of health problems that are serious and sometimes incurable. Estimates of the scope of the worldwide HIV/AIDS epidemic grow year by year, and the notion that "it can't happen to me" is slowly evolving into a different sort of national consciousness. Less visible, but also serious, are raging epidemics of other sexually transmitted diseases, including gonorrhea, chlamydia, genital herpes, hepatitis B and genital warts caused by the human papilloma family of viruses. According to recent estimates from the Centers for Disease Control in Atlanta, there are probably 9 million cases a year of these STDs in the United States; and the World Health Organization estimates that worldwide, there are more than 150 million cases annually. Since some of these conditions are linked to subsequent cases of cancer or infertility, it is clear that their ramifications are major indeed.

Fortunately, this is also a time of signal advances in the treatment of many sexual and reproductive problems. Today there are near miraculous techniques for treating infertility; a wide (and confusing) variety of treatments for problems such as impotence; more contraceptive options than ever before; and more sophisticated psychotherapeutic methods for dealing with sexual disorders than could have been imagined just a quarter-century ago. Unfortunately, up until now, the general public has not really had much guidance in sorting through this maze of high-tech, rapidly evolving treatments and diagnostic approaches.

This book specifically and skillfully fills this void. This is a well-designed, well-researched volume that avoids technical jargon in favor of clear, accessible, easy-to-grasp information. Whether you read it cover to cover or simply put it on the bookshelf for use as a reference, you will find that this is indeed a "user-friendly" book as well as a book that is loaded with immensely practical advice.

Robert C. Kolodny, M.D.
medical director, Behavioral Medicine Institute, New Canaan, Connecticut
former associate director and director of training, Masters & Johnson Institute, St. Louis, Missouri

ACKNOWLEDGMENTS

To all those busy sex therapists, doctors, researchers and scientists who shared their time and wisdom during the making of this book, my humble thanks. For efforts well beyond the call of duty, I'd like to particularly thank E. Douglas Whitehead, M.D., a director of the Association for Male Sexual Dysfunction in New York City; the wise and jovial sex therapist Jude Cotter, Ph.D., of Farmington Hills, Michigan; New York City sex therapist Shirley Zussman, Ed.D., who was always kind, patient and insightful; Howard Ruppel, executive director of the Society for the Scientific Study of Sex, ever at the ready with his amazing Rolodex and the perfect person to interview; Judith H. Seifer, Ph.D., R.N., of Wright State University School of Medicine in Dayton, Ohio, for her patient assistance in helping me understand the mysteries of female hormonal cycles; Robert Birch, Ph.D., director of the Arlington Center for Marital and Sexual Concerns in Columbus, Ohio, whose day-long presentation at a conference on human sexuality gave me invaluable understanding into sex therapy; the great, gray ghost of Dr. Alfred Kinsey, who helped me rediscover human sexuality a thousand times, in a thousand different ways; Robert Kolodny, M.D., medical director and chairman of the board of the Behavioral Medicine Institute in New Canaan, Connecticut, who read and commented upon this manuscript to ensure its accuracy; and my wonderful wife, Kae, and my kids, Lilly and Adam, who blessed me and supported me through the whole period.

I'd also like to thank my fine, ever-cheerful editor, Alice Feinstein; Bill Gottlieb, who proposed the project and got me the job; Christine Dreisbach, my tireless researcher; and my agent, Connie Clausen.

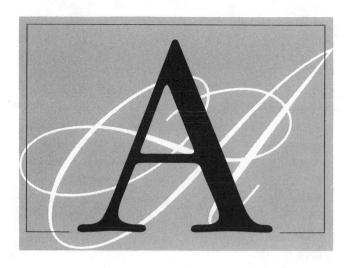

ABSTINENCE

One way of dealing with the wonderful, mysterious and sometimes rather terrifying power of one's sexuality is simply to abstain from expressing it at all. This is an option people have exercised for centuries, for brief or prolonged periods and for a variety of reasons ranging from religious conviction to lack of desire to lack of a partner.

There's nothing wrong with abstinence and no reason to believe it's harmful to one's health, according to the Kinsey Institute. But it is, perhaps, a testament to the astounding power of sexual desire that there are so few individuals who remain sexually abstinent for very long. (The body provides an "escape valve" for sexual tension, even for those who are abstinent during their waking lives—both men and women experience orgasm during sleep, although only men produce nocturnal emissions.)

Who Does and Who Doesn't

The late Dr. Alfred Kinsey found in an early survey that among men under age 31, only 2.9 percent were completely abstinent or had sex once every ten weeks or less often. Only 11.2 percent of men in this age group reported having orgasms as seldom as once every two weeks or less frequently.

Women of all ages were considerably more likely to be sexually abstinent than men, Dr. Kinsey found. And of course, as people get older, they're much more likely to become sexually inactive (although usually because of ill health or loss of a spouse, not by choice).

One recent survey of almost 2,000 men and women over the age of 60 found that 26 percent of the married men and 44 percent of the married women reported that they were no longer sexually active. (Yes, there *is* a strange discrepancy in those numbers, but it's not clear who is lying, or why.) Among unmarried men over 60, 69 percent said they were abstinent; a rather astonishing 95 percent of unmarried women that age said they were not sexually active.

The Consequences of Doing Without

What happens to your body during periods of brief or prolonged sexual austerity?

For Men: Super Sperm

In men, brief periods of sexual restraint seem to increase both the volume and the potency of semen. In a Swedish study, semen samples taken from a group of healthy men after one day of sexual abstinence and then later, after three days of abstinence, showed that when the men refrained from sex, the total volume of their ejaculate increased, as did the concentration of sperm. In fact, after three days, their total sperm count more than doubled.

Generally, guidelines for sperm donors and couples being evaluated for the treatment of infertility are to have the man refrain from ejaculation for three to six days before giving a specimen or having a sperm count done, in order to optimize the sperm count.

For Women: Vaginal Atrophy

But prolonged sexual abstinence, especially in women, may result in genital changes that make it a little more difficult to resume a satisfying sex life later on.

Older women who lose their husbands, for instance, often notice that their vaginas gradually grow drier and less elastic. In older women who are sexually abstinent for many years, the vagina even may gradually begin to close up and "undergo such severe atrophy that intercourse becomes virtually impossible," says Gloria A. Bachmann, M.D., associate professor of obstetrics and gynecology at Robert Wood Johnson Medical School in New Providence, New Jersey.

On the other hand, the best way for older women to stay "genitally healthy" is to stay sexually active. Sometimes, obviously, that may not be a realistic option. But studies have shown that "women who continue to be sexually active, either with a partner or through self-stimulation, maintain a more nearly normal state of genital health than abstinent women," Dr. Bachmann says.

In one study of 59 women aged 60 to 70, for instance, those who remained sexually active had significantly less vaginal atrophy and greater vaginal elasticity, depth and lubrication than those who had closed the book on their sexual lives. In sex, as in many other areas of human physiology, the old, crude adage applies: "Use it or lose it."

Abstinence as Ritual

Many religious orders of priests, monks and nuns require lifelong sexual abstinence of their members, but the notion that sustained sexual abstinence is a good and purifying thing probably predates modern religions. In some primitive societies, male hunters are required to abstain from intercourse for a short period before they go on a journey or a big hunt, and women must also practice abstinence before they brew beer or sow crops—otherwise, it's believed, the enterprise will fail. Anthropologists suggest that these ritual forms of abstinence may have been primitive humanity's attempt to control the forces of nature by reining in one of the wildest and most uncontrollable forces of all, thereby snatching a handful of power from the radiant realm of the spirits.

If you think that's a crazy, primitive idea, why does almost every modern-day coach or athlete have a strong opinion, one way or the other, as to the advisability of sexual abstinence on the night before a big game? One recent review of the medical literature, by the way, found virtually *no* evidence to support either idea—that pregame abstinence was good or that it was bad.

The Great Sublimation Debate

Then there's the notion that prolonged sexual abstinence can be a way of "sublimating," or diverting, energy to higher things—the dross of mere physical desire transformed into the gold of great art or literature. This notion, often ascribed to Freud, is a much more ancient human idea—but there doesn't seem to be much evidence to support it.

History does have its share of accomplished poets, artists and scientists who seem to have been sexual teetotalers—but a much greater number of famous people were known to have an enthusiastic appetite for the pleasures of the flesh.

After studying the tiny proportion of men in his sample who reported having sex twice a month or less for the past five years, Dr. Kinsey was particularly skeptical that there was anything to the idea of sublimation. Virtually all of these men were in poor health, extremely timid or inhibited, restrained by religious conviction or simply had very low levels of sexual desire. At least among this group, Dr. Kinsey found no evidence at all that any of them had successfully sublimated their lowly desires into lofty achievement.

ADDICTION, SEXUAL

Is it possible to get "hooked" on sexual pleasure, just the way people get addicted to alcohol or drugs?

In recent years, the question has become one of the hottest debates in psychology. On the one hand, many responsible sex experts claim there are a huge number of people whose craving for the "high" of sex—usually promiscuous, anonymous sex—can legitimately be considered a true addiction. In extreme cases, these addicts hunt so obsessively for illicit sexual stimulation that it wrecks their marriages, careers and physical health. Says Minneapolis family therapist Patrick Carnes, Ph.D.: "What we're talking about is a loss of control and a willingness to risk any kind of consequence for a pleasure that gets you so hooked you cannot stop." But this "pleasure," he adds, "is not about sex—it's about dissociation from pain."

On the other hand, other authorities complain that "sex addiction" is a fad diagnosis for something that cannot legitimately be considered a true addiction at all. Some believe, if anything, it's a problem more closely related to compulsions like anorexia than addictions like alcoholism. Others note that if this problem is an addiction, it's the only one whose "cure" doesn't require complete abstinence. (After all, you can live without alcohol or drugs, but it would be both unhealthy and unrealistic to ask people to live without sex.)

How Much Is Too Much?

Still other skeptics point out that in order to define what's sexually "addictive," you have to define what's not, and sexual normalcy is very much a function of our culture. On the South Pacific island of Magaia, for instance, "casual sex with different partners and frequent intercourse with multiple orgasms (as many as three climaxes nightly) are perceived as sexually normal," according to one anthropologist. In our culture, that would no doubt be considered an addiction of the highest order (although perhaps an enviable one). Or is the reason so many people are now desperately trying to "kick the habit" of promiscuity simply that they're afraid of AIDS?

Well, let's just skip all these dainty intellectual arguments. The fact remains that there are people out there whose sexual appetites have gotten desperately out of control. The most immediate question for you is, Am I one of them? How do you tell if a merely lusty libido has slipped over some indefinable line and turned into a sick, compulsive craving? And what can you do about it if it has?

Profiling the Sex Addict

Dr. Carnes, whose 1983 best-seller *Out of the Shadows* drew attention to the problem, says sex addicts usually have a recognizable psychological profile. For one thing, the vast majority are men—they outnumber women four to one, in fact. More than 80 percent have some other kind of addiction—to the bottle, to gambling, to drugs ("Cocaine is the drug of choice for sex addicts," says Dr. Carnes). They generally suffer from low self-esteem. And they almost invariably report having been abused as children. Sex addiction, in fact, may be one of the many long-range consequences of child abuse—tragedy on a slow fuse. Abused kids not only come to feel worthless, they also come to think humiliation and shame are a part of normal sexual expression.

How many sex addicts are there? Dr. Carnes estimates there may be as many as 7 to 14 million in the United States alone—3 to 6 percent of the population. The most common form of addict, he says, is the person who flits from affair to affair and may occasionally visit prostitutes, porn shops or blue movies. Although he or she feels ashamed and is secretive about such behavior, it continues even despite efforts to stop. "Second level" addicts are those whose behavior has escalated into things that could get them arrested and often involves a victim—exhibitionism, voyeurism, obscene phone calls. At its most extreme level, sex addiction can turn into the most heinous of crimes, like rape, incest or child molestation.

6

How can you tell if your sexual urges have started to run out of control? Dr. Carnes suggests that you consider the following factors. If most of your answers to the pertinent questions are yes, there may well be an element of unhealthy compulsion in your sexual behavior.

Feelings of despair. After sex, do you have feelings of shame, despair, emptiness?

Secrecy. Do you feel a need to keep your sexual behavior a secret? Do you thrive on the thrill of leading a clandestine "double life"?

Abuse. Do you engage in sexual practices that are abusive or exploitative? Do you have sex with partners who are not completely willing?

Empty relationships. Do you have sex with partners whom you don't really even know—or, worse, whom you don't even like?

Compromised values. Does your sexual behavior consistently violate your ethical values?

So many people have found themselves giving distressing answers to these questions that a nationwide sexual addiction recovery movement has emerged in the United States in recent years. Four major self-help groups, all of them modeled on the 12-step recovery program developed by Alcoholics Anonymous, have come into existence. The goal of these programs, according to one recovering sex addict, is to regain control of your life by "finding your original, authentic sexuality" under the heavy clouds of shame and sickness. But it's not easy. Another ex-addict says recovering from alcoholism is "a walk on the beach" compared with overcoming the shame and degradation of sex addiction. Still, if you've got a problem, a self-help group may be your best hope. You may wish to contact a national self-help group, which could have a local branch in your area (Sexaholics Anonymous, Box 300, Simi Valley, CA 93062; or Sex Addicts Anonymous, P.O. Box 3038, Minneapolis, MN 55403).

AFFAIRS

According to the Kinsey Institute, which recently reviewed all the major sex studies published over the past 40 years, about 37 percent of married men and 29 percent of married women have had at least one extramarital affair. That's a lot. But interestingly enough, people—especially women—

think there's a lot more hanky-panky than that going on. In the fall of 1989, the Kinsey Institute tested the "sexual literacy" of about 2,000 randomly selected American adults. When asked what percentage of married American men had had at least one affair, most women said 70!

He Does It, So . . .

"The female myth is that all men screw around," says Atlanta psychiatrist Frank Pittman III, M.D., author of *Private Lies*. In recent years, an increasing number of women have used that as a convenient rationale for having affairs of their own. "To some women, at least, men's alleged unfaithfulness makes their own screwing around only fair—it's not so much a flaw of character as a blow for liberation," says Dr. Pittman, assistant clinical professor of psychiatry at Emory University School of Medicine in Atlanta.

At the same time, he says, men seem to be having fewer affairs. The cultural ideals of masculinity have begun to shift, so the debonair affair is no longer socially acceptable behavior, no longer an admired male sport. As a society, we treat the infidelities of a Gary Hart far more harshly than we did those of JFK.

Still, despite the fact that affairs are surprisingly common, they should not be taken lightly. Marital infidelity is "the primary disrupter of families, the most dreaded and devastating experience in a marriage," notes Dr. Pittman. "It is the most universally accepted justification for divorce. It is even a legally accepted justification for murder in some states and many societies."

Passion without Personal Commitment

People who have affairs tend to be immature, have little ability to project the long-term consequences of their actions and have stereotyped ideas about gender roles, Dr. Pittman observes. They tend to "see the differences between men and women as being so determinate and absolute that members of the 'opposite' gender are essentially interchangeable. They don't have a sufficiently personal relationship with their spouse as a *person,* rather than as a man or a woman. It's easy for them to simply substitute someone else, as long as they are a member of that gender."

Despite all the talk and hoopla about affairs, people still harbor all kinds of misconceptions about them. Among the hundreds of people involved in or affected by affairs who have trooped through his office over the years, Dr. Pittman has noticed a pattern of beliefs that is rather flatly contradicted by statistics, and he undresses several of the prevailing myths.

8

Myth: Everybody has affairs. Well, that's what people who have affairs almost invariably say. But the truth is that infidelities of one sort or another occur in only about a third of marriages. And even those numbers are misleading— many affairs take place during the last year of a dying marriage. And most of those people have had only one affair, or at most only a couple. Most marital partners are faithful to their spouses, and even if they're not, surveys have shown that the vast majority of people still strongly believe in marital fidelity—for their spouses absolutely, and for themselves usually.

Myth: An affair can liven up a dull marriage. "For most people and most marriages, infidelity is dangerous," notes Dr. Pittman. Once in a great while, affairs do improve a lousy marriage, he says, but those cases are the exceptions. A discovered affair can sometimes provoke a big fight that winds up solving some long-standing problem in the marriage—but sometimes so does a car wreck or a child's illness. "To have an affair in order to trigger a crisis from which the marriage might eventually benefit is truly a screwball, convoluted approach to problem solving," he says.

Myth: Affairs prove that love is gone from the marriage. Most people who have affairs are not looking for the love they can no longer find in a marriage; more often, they're looking for friendship. Unfortunately, if the affair/friendship gets sexual, it tends to quickly degenerate into something so complicated that friendship is no longer possible.

"What is so sad, and seems so foolish, about affairs is that many of them might have been wonderful, utterly unthreatening friendships had they not been so naively sexualized by people who are overly preoccupied with gender differences," Dr. Pittman says. Many people simply don't know how to be friends with someone of the opposite sex.

One of the reasons marital infidelities are so common, he believes, is that people don't live near their relatives anymore. Without the comforting circle of family to surround them and support them through dark times, people tend to "sexualize" friendships simply out of loneliness and then are completely unprepared for the crazy-making mess that follows.

"Friendship is terribly important to marriage—much more important than romance," maintains Dr. Pittman.

Myth: The affair partner was sexier than the spouse. It's been Dr. Pittman's experience that about half the time, the person who strays from a marriage will admit that the sex was actually better at home. "Affair partners are not chosen because they are the winners of some objective sex contest," he observes. "They are chosen for all manner of strange and usually nonsexual reasons. Affair choices are usually far more neurotic than marriage choices." Maybe that's why he's noticed that affair partners are not necessarily better-looking or sexier or nicer or more accomplished than the spouse they supposedly replace. The only consistent pattern, he says, is that "the choice of an affair partner seems based on the other person's *difference* from the spouse rather than *superiority* to the spouse."

Myth: The affair is the fault of the betrayed spouse. This is an incredibly widespread belief—even among betrayed spouses and marriage counselors. But the fact is that one person cannot make another person have an affair. (Sometimes spouses *try* to do it, but it rarely works.)

"I don't find it helpful for a betrayed spouse to take responsibility for any part of the affair," says Dr. Pittman. The only thing that person can do is be available to solve whatever underlying problems there may be in the marriage. And since it's very difficult to make any progress while an affair is still in progress, the healing can begin only after the affair has stopped.

Myth: After an affair, divorce is inevitable. No question about it: An affair is a crisis in a marriage, and very often it destroys it. But it doesn't have to; the marriage usually can still be salvaged, if both partners are willing to put themselves through the pain and hard work a reconciliation will require. Therapy may help. Because although therapy often seems relatively ineffective while someone is *having* an affair, once the truth comes out and the affair is over, therapy can really work.

"I have very rarely seen a couple in therapy divorce because of an affair that is now over," notes Dr. Pittman. "It happens routinely in marriages that are not in therapy." (See also "Safer Sex.")

AGING

At least in terms of pure physical prowess—sex as athletic event—a man usually reaches his sexual peak somewhere between 18 and 20. A woman tends to reach her sexual Everest considerably later, from her mid-thirties to her early forties. But where does that leave everyone who's any older than that . . . languishing in some sexual lowland of dwindling desire?

Not exactly.

10

Sex Goes On and On and On

It's now known that while sexual response does undergo a variety of changes with age, it's also true that many men and women continue to enjoy a rich and satisfying sex life well past retirement. That may not sound like news to you, but at one time it was.

In the landmark studies of human sexuality done by the late Dr. Alfred Kinsey, his team reported that three-quarters of men over 80 are impotent—a finding that confirmed the commonly held belief that it's not only natural but right that the elderly are sweet, forgetful and sexless. But it turns out that in Dr. Kinsey's sample population, there were only three women and four men over 80. His conclusion was drawn from a grand total of *four.*

More recent studies of healthy residents of California retirement homes have shown that 62 percent of the men and 30 percent of the women over 80 reported recently having intercourse. (The figures for women would probably have been considerably higher if the ladies didn't outnumber the gents by six to one.) Perhaps more important, 87 percent of the men and 68 percent of the women reported recently having had some kind of physical intimacy with another person. No matter how old we get, few of us ever outgrow our need to touch and be touched.

It's foolish to think that aging has no effect on sexuality, but it's important to know and appreciate exactly what those effects are.

The Aging Woman

One of the most noticeable changes in the aging woman's sexual response is a decrease in vaginal wetness during sexual arousal. As a noticeable and measurable reaction, vaginal wetness is considered to be the female counterpart of the man's erection. Both the rate of production of these lubricating fluids and the volume produced decline as a woman gets older. The resulting dryness, which can cause discomfort for both partners during intercourse, can usually be remedied by using a water-based lubricating cream such as K-Y Jelly or a nonallergenic moisturizer, preferably with little or no lanolin. Both are available in drugstores.

With age, the walls of the vagina also gradually lose some of their elasticity. Many older women say their orgasms seem to come later, don't last quite as long and are less intense than they once were. Still, unlike men, women's "recovery" period between orgasms doesn't change. A sexually active woman in her sixties or seventies is just as capable of multiple orgasms as a woman in her twenties. But because her sexual responses have slowed, she and her partner will probably need to spend more time in foreplay before she's lubricated enough for intercourse.

Most women know that after menopause, their bodies dramatically slow the production of estrogen. This hormonal shift usually results in a number of changes in the body, including gradual atrophy of the vagina and a decline in vaginal lubrication. But many women don't realize that these changes are gradual and that they usually begin *before* menopause, often showing up as episodes of vaginal dryness that come and go as the body's estrogen levels fluctuate during their gradual decline, says Gloria A. Bachmann, M.D., associate professor of obstetrics and gynecology at the Robert Wood Johnson Medical School in New Providence, New Jersey.

Given the dizzying complexity of any human relationship, this minor physiological difficulty can sometimes add a few distressing new twists to a love knot, Dr. Bachmann says. Some older women may wrongly conclude that their lack of wetness during arousal is caused by a deep, dark problem in the relationship. Some men may conclude that their partner's vaginal dryness may mean she hasn't been stimulated enough, or even that she's not turned on at all anymore. Vaginal dryness is a sign of aging, not the end of love. Partners need to talk about it.

Maintaining the Flow

Estrogen replacement therapy can help maintain a postmenopausal woman's vaginal lubrication. Often, though, women are not informed by their doctors that the medications generally take about 4 to 6 months to work, and in some cases as long as 18 months to two years. (There are some health risks and considerations you should know about before taking estrogen. For more, see "Hormone Replacement Therapy.")

There's no evidence that menopause results in loss of sexual desire; in fact, in some cases, it may even result in *increased* desire. Perhaps partly because they're finally free of the fear of pregnancy, perhaps because they feel greater personal freedom after their children have flown from the nest, some postmenopausal women pass into a sort of delightful sexual renaissance. William Masters, M.D., and Virginia Johnson, of the Masters and Johnson Institute in St. Louis, have taken pains to point out that even though a woman may be getting older, "the sensual pleasure derived from sex usually continues unabated."

The Aging Man

As teenagers, men can generally get an erection in the time it takes to lick a stamp. But as they age, achieving a full, firm erection takes longer and may sometimes require a little manual help from a partner. In a study at the University of Southern California, for instance, researchers showed the same sexy movie to two groups of men, one group aged 19 to 30 and the other, 48 to 65. The younger group got erections almost six times faster than the older guys.

With age, there's also a gradual increase in the recovery time between ejaculations (the amount of time it takes to be able to have a second erection after the first one fades).

"An 18-year-old man can climax up to eight times in 24 hours; when they're 35, once every 24 hours is more the norm," says Virginia Saddock, M.D., director of the Graduate Education Program in Human Sexuality at the New York University Medical Center in New York City.

There's also a gradual decline in the expulsive pressure and the volume of semen that's expelled during ejaculation. The aging male may notice something else, too: More and more, as his arousal nears climax, he no longer feels the unstoppable urge to ejaculate. Perhaps once out of every three or four times he has intercourse, he simply lets it go without climaxing. Consider it a prerogative of age.

He has fewer morning erections as he gets older, too. And he is likely to have sex less frequently. Dr. Kinsey reported that married men between 31 and 35 average about two orgasms a week (whether by intercourse or masturbation); men between 56 and 60 average about two a month.

As he ages, a man's testosterone levels also begin to decline, but very gradually — and that doesn't seem to be what causes his gradual decline in sexual desire. In fact, men who have gotten experimental injections of testosterone have a few more sexual fantasies, but the hormones don't produce any startling blast of libidinous desire, nor do they enhance the ability to produce an erection. When testosterone levels in an aging man are subnormal, however, injections may prove helpful. (See "Testosterone.")

The Plus Side of the Score Sheet

All of this may sound like a catalog of unmitigated mortal decline, but it doesn't have to be. After all, as a man's sexual responses begin to throttle down with age, he finds it easier to last longer before ejaculation and therefore easier to satisfy his lover. At the same time, his mate is inclined to require more foreplay before she's sufficiently lubricated for entry.

The dalliance of age can make for sex that's all the sweeter for being slower. Says Paul A. Fleming, M.D., former editor of the newsletter *Sex after Forty:* "You may not be able to have sex three times in an hour, but you'll be better equipped to do it once and make it last an hour. So much for the myth of sexual decline!"

It was once thought that the physiological changes wrought by age were entirely inevitable; as you got older, you started falling apart, and that was that. But it's now known that many of those creaks, rattles and groans are the result not of mere age but of ill health or inactivity. And the same principle applies to a person's sexual life.

In one survey of 225 older men, chronic illness and poor health turned out to be practically as significant a cause of sexual decline as aging itself. In fact, the middle-aged men in this study (median age: 59) who considered themselves "in poor health" compared with other men their age were *6 times* as likely as healthy men to be having some kind of sexual difficulty. Among men over 75, the connection was even more dramatic: Poor health made them 40 times more likely to be having sexual problems.

Pleasure Lasts

By contrast, people who keep themselves physically fit and sexually active can go on enjoying the sweet feast of satisfying sex almost to the very end of their lives.

For instance, one study of 160 male Masters swimmers between the ages of 40 and 80 showed a strong correlation between vigorous physical conditioning and sexual frequency and pleasure. These robust men, hungry for life and pleasure, reported a frequency of intercourse similar to that of men 20 to 40 years their junior.

Another study of 800 men and women ranging in age from 60 to 91 revealed that most people over 60 are very interested in sex. Most say that they enjoy sex as much as they did when they were younger—in fact, most say that they enjoy it even more. One 72-year-old woman told gerontological researchers Bernard Starr, Ph.D., and Marcella Weinter, Ed.D.: "Our sex is so much more relaxed, I know my body better, and we know each other better. Sex is unhurried and the best in our lives!"

AIDS.

See Safer Sex

ALCOHOL

Shakespeare seems to have had the last word on just about everything, including the effect of alcohol on sex. In *Macbeth,* a sly porter observes about drinking: "... it provokes, and unprovokes; it provokes the desire, but it takes away the performance."

Although researchers have filled in a lot of the physiological details since Shakespeare's day, that's still about the size of it.

Free Up Inhibition, Close Down Performance

A sip of spirits—especially champagne, with its ejaculatory pop of the cork—is probably the best known of all aphrodisiacs. In moderation, it casts a seductive glow over everything at the same time it loosens the buttons of inhibition. One *Psychology Today* questionnaire showed that 45 percent of male respondents and 68 percent of female respondents reported that alcohol "greatly or somewhat" enhanced their sexual enjoyment.

But the odd fact is that beyond a drink or two, alcohol seems to have precisely the opposite effect. In men, studies have shown that low levels of alcohol mildly enhance sexual arousal, as measured by swelling of the penis in response to erotic stimulation. However, once the guy's blood alcohol concentration (BAC) tops about 0.05, all the physiological measures of sexual arousal begin to droop. (A BAC of 0.05 is roughly the level a 150-pound man would reach after consuming three mixed drinks in the space of 1 to 2 hours.)

In one study, men were asked to consume varying amounts of alcohol before masturbating. Volunteers with a BAC of 0.06 took significantly longer to ejaculate, and at 0.09, many subjects were unable to ejaculate at all. This less-than-impressive performance is undoubtedly related to the fact that a few stiff drinks are also known to cause a dramatic drop in blood levels of testosterone, the hormone that ignites male libido.

Alcohol seems to affect women similarly. Studies have shown that even at BAC levels as low as 0.04, women's level of sexual arousal is reduced (as measured by blood circulation to vaginal tissue, which is considered a good general measure of sexual excitation). Other studies have shown that alcohol increases the amount of time it takes women to achieve orgasm by masturbation and also reduces the intensity of their orgasm. So from a strictly physical point of view, anything beyond the third drink is a sexual downer.

The Whoopee Factor

Still, human sexual response is not solely a physical phenomenon; the subjective sensation of arousal—the ghost in the machine—is part of it, too. And *that's* where it all gets a bit confusing.

Studies have shown that as men get drunker and their sexual responses grow duller, their subjective sense of arousal also diminishes. But women seem to be dancing to a different tune: As they steadily get more drunk, causing all the physiological measures of arousal to steadily decline, they just go on feeling more and more aroused. You figure it out; so far, the researchers can't.

Male alcoholics also demonstrate this puzzling contradiction between the *feeling* of arousal that alcohol causes and the performance-inhibiting physical changes it brings about. In several studies, when male alcoholics were shown erotic films while drinking, they demonstrated the predicted decline in physical arousal. Even so, both before and after the experiment, they predicted that the booze would have either no effect or a positive one on their ability to perform sexually. When it comes to sex, alcohol has a way of telling the mind something different from what it's telling the body.

For Men: Calamity in the Making

When it comes to the *long-term* effects of chronic, heavy drinking, alcohol's effect on sex is not puzzling at all. It's plain, flat-out disastrous.

Studies of aging alcoholic men have shown that prolonged drinking damages the body's sexual capacities in a whole variety of ways. It destroys the cells in the testes that manufacture testosterone, dampening sexual desire and interfering with all the complicated hormonal chemistry of testosterone metabolism.

At the same time, alcohol also decreases one's ability to have a full, firm erection. One researcher has estimated that 70 to 80 percent of male alcoholics have decreased sexual desire or potency, or both. Male alcoholics also often report having problems ejaculating. And chronic alcohol abuse also damages the intricate plumbing of the male reproductive system, reducing a man's ability to produce normally formed sperm cells.

At the end of this dreary road lies a tragic irony. Although heavy drinking tends to be associated with swashbuckling masculinity—what's a western without a good bar fight?—in practice, it has exactly the opposite effect.

Chronic alcohol abuse disrupts men's hormone levels—increasing the female sex hormones (estrogens) in both the liver and the testicles—so that some hard-core male alcoholics may wind up with estrogen levels similar to those of women. And they may even begin to acquire female sex characteristics. They begin to lose their body hair. Their breasts swell—a strange and uncomfortable trans-formation called gynecomastia. Their muscle mass begins to shrink. They may even develop something researchers have given the terrifying name *alcoholic hypogonadism*—shrinkage of the penis and testicles.

For Women: Double Disaster

Alcoholic women have not been studied as intensively as men (perhaps because there aren't nearly as many of them), but heavy drinking is no less harmful to them. It can lead to reduced interest in sex, reduced sexual arousal and less pleasurable orgasm. Alcohol can also move through a woman's reproductive system with all the delicacy of a wrecking ball, disrupting menstruation and ovarian function, decreasing fertility and causing the female version of hypogonadism—shrunken breasts and malformed genitals. And of course, drinking during preg-nancy can cause irreparable harm to the developing fetus.

Need any more be said?

ALLERGIES

Nothing could be more unromantic than a runny nose, an itchy rash or a fit of uncontrollable sneezing every time you make love. It's bad enough when you have a cold, but some lovers have to suffer through these withering indignities because of allergic reactions to some substance with which they're coming into contact during sex.

Reacting to Rubber, Spermicide

Occasionally, someone is allergic to the rubber in diaphragms or condoms. Much more common are allergic reactions to nonoxynol-9, the spermicide that's a key ingredient in many forms of birth control sold in the United States, including the contraceptive sponge, jellies made for use in diaphragms, foaming tablets and vaginal suppositories. In fact, about 5 percent of people who use nonoxynol-9 experience some localized allergic reaction to it, says Philip Darney, M.D., associate professor of obstetrics and gynecology at San Francisco General Hospital.

Luckily, says Dr. Darney, "the reaction is generally very mild and self-limiting. Men will experience a mild rash with itching, and women will notice a burning sensation and vaginal itching, much like a contact dermatitis."

The symptoms are usually considerably less severe than the worries they provoke—many people with such reactions fear that they may have vaginitis or an infection or that they've caught a sexually transmitted disease. "The fact that they have an allergy comes as a very pleasant surprise to most people," says Dr. Darney.

The problem affects men and women about equally, and it may sometimes cause an annoying reaction in one partner and absolutely no symptoms at all in the other.

Block That Reaction

If you're a man who reacts to nonoxynol-9, you can probably solve the problem simply by wearing a condom to protect your skin from the offending ingredient. Just make sure that the condom itself is not lubricated with the spermicide. If you think you may be reacting to rubber, you might try switching to condoms made from sheep gut. You should be aware, however, that while condoms made of animal skin work as birth control devices, they do not provide protection from the virus that causes AIDS. (See "Safer Sex.")

If you're a woman, you might first try changing the brand of spermicide you use, since it may be that you're allergic not to nonoxynol-9 but to some other ingredient in the foam, cream or jelly.

If you still react, you'll probably have to find a new form of birth control. (There may be another alternative for women available sometime soon. A new spermicide called menfegol, currently used in Japan, may soon be approved for use in the United States. It appears to cause fewer allergic reactions.)

What If You're Allergic to Him?

A woman also may sometimes have an allergic reaction to her lover's semen (a terrible omen, but one that has nothing to do with the potential of their relationship). Within minutes after intercourse, women who have these allergies will experience mild vaginal irritation, break out in hives or even begin having trouble breathing, as their bodies slip into potentially life-threatening anaphylactic shock.

"We don't have any real numbers on it, but it's a lot more common than people think," says Leonard Bernstein, M.D., codirector of the Allergy Research Laboratory at the University of Cincinnati College of Medicine in Ohio. "I talked about this on a Phil Donahue show one time, and afterward I got thousands of letters. Probably 10 percent of these women sounded like they could have semen allergies.'' Many women are too embarrassed to talk about it, Dr. Bernstein says, and others actually believe that breaking out in hives is a normal part of orgasm! Love is wonderful, but this is ridiculous.

A simple way to test whether it's his semen you're allergic to is to try having him use a condom. If you're still in doubt, see an allergist, since high-tech lab tests are the only reliable way to pinpoint the source of a reaction. If semen is the source, the problem can successfully be treated with immunotherapy, in which the woman is desensitized to her lover's ejaculate by a series of shots made from protein fractions taken from it. ''It's a fairly complicated and expensive procedure, but it only takes a few days, and it works,'' says Dr. Bernstein. ''Repeated exposure builds up a tolerance to the allergen, and as long as the couple has regular intercourse, the tolerance will be maintained.'' Then they can return to making each other happy without making each other sick.

In a few fairly rare cases, women who have allergic reactions to their lover's semen turn out to be reacting to something *in* the semen, such as substances from food or chemicals he ate or medications he's been taking (like penicillin or sulfa drugs). Once he stops eating the food or taking the medicine, the symptoms go away. In some other cases, women develop what appears to be vaginitis (itching, burning and discharge) after intercourse. Actually, though, it turns out to be a nasty reaction to antibodies in her lover's semen produced by *his* allergies. The physiology is rather complicated, but the solution is simple: Try using a condom.

Not Tonight Dear, I've Got A-Chooo!

In some other cases, people will cough, sneeze, itch and break out in hives after sex—not because of a physical allergy but because of an emotional one. These distressing symptoms, which perfectly mimic a real allergic reaction, can be caused by unexpressed anxiety, fear of intimacy or any number of other powerful emotions evoked by a sexual encounter.

''Our bodies react to our feelings, and those feelings *must* be expressed. If your mind and mouth don't bring them up, your body will,'' says New York City marriage and sex therapist Natalie Wayne.

Such people, says Wayne, often make the rounds of every specialist in town, subjecting themselves to every allergy test in the book, before they can be convinced that their problem is not a purely physical one. That's not to say that it's any less real—only that they need a therapist, not an allergist.

''We all experience some degree of anxiety when we allow ourselves to become intimate with someone else,'' says Wayne. ''It's perfectly normal. If you can talk to the other person and express your feelings, you'll probably never experience this kind of a reaction." But feigning sexual confidence when you're quaking inside can provoke what looks and feels for all the world like a first-class allergic explosion.

Better Than Aspirin

All this talk of allergy seems to add up to one great long litany of human desolation and misery. But there's at least one bright spot: For some people who suffer from allergies, sex may be not the *cause* of itchy rashes but their *cure*.

"Sex, for me, will totally stop a reaction for several days," explains one highly allergic patient of San Francisco allergist Alan Scott Levin, M.D. "When I was really sick and nothing else helped, I could always count on sex." And she's not alone. Dr. Levin says that other patients also report that their symptoms disappear, "almost miraculously," during and after sexual intercourse.

Sure, Dr. Levin says, having sex tends to take your mind off your hives, "but there is a physiological reason for feeling better, too. Sex stimulates the flow of adrenaline, the hormone secreted by the adrenal gland in times of stress. That adrenaline relaxes the bronchial tissue and raises the blood pressure, increasing the flow of blood from the head and decongesting the nasal passages."

For some allergy sufferers, it's better than a blast from a bronchodilator.

ANAL INTERCOURSE

Art dating back to ancient times suggests that the prac- tice of anal sex—stimulation of the anorectal area, including penile penetration— has been around for many centuries. In fact, some might find it surprising how common a practice it is among heterosexual couples today. In one survey of 100,000 female readers of *Redbook* magazine, 43 percent of the women said they'd tried it with their partners at least once. Of that number, 40 percent said they found it somewhat or very enjoyable. (That is, about a quarter of the total number of women surveyed said this.) Forty-nine percent said they didn't care for it, and 10 percent said they had no strong feelings one way or the other. While not a controlled scientific study, this survey roughly parallels the findings of many other sexual surveys.

Something else that may come as a surprise to many: While a fair number of heterosexuals engage in the practice, not all homosexuals do. In a review of the existing data on the subject, the Kinsey Institute concluded that between 59 and 95 percent of male homosexuals had engaged in anal sex at least once.

In the age of AIDS, anal sex has received a lot of bad press—and for good reason. Unprotected anal intercourse is the single most risky behavior in terms of exposure to the dread disease. (See "Safer Sex.") It bears mentioning, however, that if neither you nor your partner is already infected with HIV (human immuno-deficiency virus), you cannot get AIDS from anal sex. This may seem self-evident, but in a nationwide sex survey conducted by the Kinsey Institute, half of the American adults questioned said they thought you could get AIDS through anal intercourse, whether or not one partner was infected. This is simply not true.

What is true is that having anal intercourse with an infected partner, without using a condom, is the kind of sex behavior most likely to transmit AIDS. That's probably because the sensitive lining of the rectum is likely to tear during intercourse, allowing AIDS-infected blood or semen to pass directly into a sex partner's bloodstream. In fact, the evidence for this mode of AIDS transmission is so clear—and AIDS itself is so scary—that doctors now recommend against having anal sex with anybody, under any circumstances.

If you insist on trying it anyway, take two precautions: The vagina is naturally elastic and moistened by its own natural lubricants, but the rectum is not. Therefore, before attempting anal penetration, it's important to use a water-based lubricant like K-Y Jelly. Also, before entering the vagina after anal intercourse, be sure to thoroughly wash the penis. Otherwise, it's likely to transfer bacteria from the rectum, which may cause vaginal infections.

ANXIETY

Lots of people who suffer from anxiety disorders also have sexual troubles. It stands to reason: Sweet sex involves deep physical relaxation, and if you're chronically tense and anxious, it's difficult to either give or receive sexual pleasure.

Everybody feels a little anxious from time to time. What we're talking about here is a feeling of vague uneasiness or dread so severe and so persistent that it qualifies as a psychiatric syndrome. People who suffer from anxiety disorders often complain that they're so keyed up they can't sleep and that they are unable to relax and can't concentrate. Occasionally they have other distressing physical symptoms like heart palpitations, dizziness or shortness of breath.

Sidestepping Side Effects

There are a variety of prescription drugs that psychiatrists often use to soothe the frazzled nerves of anxiety patients, but unfortunately many of these medications also can adversely affect their patients' sex lives. One new anxiety-reducing drug, however, may be different. Recently two psychiatrists at the University of Kansas Medical Center in Lawrence discovered that the drug buspirone (BuSpar) can reduce anxiety at the same time it actually *boosts* sexual desire in many patients.

The doctors tested the drug in nine anxiety patients who also complained that their sex drive was flagging. One woman, in fact, confessed that she was so concerned she wasn't being a "good wife" that she feared her husband would leave her. After four weeks on the drug, eight of them not only felt less anxious but also had returned to normal sexual functioning. (The psychiatrists noted that the drug seemed most effective at the fairly high dosage of 60 milligrams a day, the manufacturer's daily maximum.)

If you suffer from chronic anxiety, you might consider discussing this drug with your doctor. Don't forget, of course, that therapeutic drugs may not be the only answer. Also try looking into drug-free therapies such as biofeedback, meditation, progressive muscle relaxation and guided imagery, which can soothe your soul without disturbing your biochemistry. (See also "Painful Intercourse," "Performance Anxiety," "Sex Therapy" and "Vaginismus.")

APHRODISIACS

Ever hear the one about the farmer who had a bull that wouldn't breed? The vet gave him some medicine, he fed it to the bull, and that same afternoon, the beast went out and serviced four cows. A neighbor, noticing the goings-on, leaned over the back fence and asked the farmer what was in the medicine. "I don't know," the farmer said, "but it tasted like licorice."

Hope Springs Eternal

Potions that heighten sensual love or enhance sexual prowess have been sought after for thousands of years. Almost any food, drug or drink you can imagine has at one time or another been used to call down the gods of love—from substances as utterly ordinary as an apple to those as profoundly weird as hippopotamus snout. In fact, several species of plants and animals have been driven to the brink of extinction after word got around that their leaves or their livers had the power to arouse.

How does anything develop a reputation as an aphrodisiac? Sometimes it's for embarrassingly obvious reasons, like its shape (bananas, carrots and asparagus spears have all been used as love potions). Or somebody makes a pseudoscientific observation: After Ireland's population boomed, the English concluded that the potato must be an aphrodisiac. Sometimes the mere fact that something is exotic, rare or expensive may be enough: When the Europeans discovered tomatoes in South America, they decided the deep red globes must be the forbidden fruit of Eden and dubbed them "love apples."

But practically speaking, does any of this stuff actually work? Well, the Food and Drug Administration (FDA) has taken a pretty humorless approach to the question and, in a ruling effective January 6, 1990, banned the interstate commerce or over-the-counter sale of "any product that bears labeling claims that it will arouse or increase sexual desire or that it will improve sexual performance." In the FDA's view, there is no over-the-counter food, lotion, potion or medication that fits that bill.

Orgasmic Chocolates and Other Delectables

Still, taking a more mild-mannered approach to the question, it could be argued that there are some things that really do seem to arouse some people, at least sometimes. Strictly speaking, no food has ever been proven to be an aphrodisiac. But there are still reasons why some foods may enhance one's sexual pleasure.

Chocolate, that much-loved Valentine's Day gift, contains a substance that accumulates in the pleasure centers of the brain and thereby mimics what occurs during sex, says George Armelagos, Ph.D., an anthropologist at the University of Florida in Gainesville and author of *Consuming Passions*. Other foods long associated with love—like oysters, eggs and caviar—may enhance sexual desire simply because they are good sources of protein and may therefore tend to contribute to a general sense of health and well-being.

Still, adds Dr. Armelagos: "Almost any food has the properties of an aphrodisiac because the very act of eating causes an increase in the pulse rate and the blood pressure, raising body temperature and sometimes even producing sweating— changes that occur with orgasm."

Substances with a . . . Ahem . . . Reputation

Sexual arousal is not triggered solely by plumbing and physiology, any more than love is triggered by hormones. If truffles and champagne seem to put you in the mood, who's to say they don't?

"The brain," notes Dr. Armelagos, "is the most important sexual organ. If you think saltines will work, then you've got a good, cheap aphrodisiac."

But there are a few other substances that *may* work a little better.

Barking Up the Right Tree

Yohimbine, a chemical derived from the bark of the African yohimbe tree, has a long folk history as a love potion. Maybe all those "folks" were on to something—it really does seem to work in about a third of the impotent men who try it. It recently has even become a respectable prescription drug for the treatment of male impotence. But there's so much to be said about yohimbine that we discuss it separately. (See "Yohimbine.")

Getting to the Root of the Matter

For 5,000 years, the Chinese have sworn by ginseng, a gnarled woodland root, as a sovereign remedy for more illnesses than you probably knew existed. And for just as long they've touted it as an aphrodisiac. (One recent computer search found that ginseng is listed as a folk remedy for 82 different disorders, ranging from diabetes to poisonous centipede stings. In fact, the "panax" in Chinese ginseng's scientific name, *Panax ginseng,* means "cure-all.")

U.S. farmers and "sangers" (woodland gatherers) still export $40 million worth of American ginseng a year to the Orient, where people chew the stuff even if they're not sick, in the belief that it will increase their feeling of general vitality and well-being.

There is some bona fide scientific evidence suggesting that ginseng can reduce the stress effects of temperature extremes, strenuous exercise, weird diets and other unpleasantries. It's also been shown to have some positive effects on conditions ranging from depression to ulcers. But does it really work as an aphrodisiac? Well, rats fed ginseng extract do demonstrate stepped-up mating behavior—but it's not clear whether that has any relevance at all to human behavior. One modern herbalist, Varro E. Tyler, Ph.D., of Purdue University, says flatly in *The New Honest Herbal:* "There is no evidence of enhanced sexual experience or potency resulting from its use."

On the other hand, it's difficult to completely dismiss 5,000 years of human experience. It could be that ginseng exerts an *indirect* effect on one's love life simply because it fights fatigue and makes you feel a little spunkier. (Studies have shown, for instance, that it increases running speed in soldiers and reduces drowsiness in night-shift workers.)

"Any improved sense of well-being would certainly tend to make one feel more sexual," observes Gordon S. Walbroehl, M.D., assistant professor in the Department of Family Practice at Wright State University School of Medicine in Dayton, Ohio. "If a patient wishes to use ginseng in modest amounts, I would not see any problem." But strictly speaking, it's not really an aphrodisiac, he notes.

One caution: Chinese ginseng (*P. ginseng*, which is more potent than the American variety, *P. quinquefolius*) is so expensive, and quality control is so poor, that you can never be sure what you're getting when you buy "ginseng" tea, powder or capsules. In one study of 54 commercial ginseng products, 60 percent of the stuff analyzed was worthless, and a quarter contained no ginseng at all.

Vitamin E: Don't Get Your Hopes Up

Alpha tocopherol, or vitamin E, has a widespread but ill-deserved reputation as an aphrodisiac. Why?

Perhaps, suggests June Reinisch, Ph.D., director of the Kinsey Institute, it's because of widely reported studies that showed that the testicles and ovaries of rats deprived of vitamin E begin to atrophy. When the animals are returned to a diet rich in vitamin E, their genitalia return to normal.

But does that make vitamin E an aphrodisiac? Not by a long shot. Humans whose bodies are deficient in vitamin E do tend to have reduced sex drive—but if your vitamin E levels are normal, adding supplements to your diet will have absolutely no effect on your sex drive, Dr. Reinisch says.

Love Potions by Prescription

In recent years, pharmaceutical research labs have begun the search for reliable "love drugs," and some of the medications they've developed really do work. Unfortunately, most of them are available only by prescription (if they're available yet at all) and tend to be used mainly as treatments for sexual disorders rather than as tonics to enhance an already zesty sex life.

Far from Depressing

One antidepressant, Wellbutrin, has been found to warm up the libidos and improve the sexual performances of many of the men and women who take it. (Many other antidepressants do just the opposite.) In one study conducted at the Crenshaw Clinic, a sex therapy clinic in San Diego, more than 60 percent of the depressed patients who took the drug reported positive effects. Follow-up studies at other clinics haven't been quite so rousing, however. Out of 62 patients given the drug by a Philadelphia psychiatrist, for instance, only a dozen or so found it added any octane to their sex lives.

Don't forget, of course, that these people were all clinically depressed and suffering from low sex drive when they started taking the drug. If you have a normal, robust sex drive, says Washington, D.C., psychiatrist Elmer Gardner, M.D., Wellbutrin won't improve it. It also won't have any effect on men whose impotence is caused by physical rather than psychological difficulties. On the other hand, if you are depressed and feel sexless, you might consider asking your doctor about it.

Injecting Performance

Prostaglandin-E is a vasodilator, meaning that this drug works its wonders by causing blood vessels to dilate, thereby boosting blood flow to a specific bodily neighborhood. When it's injected directly into the penis, it can produce a triumphant erection within 5 minutes. *Injected?* Sorry, but yes. Prostaglandin-E is one of a small class of new drugs now being used to treat male impotence that must be delivered directly to the member in question in order to work.

"It really doesn't hurt," claims University of California, Irvine, endocrinologist Grant Gwinup, M.D. "The needle is tiny and lubricated with silicone, so you get only the slightest discomfort."

For men suffering from physical or psychological impotence, the inconvenience may be worth it. Dr. Gwinup says it's helped all but 2 of the 50 patients he's prescribed it for, and after several years of fairly widespread use, no serious side effects have been reported. (For more on two similar injectable impotence drugs, papaverine and phentolamine, see "Erection Problems.")

Biochemistry to the Rescue

Sexual arousal is a marvelously complicated chain reaction of chemical and physiological changes. But the very last neurotransmitter in the chain, the thing that actually puts the icing on the cake—producing vaginal wetness in women and erection in men—is a mild-mannered biochemical called vasoactive intestinal peptide, or VIP. If it was possible to create a synthetic version of VIP in the lab, then apply it directly to the vagina or the penis, would it simulate sexual arousal?

Apparently so—at least, that's the way it looks in preliminary studies conducted by a small California biotech company called Senetek, which has been testing a couple of VIP concoctions to do just that. (The company makes it clear, though, that these drugs simulate physical arousal only, not sexual desire.)

For women, VIP is delivered in the form of a vaginal cream, which provides a more "natural" lubrication than other gels and creams, according to information provided by Senetek. For men (unfortunately) the drug must be delivered via a small injection at the base of the penis. In clinical studies conducted in Denmark involving 200 men, the shots helped those with impotence caused by vascular problems (38 percent got erections), diabetes (50 percent), psychological problems (78 percent) and damage to nerves (88 percent).

Not Just for the Heart

Nitroglycerin, well known as an angina drug, produces an erection within a few minutes. To work this wonder, it must be applied directly to the penis in the form of a paste. There is no need for an injection of any kind. (Taking it in pill form doesn't seem to work.) Physiologically, the drug works as a vasodilator, boosting blood flow to the penis. In one study conducted by pharmacologist James Owen, Ph.D., of the Kingston Psychiatric Hospital in Kingston, Ontario, it produced erections in 25 of 26 impotent men who hadn't been visited by a single erection in the three months prior to the study.

But don't get too excited just yet. These experiments were conducted in a controlled clinical setting—the men were surrounded by an array of measuring devices and guys in white coats. And they did not actually put these nitro-erections to use by having intercourse with a woman.

"We just have no idea if this drug would really be useful in an actual partner-to-partner situation, since the partner would absorb the drug through the skin and might not tolerate it as well as the man does," says Dr. Owen.

It's been reported, for instance, that at least one woman got a tremendous headache after having sex with a man using nitroglycerin paste. (Nitro can cause headaches in people who use it as an angina drug, too.)

Other drawbacks: Nitroglycerin may interact in unknown ways with other medications a person is taking, which is part of the reason it's available only by prescription. And so far, it hasn't officially been registered for use in impotence, so your doctor couldn't prescribe it for that purpose. On the other hand, you should definitely *not* try whipping up your own do-it-yourself concoction of nitro paste.

"It's a powerful drug that can cause profound side effects, including a serious drop in blood pressure," says Dr. Owen.

The bottom line here, at least for now: Have a love apple instead.

ARTHRITIS

Here's the good news: People with arthritis who go ahead and have sex, despite the pain in their joints, often report that their joints are pain-free for more than 6 hours afterward. Researchers believe that sexual arousal touches off a cascade of blissful hormonal changes, boosting the production of corticosteroid, a hormone that reduces pain and inflammation in the joints, as well as endorphins, the body's natural opiates. (By some lights, falling in love is the best arthritis medicine of all. Heart surgeon Christiaan Barnard, for instance, suffered from rheumatoid arthritis for years before he married a ravishing young woman named Barbara. "For several years after the wedding," he reported later in a book, "I virtually ceased to be a sufferer.")

Communicate Your Needs

Okay, now here's the bad news: About half of the 36 million Americans who suffer from some form of arthritis also complain that it interferes with their sex lives. In fact, people with rheumatoid arthritis, a severe form of the disease much more likely to affect women than men, have a higher divorce rate than people with most other kinds of chronic disease.

Usually it's pain and stiffness in the hips, knees or lower back, rather than any loss of desire, that get in the way. Sometimes feelings of weakness or fatigue also interfere. That's why sexual communication—letting your partner know what feels good and what doesn't—is so important. Good communication is important in *any* sexual relationship, of course, but when you've got arthritis hanging over the bed, there's a great potential for hurt feelings.

"The person who has arthritis often feels insecure and sometimes misinterprets concern on the part of the partner as distaste," observes George Ehrlich, M.D., an adjunct professor of clinical medicine at New York University School of Medicine in New York City. "Or a spouse may avoid sexual overtures for fear of hurting the arthritic partner; this may be perceived by the patient as a sign of revulsion." So be kind, and be specific. Let your partner know what feels good and what hurts.

Or if you feel too squeamish to talk about sex, try taking turns giving each other a gentle massage. When your partner's hand gets near a painful place, just redirect it toward a place where you enjoy the touch most. A sensitive partner should understand what you mean. The Arthritis Foundation also suggests having a clear, preset signal to let your partner know if you really have severe pain. That way, your partner can stop quickly without completely ruining the mood.

You *Can* Enjoy Sex

Here are some other ways to make sex more painless and pleasurable.

Get ready. An hour beforehand, take whatever pain-relieving medication you're using. Avoid painkilling narcotics or other drugs that have sex-inhibiting side effects. Corticosteroids, for instance, may relieve pain in men, but they also suppress erection.

Loosen up. While you relax and get in the mood, try doing a few gentle range-of-motion exercises to limber up your joints.

Warm up. Take a warm bath or shower in preparation—or better yet, invite your partner to join you. Turn it into a slow, soapy, delicious form of foreplay.

Stay toasty. Try an electric blanket—it may keep you limber while it keeps you warm. Or what about a heated waterbed? Some arthritis sufferers say it makes all the difference.

Don't forget to touch. Don't forget that physical love doesn't only mean intercourse—there's always kissing, hugging, caressing, stroking, massaging and a thousand other variations on the ecstasy of touch.

Lubricate. Sometimes women who have arthritis also suffer from Sjögren's syndrome, an unpleasant side effect that causes dryness of the mucous membranes around the eyes, mouth and vagina. It may help to use a germ-free, water-soluble suppository lubricant like K-Y Jelly, Lubrin or Steri-lube, which are available without a prescription in drugstores. (Petroleum jelly products and other oily substances should not be used, because they may harbor germs and cause infection.)

Experiment with times. Most people with rheumatoid arthritis have their most severe symptoms in the morning when they awaken. Symptoms are often lowest in midafternoon and tend to worsen later in the day. Try adjusting your timetable for lovemaking to coincide with the periods during which symptoms are less severe.

Experiment with positions. The usual missionary position may be very uncomfortable if the woman has arthritis in her hip or the man has it in his knee, leg or arm. The Arthritis Foundation puts out a nice little booklet about sex and arthritis called *Living and Loving,* which (among other things) describes seven positions likely to be more comfortable.

For instance, when the woman has hip problems, you might try a position in which both partners lie on their sides and the man enters from behind. Sometimes it feels better if the woman has a pillow between her knees. If the man has back problems, try lying face-to-face, both of you on your sides, with the woman providing most of the hip movement. Or if the man has hip or knee problems, he can try lying on his back, perhaps using pillows to cushion his head, with the woman sitting on top, supporting her own body weight with her elbows or knees.

To order the booklet on sex and arthritis from the Arthritis Foundation, call 800–283–7800.

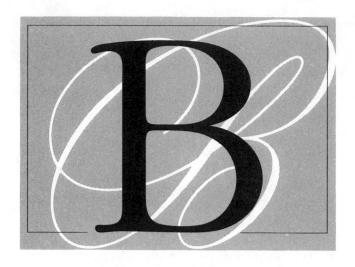

BACK PAIN

At some point in their lives, eight out of ten Americans are laid low by low back pain. It's the sort of pain that can deal a crushing blow to your sense of pride and immortality—and also, sometimes, to your sex life. When you're in acute pain, making love hurts too much to attempt.

Chronic back pain, of the sort that lasts months or even years, can be worse: It tends to reduce your desire for sex altogether, at least partly because it often becomes intermingled with psychological depression, says Irene Minkowski, M.D., San Francisco physiatrist and cofounder of the Physician's Back Institute. (Fortunately, almost all low back pain goes away within two weeks.)

Better Than a Back Rub

The irony is that making love can sometimes help *soothe* a suffering back. Lovemaking triggers the release of endorphins, the body's homegrown painkillers, which can do wonders to snuff out the pain. (The effects of this natural narcotic are relatively short-lived, however; they don't alter any underlying damage to disks or joints.) The deep relaxation that follows satisfying sex also can sometimes help relieve the pain.

"What we've discovered is that people with acute back pain will develop what are known as 'tender spots' elsewhere in the body—in the abdominal region, in the buttocks, over the pubic bone," Dr. Minkowski explains. "These spots, which are not acutely painful unless they're pressed, nevertheless send a message to the brain that the back pain is still there. We treat them with an osteopathic muscle technique in which the muscle is put in a slack position, or relaxed, for about 90 seconds, which is enough to 'reprogram' the brain's memory engram of pain—which in turn soothes the back pain. Lovemaking can soothe back pain by the same mechanism, apparently just because it deeply relaxes the muscles in those tender spots."

In order to soothe the pain and inflammation of a sore back, doctors often prescribe medications from the large class of drugs called nonsteroidal anti-inflammatory drugs. These medications are generally free of sexual side effects. However, the first report of sexual dysfunction apparently caused by one of these drugs, indomethacin (Indocin), has appeared in the medical literature. A 60-year-old man with a long history of back pain became impotent and lost his sex drive after taking indomethacin for two or three weeks. As it turned out, this wasn't a terribly serious problem; his sexual prowess returned within a week after he quit taking the drug. If taking this drug seems to give you problems in the potency department, let your doctor know.

Play around the Pain

Sometimes the best you can do is just try to make love in the least painful way possible. Listen to your body, says Dr. Minkowski; pain is your body telling you, quite plainly, which positions to avoid. People with ruptured disks, for instance, would be better off taking the bottom position during sexual intercourse because being on top requires bending forward, which can be painful, advises Augustus A. White III, M.D., professor of orthopedic surgery at Harvard Medical School and a leading back specialist. (If there is a significant weight difference and the person on top is very much heavier, a side-by-side position might be a better idea.) Also try to avoid positions that involve extreme arching of the back, which puts tremendous pressure on disks and joints in the low back. It's also a good idea to avoid overzealous pelvic thrusting, he says.

In his book *Your Aching Back,* Dr. White describes several lovemaking positions likely to minimize backache as well as the aggravation to underlying disks and joints.

In one back-saving position, both partners lie on their sides, nestled together like spoons, and the man enters from behind. The man and woman should both keep their hips and knees slightly bent. This way, neither partner has to support his or her own weight, or the partner's weight, and the strain is taken off joints and muscles. This is the best position for making love when in acute pain, whether it's the man or the woman who's hurting, Dr. White says.

When the woman has a backache, the couple might try a sort of modified missionary position. The usual missionary position, with the man mounting the woman while she lies prone, can be painful for her. In the modified position, the woman lies on her back, and the man kneels between her spread legs. The woman drapes her legs *over* his thighs. (His knees are spread about 2 feet apart.) Her upper body should be supported by pillows, and her thighs, by her partner's thighs. The man may also support her lower back a little with his hands. In this position, Dr. White explains, the psoas muscle, which supports the lower back, is relaxed, releasing the strain on her back.

Here's another good position for a woman with back pain: The man lies on his back, and she mounts him, supporting her weight by bending over and putting her hands beside his shoulders. Her legs are spread, her knees bent. This way, her hips are flexed, she avoids arching her back, and she can support her own weight. For spice, she can try turning around so that she's facing his feet, supporting herself by putting her hands on his knees.

A man with back pain can try this position: The woman lies on her back with her legs extending over the edge of the bed and her feet flat on the floor. He kneels on the floor between her legs and enters. He can take some of the weight off his upper body by leaning his elbows on the bed, Dr. White suggests.

Bicycling

Like almost any kind of sustained aerobic exercise, bicycling tends to make people feel trim, taut—and randy. These delightful benefits of participating in the popular sport surfaced in a 1989 survey of the readers of *Bicycling* magazine. Of the more than 1,600 (mostly male) cyclists surveyed, 66 percent reported they believed bicycling made them better lovers, and 44 percent said it increased their sex drive. Fourteen percent even reported having had sex during a bicycling rest stop. The survey also added a bit of cannon fodder to the sex wars: Men reported that they were more likely to think about sex while they were cycling, and women, that they were more likely to think about cycling during sex.

The Perils of Pedaling

These recreational riders also reported one mildly bothersome sexual side effect of riding. More than half admitted having experienced a little bit of genital numbness after a long ride. This is a relatively minor inconvenience, of course, far outweighed by the benefits of riding. But it's worth noting that in some extreme cases, it can make some male cyclists at least temporarily impotent.

In one such case reported in the medical literature, a 55-year-old doctor who was also an enthusiastic exerciser began noticing a sensation of tightness around the head of his penis after his daily 12-minute bouts on a stationary bicycle. This rather distressing sensation went away a few minutes after he got off the bike, but something much more worrisome also began happening: During lovemaking, he noticed his erections were slower in coming and more difficult to maintain. The numbness in his penis went away after he lowered the bicycle seat, but after pumping up his penance to 20 minutes a day, the doctor's ability to achieve an erection gradually wilted away until he was almost totally impotent.

The doctor who examined the fit physician, finding nothing else wrong, recommended that the man simply stop riding the exercise bike. A month later, his potency had returned to normal.

The examining doctor theorized that the man's problems were caused by sustained pressure on the perineum, the area between the anus and genitals. The hard, narrow bike seat had apparently squeezed off the blood flow to the man's penis, causing the sensations of numbness. But it was compression of the pudendal nerves, which service the genitals, that caused his impotence.

Don't let this minor-league horror story dissuade you from biking. But do remember these tips from experts: When you're in the saddle, try not to put so much weight on the forward, pubic area rather than the rearward, sitting area. For men, the bike seat should be level and at a height that allows the knees to be slightly bent at the bottom of each pedal stroke.

BIRDS AND BEES

How do you teach your kids about sex and then teach them to be sexually responsible?

Surely it's one of the most critical tasks of parenthood, but an astounding number of parents manage to think of some excuse to avoid the whole thing altogether.

"Parents still hold on to the false hope that if they don't mention sex, and the child doesn't hear about sex, somehow the child won't have any idea that sex even exists," says Jacqueline Forrest, M.D., vice president of research at the Alan Guttmacher Institute in New York City.

That's like assuming they'll never notice the sky unless you tell them to look up. Sex, of course, *does* exist, and kids' bodies tell them about it soon enough. They tumble headlong into their sexual awakening, frightened and confused, their hormones aflame, their bodies surging and swelling with alarming new urges—whether you're there to help them through it or not.

Urgent Need for Information

Today, the average age at which a typical American first has intercourse is 16 or 17, according to a survey done by the Kinsey Institute. Another recent survey showed that 35 percent of 15-year-old boys, 49 percent of 16-year-old boys and 61 percent of 17-year-old boys have had sexual intercourse. All that raging teenage testosterone adds up to another somber statistic, too: About a million American teenage girls get pregnant every year, about three-quarters of them unintentionally.

But perhaps the scariest numbers of all are those that apply to the spread of AIDS among the young. Around 20 percent of all people diagnosed with AIDS in 1988 were in their twenties—and since the incubation period of HIV (human immunodeficiency virus, the virus that causes AIDS) is thought to be eight to ten years, researchers conclude that this means those infections occurred when these young people were teenagers. The U.S. Surgeon General has concluded that teenagers are "especially vulnerable" to AIDS because of their curiosity, their raging hormones and their general foolishness.

They Want to Hear It from *You*

But won't kids learn about AIDS, safe sex and all the rest of it in school? Unfortunately, the quality and completeness of sex education in public schools varies dramatically from place to place. "In general, we think it's horribly inadequate—less than 10 percent of American kids get what we feel is adequate sex education in school," says Deborah Haffner, executive director of the Sex Information and Education Council of the United States.

But more than that, kids would really rather hear it from *you.* When teenagers are polled about where they'd *like* to learn about sex—from friends, school counselors or their parents—nine out of ten say they would prefer to hear about it from Mom and Dad. It's *your* job. And it could be your finest hour. Why not rise to the occasion? Here's some good general advice about how to go about giving your child helpful, accurate and potentially lifesaving information about sex.

The big talk doesn't work. Many parents still picture themselves (someday) sitting down with their teenage son or daughter, awkwardly clearing their throats and launching into a 2-hour keynote address about the joys, sorrows and physiological complexities of sex. No wonder they never get around to doing it! Just *thinking* about it is embarrassing. (Also, not many of us know enough about sex to last that long.)

But the plain fact is "the big talk doesn't work," says Howard Ruppel, executive director of the Society for the Scientific Study of Sex. That's simply not the way kids (or anybody else, for that matter) really learn things. We absorb information in little snippets, over time, rather than having a dump truck–load of it poured on our heads all at once. The "big talk" quickly turns into information overload, and the child hardly remembers anything. After all, when you were in school learning mathematics, you didn't learn it just once—you spent years at the task.

The earlier, the better. A much better approach is to think of your child's entire childhood as a time of learning—about trees and animals, about the exports of Venezuela and about sex. And the earlier you begin, the easier it is for everybody, say a host of experts.

What's *too* early? "When is it too early to teach a kid about red wagons, or how chicks hatch out of eggs?" Ruppel responds. "What families need to do from the cradle onward is treat reproduction as just another part of life and establish an easy, natural communication about it."

Parents who worry that they may be giving their kids too much, too early, should relax—kids tend to process only what they're ready for. "If they're too young to understand it, it just goes in one ear and out the other. They don't even remember it," says Jean Brown, developer of an innovative sex education program called the Parent-Child Sexuality Education Program. But if they're ready, it sticks.

Don't be embarrassed. Parents often have trouble talking to kids about sex, at least partly because they're embarrassed about it themselves. But the *kids* aren't—at least not while they're still young. Research has shown that kids don't usually feel uncomfortable talking about pregnancy and childbirth until sometime between the ages of eight and ten, which is one more reason why starting early makes the whole thing easier for everybody.

Become a masterful question-answerer. Take the opportunity, whenever it presents itself (say, a pregnancy or birth in the neighborhood, or a trip to the zoo or the farm), to tell them a little about "the birds and the bees." If you're unsure about your child's level of comprehension, start out by asking them what their ideas of childbirth are. That way, you can get a better feel for where they stand and tailor your responses accordingly.

If they ask questions, respond calmly, honestly and simply. Don't make things up and don't evade. Becoming a masterful question-answerer—whether the subject be sex or the seaworthiness of the Santa Maria—is one of the great marks of successful parenting, say the experts.

Buy time. Kids have a way of picking totally inappropriate moments to ask profound or embarrassing questions. In the supermarket checkout line, scanning the latest headlines in the tabloids, they'll turn and ask, "Mommy, what is rape?" At moments like these, you feel you really must give the child a fair and honest answer—but not now! The solution, says Brown, is just to buy time. Don't ignore the question or give an evasive answer, but promise the child you'll talk about it later—in the car on the way to soccer practice, for instance. "Parents don't need to feel that they must always have a ready answer for questions about sex," says Brown. "Give yourself a little time to think about it first."

Call a spade a spade. When kids ask you questions about sex, give them answers that are both honest and accurate. *Don't* make up dumb, cutesy names for body parts. Human reproduction is as lovely and perfect a thing as the ocean by moonlight or the aurora borealis, and there's no reason to be ashamed of it. Call a penis a penis, not a wee-wee, a pee-pee or a "thing."

"If you were telling a kid not to cross the street until he looked for cars, you wouldn't call a car a bippy, would you?" asks Ruppel. "We don't use made-up names for anything else, so why do we use them when we're talking about sex?"

Made-up names simply force kids to relearn the right names later—and somehow it communicates the message that we think talking about the body is nasty or wrong.

Decide what your sexual values are. Sex education is very value-laden, and it should be. Kids need to know not only the physiological facts of sex but how you *feel* about them.

"The fundamental question is, What sexual values do I want to teach my kids?" says Haffner. What values you decide to teach them is a matter of personal conscience. But very often, even people with fiercely held religious or moral convictions have not *clearly* thought out what sexual values they'd like to communicate to their kids. It's important to *think* about this and to precisely and consciously decide what they are to be.

"With our whole society in such a state of flux, most people are completely at a loss about what sort of sexual values to pass down to their kids," says Ruppel. "Usually they just recycle their parents' values, or they fall back on the old myths—stuff about storks and cabbage patches and getting hair on your hands. Neither solution is really adequate. You have to think it through for yourself."

If you say nothing, you're saying something. You communicate powerful messages about love, physical affection and sex to your kids all the time, whether you know it or not. When you come home from work and give your spouse a hug and a kiss—or don't—you're communicating a message to kids about whether physical affection is permissible. When you allow their childhoods to slip by without ever uttering a word about sex—that, too, is a powerful message, and kids get it loud and clear.

"I teach a sex education course at the University of Iowa, and every year I have my students write an autobiography," says Ruppel. "Every year, nearly all of them write, 'I received no sex education in my home.' And every year, I have to say to them 'No, you received a *lot* of sex education at home—what you learned was: Don't ask any questions.' "

Adds Haffner: "When you say to a small child 'Here's your nose, here's your belly, here's your knees, and here's your toes,' you've just taught the kid that there's a part of the body that has no name—a part that is not spoken of."

Try to become conscious of the *nonverbal* ways you transmit negative messages about love and sex, through all the things you *don't* say and all the things you *don't* do. Try to turn those errors of omission into a continual demonstration of what it means to be a loving, mature and sexually responsible adult. It's the best way to teach kids about the birds and the bees.

"I have come to believe," says Haffner, "that the best sex education would simply be to have two parents who love each other."

BIRTH CONTROL.

See Cervical Cap, Coitus Interruptus, Condom, Contraceptives, Diaphragm, Intrauterine Device (IUD), Norplant, The Pill, Rhythm Method, Spermicides, Tubal Sterilization, Vasectomy

BISEXUALITY

People tend to think that a person's sexual orientation is a sort of black-or-white affair: Either you're heterosexual or you're homosexual, and that's that.

But the matter is just not that simple. Human sexual desire is both enormously mysterious and bewilderingly diverse—it's more like a vast spectrum of color than a simple division between black and white. A huge number of people are exclusively heterosexual during their entire adult lives; a far smaller number are exclusively homosexual. But there's also a vast number of people who fall somewhere in between—people whose sexual desires are aroused, either often or occasionally, in fantasy or in fact, by *both* men and women.

Drawing the "Bi" Line

People in this group are known as *bisexuals*—although even sex researchers are not exactly sure how to define this term. Are you a bisexual *only* if you've actually had sex with both male and female partners? What about someone who has a fleeting homosexual encounter as an adolescent but never repeats the experience as a heterosexual adult? What about those who sometimes fantasize about having homosexual sex while they're making love to their spouse? (In fact, researchers have found that this is one of the most common fantasies of heterosexuals.)

Taking all this into account, Dr. Alfred Kinsey and his colleagues devised a seven-part scale, later to become known as the Kinsey scale, in order to give a more accurate picture of the full scope of human sexual orientation. Thousands of men and women were ranked on this scale after being extensively interviewed about their lifelong sexual experiences and their feelings of sexual attraction since puberty. At one extreme were people who were exclusively heterosexual, and at the opposite extreme, those who were exclusively homosexual. In between, there were five different categories to include everyone who might be considered bisexual to one degree or another.

After examining the resulting data, Dr. Kinsey made this rather amazing pronouncement: "Since only 50 percent of the population is exclusively heterosexual throughout its adult life, and since only 4 percent of the population is exclusively homosexual throughout its life, it appears that nearly half (46 percent) of the population engages in both heterosexual and homosexual activities, or reacts to persons of both sexes, in the course of their adult lives." Alex Comfort, M.D., Ph.D., in *The Joy of Sex,* goes even further, suggesting that "all people are bisexual—that is to say, able to respond sexually to some extent to people of either sex."

Still, if you define bisexuality a bit more narrowly and include only those people who have actually had sex with both men and women over a period of years and not just people who occasionally fantasize about same-sex encounters, only 10 or 15 percent of the population would qualify, the Kinsey Institute recently reported. Interestingly enough, a number of different studies have also discovered that about twice as many men as women fall into this "in-between," bisexual category, although it's still not clear why. And as if to make the whole picture even murkier, other studies have shown that over 60 percent of adult men who consider themselves homosexuals and over 70 percent of adult women who consider themselves lesbians have at least occasionally made love with partners of the opposite sex.

And you thought you had it all figured out! (See also "Safer Sex.")

BOOKS ON BETTER SEX

There's no end to what you can learn about sex. Besides being inherently fascinating, learning more about sex may just enhance your pleasure and that of your partner as well. Here's a short list of good books about sex and sexuality.

General

Human Sexuality, 3rd ed., by William H. Masters, M.D., Virginia E. Johnson and Robert C. Kolodny, M.D. (Scott, Foresman, 1988). This is actually a textbook, but a comprehensive and interesting one.

Human Sexual Response by William H. Masters, M.D., and Virginia E. Johnson (Little, Brown, 1966). The writing is dense and difficult, but the subject is fascinating. This is the first scientific report on human sexual response.

The Illustrated Kama Sutra, Ananga-Ranga and Perfumed Garden: The Classic Eastern Love Texts (Park Street Press, 1987). The Sir Richard Burton, F. F. Arbuthnot translation of the ancient erotic treatises, gloriously illustrated.

The Kinsey Institute New Report on Sex: What You Must Know to Be Sexually Literate by June M. Reinisch, Ph.D., with Ruth Beasley (St. Martin's Press, 1990). Authoritative and far-ranging, this book, coauthored by the director of the Kinsey Institute, leaves almost no stone unturned.

Masters and Johnson on Sex and Human Loving by William H. Masters, M.D., Virginia E. Johnson and Robert Kolodny, M.D. (Little, Brown, 1986). This is probably the most readable, and practical, of the many books written by Masters, Johnson and colleagues.

The New Joy of Sex: A Gourmet Guide to Lovemaking for the Nineties by Alex Comfort, M.D., Ph.D. (Crown, 1991). First published in 1972, this old standby—the wittiest, warmest, most explicit sex manual ever written—has been newly updated for the age of AIDS.

Sex in History by Reay Tannahill (Stein & Day, 1980). All about sex through the ages, this easy-reading overview is really a delightful romp.

Sexual Behavior in the Human Male (W. B. Saunders, 1948) and *Sexual Behavior in the Human Female* (W. B. Saunders, 1953) by Alfred C. Kinsey and colleagues. These are really basic texts—a little dense, a little outdated, but still worth reading after all these years.

The Sexual Pharmacy: The Complete Guide to Drugs with Sexual Side Effects by M. Laurence Lieberman (New American Library, 1988). Written by a pharmacist, this volume lists over 200 drugs that can affect sexual performance (not all of them for the worse).

Sexual Practices: The Story of Human Sexuality by Edgar Gregersen, Ph.D. (Franklin Watts, 1983). This book is an anthropologist's fascinating account of sex in cultures across the globe.

For Women

Becoming Orgasmic: A Sexual Growth Program for Women by Julia Heiman and Joseph LoPiccolo, Ph.D. (Prentice-Hall, 1988). This is a practical program designed by therapists.

For Each Other: Sharing Sexual Intimacy (New American Library, 1984) and *For Yourself: The Fulfillment of Female Sexuality* (New American Library, 1975) by Lonnie Barbach, Ph.D. These two great books about female sexuality are often recommended by therapists.

The G-Spot and Other Recent Discoveries about Human Sexuality by Alice Kahn Ladas, Beverly Whipple and John D. Perry (Dell, 1982). This book makes a convincing case for the existence of the G-spot, female ejaculation and a few other things that make women mysterious.

For Men

BioPotency: A Guide to Sexual Success by Richard E. Berger, M.D., and Deborah Berger (Rodale Press, 1987). This is a thorough but readable explanation of the causes of, and cures for, male impotence.

How to Overcome Premature Ejaculation by Helen Singer Kaplan, M.D., Ph.D. (Brunner/Mazel, 1989). This book explains an effective method so clearly that you may not need a therapist at all.

The Male by Sherman J. Silber, M.D. (Charles Scribner's Sons, 1981). This is a breezy, popular book written by a leading urologist and microsurgeon.

Male Sexuality: A Guide to Sexual Fulfillment by Bernie Zilbergeld, Ph.D. (Bantam, 1978). This is probably the best book on the subject in print.

Sexual Solutions: A Guide for Men and the Women Who Love Them by Michael Castleman (Touchstone Books, 1980). Here's a calm, warm self-help book about men's sex problems and their cures.

42

Birth Control

Contraceptive Technology 1990-1992, 15th rev. ed., by Robert A. Hatcher, M.D., and colleagues (Irvington Publishers, 1990). This volume is considered the bible of birth control, written by doctors and specialists and updated every other year.

Illness

Sexuality and Chronic Illness: A Comprehensive Approach by Leslie R. Schover, Ph.D., and Soren Buus Jensen, M.D. (Guilford Press, 1988). For people suffering from chronic conditions like cancer, cardiovascular disease or diabetes, this book (although fairly technical) offers a serious look at the sexual side effects and how to overcome them.

Aging

Love and Sex after 60, by Robert N. Butler and Myrna I. Lewis (Harper & Row, 1988). Here's a frank discussion of sex and aging.

Menopause: A Guide for Women and the Men Who Love Them by Winnifred B. Cutler, Ph.D., C. R. Garcia and D. A. Edwards (W. W. Norton, 1983). This volume is useful, authoritative and written in plain English.

Prime Time: Sexual Health for Men over Fifty by Leslie R. Schover, Ph.D. (Holt, Rinehart & Winston, 1984). Here's some practical advice for boosting male sexual longevity.

BREASTS

There's probably never been a culture in history that was entirely blind to the beauty of the female breast. "Thy breasts are like two young roes that are twins, which feed among the lilies," sang the psalmist of Solomon. The womanly breast probably deserves such reverence, having suckled civilization— but it's also, of course, a potent trigger of sexual arousal and sexual pleasure.

The breast, nipple and areola (the darker ring that encircles the nipple) are richly endowed with nerve endings, which is why they're so sensitive to all kinds of stimulation. In fact, William Masters, M.D., and Virginia Johnson, of the Masters and Johnson Institute in St. Louis, discovered that a tiny fraction of women (about 1 percent) are actually able to masturbate to orgasm simply by touching and stroking their nipples and breasts. (How on earth do they *do* that?) "Women have a much higher ability than men to 'erogenize' areas of the body far away from the clitoris and vagina," explains Dr. Masters.

On the other hand, many women really don't respond to having their breasts kissed, sucked or stroked. Studies have shown that although 90 percent of women say their partners like to fondle their breasts during sex play, only about 50 percent of women actually like it. Some women find it uncomfortable or even painful, especially just before or during menstruation, when the breasts tend to become tender. For many women, says Dr. Masters, "the only real stimulation in breast play is watching the man enjoy it." Either way, it's important to communicate with your partner. If you're a woman, tell your partner if you enjoy it or not; if you're a man, ask her if she does or doesn't.

Changes during Arousal

The changes a woman's breasts undergo during sexual arousal depend partly on whether she has previously breastfed a baby, explains Dr. Masters. In a woman with unsuckled, "virginal" breasts, nipple erection is usually the first sign of arousal. (Not all women get erect nipples, though—and if your nipples don't stand at attention when you're aroused, you shouldn't worry that you're frigid. Also, some women have inverted nipples—"innies" instead of "outies"—which are quite normal but make nipple erection impossible.) Then the areolas swell, often so much that "frequently it looks as if she's lost her nipple erection," says Dr. Masters, who has probably observed the process more often than any man in history. Then the breast itself, engorged with blood, begins to swell—sometimes by 20 or 25 percent. It becomes so swollen that the blue traceries of veins can be seen, and it looks "just like a nursing breast," he says.

The breast of a woman who has suckled a child goes through the same changes during arousal, except that it doesn't swell. (The circulatory demands of nursing result in a changed pattern of blood flow.)

The Parade of Puberty

Breasts are probably as much a symbol of womanliness to women as they are to men, at least partly because breast enlargement is usually the first sign of puberty in girls. Usually the breasts begin to bud sometime after the age of 12, but some girls, probably because of an overeager endocrine system, may begin showing breasts as early as 8. Budding breasts are the first proud announcement of a dizzying parade of changes that accompany puberty, usually followed (in order) by the appearance of straight pubic hair, then a generalized growth spurt, kinky pubic hair, menstruation and finally the growth of hair beneath the arms.

But even after the hormonal tides of puberty have abated and a woman is a full-fledged adult, she's likely to be unsatisfied with her breasts. Many women worry that their breasts are not the same size, for instance. But the truth is that just as no two pairs of feet are precisely matched, no woman has a perfectly matched pair of breasts. In fact, some researchers now estimate that more than half of all American women have breasts that vary so much in size that it's readily noticeable to the naked eye. Nearly a quarter have one breast that is at least 20 percent larger than the other, reports the Kinsey Institute.

Bigger Does Not Equal Better

Many women also long for bigger breasts, presumably because they believe men will find them more attractive. (To be fair, one has to admit that our whole *culture* seems obsessed with big breasts.) Yet it may be that men are not actually as infatuated with the Dolly Parton School of Female Beauty as women think they are. The Kinsey Institute reports that at least one study of what men find most sexually attractive about women showed that only half of them even mentioned breasts at all, and of those, half said they preferred *small* ones.

But scientific studies have never done much to dissuade people from their original beliefs or their behavior. Sales of hormonal breast creams, breast pumps and breast-boosting exercise schemes will no doubt continue at a steady clip. Does anything actually work? Except for breast augmentation surgery, says Dr. Masters, "the short answer is no."

Breast exercises may strengthen the underlying pectoral muscles but will not alter the size or shape of the breast itself. One study done at the University of Arizona Exercise and Sports Sciences Laboratory carefully monitored changes in bust size in a group of women who underwent a 21-day "bust development program" (a series of upper body exercises using a spring-loaded plastic paddle device). At the end of the study, after every conceivable kind of measurement was taken, the researchers could find no increase in the women's bust sizes whatsoever. (In fact, many of the women registered tiny *decreases* in breast size.)

Breast Implants: The Safety Question

If she's not blessed with them by birth, implant surgery is really the only thing that can give a woman those high, full, firm breasts our culture so adores.

Breast augmentation surgery, which first became available in the early 1960s, involves implanting a half-moon-shaped envelope of silicone or polyurethane, filled with silicone gel or saline solution, directly into the breast. The implant is slipped through a small incision made at the crease along the underside of the breast and normally leaves only a tiny scar. Over a million American women have had breast implants, 80 percent of them for cosmetic reasons and the rest to restore breasts damaged by cancer surgery.

Even so, in recent years an increasing number of questions have been raised about the long-term safety of breast implants. Some medical studies have suggested that the silicone gel may leak out of the envelope and migrate to other parts of the body, causing pain, infections and a hardening of skin and tissue called scleroderma, and perhaps increasing the risk of autoimmune disorders. Silicone and some of its breakdown products have been shown to cause cancer in lab animals (although—at least so far—there's no convincing evidence that it causes cancer in humans).

There's also a concern that implants may make early detection of breast cancer more difficult by interfering with mammograms. The American College of Radiology recently issued a consensus statement that "women contemplating augmentation be informed that mammography may be more difficult to perform and may be less effective." (Other radiologists dispute this claim, but the controversy lingers.)

Many of these long-simmering claims and questions came to a head in 1992, when the Food and Drug Administration (FDA) reviewed mountains of data on the safety of implants. (Implants first came on the market before the FDA was given authority to regulate medical devices; this was the first time a sweeping review of the data had been conducted.) FDA scientists concluded two things. First, although the evidence was sketchy and inconclusive, there were enough reports of health problems associated with implants to be worrisome. And second, there simply were not enough hard scientific data to conclude that they were completely safe. As a result, the FDA has called a moratorium on selling and implanting the devices until further studies can be conducted.

So for now, at least, that's one option that won't be available to most women. If you already *have* breast implants and they're giving you no trouble, there's no reason to have them removed, stresses FDA Commissioner David A. Kessler, M.D. But women who are troubled by symptoms they suspect are related to their implants (such as joint pain, muscle pain or fatigue) should not hesitate to see their doctor.

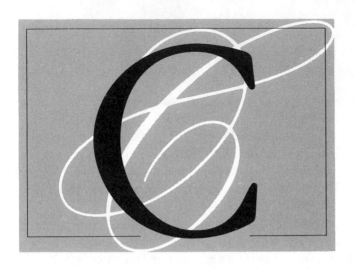

CAFFEINE

Go ahead, enjoy your coffee. Over the years, a vast array of studies have explored the connection between caffeine, sex and reproduction. Researchers looked into whether caffeine causes birth defects or increases the risk of breast cancer. And for the most part, your steaming cup of java has been cleared of reproductive wrongdoing, as long as you drink only a cup or two.

One recent review of the literature concluded that "no evidence has yet been offered that caffeine consumption at moderate levels by pregnant women has any discernible effect on their fetuses." Other studies seem to have ruled out any connection between caffeine and breast cancer, which was a worry at one time.

But what about sexual performance? Another group of studies has shown that caffeine can deliver a performance-boosting jolt to sperm cells, increasing both their velocity (speed) and motility (liveliness). But don't imagine that Folger's Mountain Grown will become the next fertility drug—in these studies, massive amounts of caffeine were applied directly to semen samples wriggling in laboratory dishes. Practically speaking, the only value of this finding is to suggest a way of improving the chances of conception during *in vitro* fertilization.

Look Who's Still Perking

But probably the most intriguing new discovery emerged as an unexpected surprise in a survey of the sexual activities of elderly residents of a sample neighborhood in Michigan. A team of researchers from William Beaumont Hospital, in the Detroit suburb of Royal Oak, interviewed almost 2,000 men and women over the age of 60. They asked about things such as whether the men had trouble getting an erection and whether the women were still sexually active.

After the data were analyzed, the team was surprised to discover that the elderly householders who drank at least one cup of coffee a day were considerably more likely to be sexually active than those who were coffee abstainers. Sixty-two percent of the married women who drank coffee reported they were sexually active, compared with only 40 percent of the married women who didn't imbibe. Among men, the researchers found a similar connection: 36 percent of the coffee drinkers admitted they were sometimes impotent, compared with 59 percent of those who didn't drink coffee.

What's going on here? It's not exactly clear. In their report in the *Archives of Internal Medicine,* the researchers point out that the caffeine in coffee belongs to a group of substances known as methylxanthines, a powerful central nervous system stimulant and smooth-muscle relaxant that is also known to enhance the response to sensory stimulation. But unfortunately, since it was aging, not coffee, that was the real subject of this study, the researchers failed to ask if these folks were drinking caffeinated or decaffeinated coffee—meaning that caffeine may not have been the active ingredient at all (if there even was one). It's possible, they suggest, that the coffee drinkers in this particular group just happened to be a little sexier than the rest.

CANCER

Doctors usually assess the value of cancer treatments like chemotherapy or surgery from the point of view of survival rates alone. But for the patient, other considerations may be nearly as important—like the overall quality of life, including sexual life. And cancer, even if you survive it, can often have a dispiriting effect on that prized, private part of life.

From a strictly physiological point of view, cancerous tumors can interfere with the mechanics of sexual arousal by damaging nerves, blood vessels, hormonal systems or the genitals themselves. But it's even more likely that the *treatments* you get for cancer will have a negative effect on your sex life. Surgery may leave you with unsightly scars; chemotherapy gives you (at least temporarily) an unhealthy-looking pallor, makes your hair fall out and makes you nauseous; and cancer drugs can have other unpleasant side effects. Is it any wonder that cancer patients often struggle with feelings that they're physically unlovable at the same time they're struggling to overcome the disease itself?

Problems for Women

For women who have cancer surgery or radiation treatments, the most common sexual problem is pain during intercourse, says Leslie R. Schover, Ph.D., staff psychologist at the Center for Sexual Function at the Cleveland Clinic Foundation in Ohio. The same chemotherapy drugs that cause painful blisters inside the mouth can also irritate the lining of the vagina.

"The discomfort can often be alleviated by trying different positions for intercourse, using estrogen replacement therapy or water-based vaginal lubricants or dilating the vagina on a regular basis," says Dr. Schover. She advises women to try positions that allow them to control the depth and angle of penis penetration.

The vaginal dilator, a dildolike device, is often given to women who have had radiation therapy or pelvic surgeries in order to keep the vagina stretchable and soft. (One side effect of radiation therapy and some surgeries in the pelvic area is pelvic fibrosis, a gradual buildup of stiff fibrous material in the vagina.) Many women are embarrassed about using a dilator, perhaps feeling that it's really a kind of masturbation. Still, says Dr. Schover, a woman who isn't having sex a couple of times a week should use a vaginal dilator up to three times a week for the first few months after surgery and "probably for the rest of her life, since pelvic fibrosis is a slow process."

Pain during intercourse can also be caused by premature menopause, which is induced when women have their ovaries removed during cancer surgery or have chemotherapy or radiation treatments in the pelvic area. (Women who've had *both* chemotherapy and radiation treatments are especially likely to experience premature menopause, as well as menstrual irregularities.) To many women, this may come as a surprise, since doctors often fail to adequately warn female patients of the treatments' sexual side effects. Yet this artificially induced menopause is "often more abrupt and severe than the effects of natural menopause," says Dr. Schover.

Problems for Men

For men, the most common sexual complaint after cancer treatment is the inability to get a serviceable erection. It's a distressing problem, but at least it's less common than it once was. In the old days, surgery for prostate cancer caused impotence about 80 percent of the time; nowadays, nerve-sparing versions of the old operation may result in impotence less than half the time. Also, a new generation of hormonal drugs for prostate cancer (called nonsteroidal antiandrogens) is less likely to cause impotence than the old drugs. And even if treatment does result in impotence, there are a whole variety of promising new options available—from inflatable implants to injectable drugs—that may help restore functioning. (For more, see "Erection Problems.")

Terrible Fears, Crazy Ideas

But if cancer has a profound effect on the physical aspects of sex, it can have an even more complex impact on the emotions. Sex and cancer, after all, are two of the most potent forces we ever encounter, and when they explode in the subconscious at the same time, you often get a potent brew of terrible fears, dark foreboding and frankly crazy ideas. In some cases, simply telling a man he has cancer is enough to cause impotence, due to the depression and anxiety this news engenders. Other people can't seem to shake a feeling that the cancer has made them untouchable, repulsive, damaged—or that their partners feel this way—and these feelings can put a swift and terrible end to a sexual relationship.

Researchers have found that even people who should know better sometimes come to believe strange things about their cancers. Some come to feel that genital cancers are punishment for some imagined sin like masturbation, an abortion or an affair. A surprising number of people still think that genital cancers are caused by promiscuity or that they are contagious and can be passed on to a sex partner. After her cervical cancer was diagnosed, for instance, one of Dr. Schover's patients was accused of sexual promiscuity by her mother-in-law. Other cancer patients find themselves vowing to give up sex in exchange for survival, no matter how crazy that may sound.

The good news is that several studies have shown that divorce or separation is no more common among cancer patients than it is among anybody else.

Marriages that crumble under the strain of cancer are usually those that were ready to crumble anyway; those that survive often grow deeper and more meaningful.

To help restore your sex life to what it was before the cancer was diagnosed, Dr. Schover says, it helps to change maladaptive beliefs—such as the idea that sex has to occur spontaneously. If you can get comfortable with the idea that lovemaking will take a little more planning—you may have to schedule it for times when you're not fatigued or uncomfortable—you're likely to have sex more often. Also, with your doctor's guidance and advice, make a gradual return to sexuality. Rather than jump-starting a love life that's lain dormant for months, start with kissing, cuddling and genital caressing before moving on to the full show. Women have less pain if they learn to relax the muscles that control the vagina with Kegel exercises. (See "Kegel Exercises.")

And don't forget to thank your spouse.

"Having a warm and supportive partner is the single most helpful factor in sexual rehabilitation after cancer treatment," Dr. Schover says.

CANDIDA ALBICANS.

See Yeast Infections

CASTRATION

Here's a sure cure for male pattern baldness—in fact, it's the only sure cure known: Get yourself castrated before you reach puberty. Well, yes—it's a bit of a high price to pay for the just-stepped-out-of-the-salon look, but it works. It also suggests something about the wonderful complexity of male sexual development and the oddities of the strange practice known as castration.

The Palace Punishment

In ancient days, castration was known as "the palace punishment" because shearing off the genitals of male slaves, captured enemies or other unlucky young men was thought to be the only way to make them safe for service in the harem. There were several variations on this odious operation. Some castrati, or eunuchs, as they were called (in Greek, the word means "he who has charge of the bed"), were simply shaved of all their external sex organs, so that they had to urinate through a quill. Others were relieved of only their penises, leaving the testes intact; sometimes only the testes were removed. Whatever method was used, the risk of infection and death was high. In fact, in Reay Tannahill's *Sex in History,* a delightful romp through five millennia of sexual practices, she reports that "in the seventeenth century on the Upper Nile, the main source of supply for fully shaved eunuchs in the West, only one in four could be relied on to survive."

But although lost, the severed genitalia were not forgotten. Chinese eunuchs treasured their dismembered members like small children who've lost a tooth, secreting them carefully "in common pint measures hermetically closed, and placed on a high shelf." Even in the late nineteenth century, Tannahill reports, in order to show that he was qualified for a palace promotion, the aspiring eunuch might have to present his "pickled precious" to the chief eunuch in order to demonstrate his fitness for the job. Sometimes they were even buried with the poor fellow in his coffin.

Is There Life without Testosterone?

If a male was shorn of his genitals (and his testosterone, which is manufactured primarily in the testes) while still a boy, he never went through puberty. All the secondary sex characteristics that we associate with adult males—the deep voice, body hair and beard, muscle mass, large physical size—never got a chance to happen. All of these masculine attributes are triggered by testosterone, that potent hormone that also fires up the male libido. Instead, the palace eunuchs who were castrated as boys had long, spindly arms and legs with very little muscle mass. They didn't go through the tremendous growth spurt most boys experience at around age 12, and they kept their angelic, preadolescent voices for life. (In fact, until 1878, eunuchs were employed in the Papal Choir of the Sistine Chapel for that reason.)

Their bodies were also almost completely innocent of hair, and they were beardless—but they usually had thick, luxuriant hair on top of their heads. Why? Because, in a strange hormonal irony, it's male hormones that trigger male pattern baldness (at least in those men who are prone to it), and it's also male hormones that encourage the growth of body hair. That same testosterone that gives you a hairy chest also makes you bald.

What happens to men who are castrated *after* puberty? They simply retain the deep voices, heavy beards and other secondary sex characteristics that they developed during puberty, looking in every way like normal adult males, reports Sherman J. Silber, M.D., renowned urologist, microsurgeon and author of *The Male*. What happens to the sex drive of these men? Well, says Dr. Silber, it varies widely: "Most castrated men do retain their libido for a certain period of time. It tends to diminish gradually, and eventually in most cases the desire for sex goes away completely."

This is not exactly news. Tannahill reports that "it had been known from Greek times, and probably before, that castration did not eliminate sexual desire and that a castrate who had preserved his penis was, under certain circumstances, capable of having erections for some time afterwards. . . . Richard Burton, the Victorian traveler, reported that a eunuch's wife had told him that her husband could even be aroused to a kind of ejaculation (presumably of fluid from the prostate) after a protracted period of erotic stimulation."

Castration as Cure

But castration is not always a crude ancient rite of death and domination; in modern medicine, it's used to save lives. In 1941, a urologist named Dr. Charles Huggins made the amazing discovery (which later won him a Nobel Prize in medicine) that most prostate cancers depend on testosterone to continue growing. Today many older men whose prostate cancer has spread throughout their bodies are shorn of their testicles (the operation is called an orchiectomy) in order to slow the spread of the disease. Sometimes the results are dramatic. Dr. Silber reports: "Patients who appeared to be on their deathbed, in miserable pain and nearly comatose, will after castration improve overnight, wake up the next day bright and cheerful and go home within the week." (For more, see "Testosterone.")

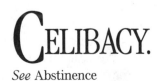

CELIBACY.

See Abstinence

CERVICAL CAP

The cervical cap is a contraceptive device for women that looks like a tiny rubber top hat or a miniature diaphragm. It fits directly over the cervix (the bulbous lower end of the uterus, at the deep end of the vagina) and seals off the womb from invasion by sperm. Cervical caps have to be prescribed and fitted by a doctor, because it's important that they form a snug seal around the cervix and aren't dislodged during intercourse. A few women (less than 10 percent) can't use caps because the shape of their cervixes makes a proper fit impossible.

Shortly before intercourse, the cervical cap is one-third filled with spermicidal cream or jelly and then slipped into the vagina over the cervix. Some experts recommend allowing half an hour between insertion and intercourse, so a nice tight suction develops. The cap should provide good protection for the next 48 hours, no matter how often you make love in the meantime, although it should be removed and carefully cleaned within 72 hours.

Casanova's Invention

Although cervical caps have been available in Europe for years, they were approved by the Food and Drug Administration for use in the United States only in 1988 and are still not widely available here. Yet cervical caps of one sort or another have been around for over 300 years. The amorous scoundrel Casanova is supposed to have slipped hollowed-out lemon halves over his lovers' cervixes, and early doctors used caps made of molded beeswax, silver or copper. The globe-trotting birth control advocate Margaret Sanger, after having discovered a kind of cervical cap called a pessary being used in France, described it in one famous 1914 pamphlet as "the surest method of absolutely preventing conception." This is no longer true.

In terms of effectiveness, "the vaginal contraceptive sponge, diaphragm and [cervical] cap methods all provide similar contraceptive efficacy," according to *Contraceptive Technology 1990-1992,* the doctors' bible of contraception. Studies have shown that of every 100 women who use cervical caps or diaphragms, about 18 will get pregnant during the first year. Actually, though, in various studies, pregnancy rates for women using cervical caps have ranged anywhere from 8 to 27 per 100 during the first year of use. What can increase your odds of getting pregnant while using a cervical cap? Several things:

- Frequent intercourse (more than four times a week)
- Being highly fertile (younger than 30)
- A personal sexual style that makes it hard for you to use the cap consistently
- Having previously gotten pregnant while using birth control (of any type)
- Ambivalent feelings about whether or not you want to get pregnant

For instance, a woman's risk of getting pregnant while using a cervical cap is roughly *doubled* if she is less than 30 or makes love more than four times a week. On the other hand, you can *increase* the cap's effectiveness by using one or even two additional kinds of birth control (like condoms or the Pill). Also, be especially careful during the most fertile times of the month—which usually begin about four days before ovulation.

Better Not Use Butter

One important note: It's probably not a good idea to use oil-based lubricants with a cervical cap. Why? Because recent studies have shown that latex condoms significantly deteriorated after an hour's contact with oil-based lubricants like mineral oil, baby oil, suntan oil, vegetable oil and butter. Obviously, a condom is not a cap, but they're made of similar materials, and it's reasonable to be concerned that the same thing might happen. These same studies also showed that some vaginal medications (like Femstat cream, Monistat cream, estrogen cream and Vagisil) could rapidly damage a latex condom. If you need more lubrication during intercourse, try saliva, a few squirts of a vaginal spermicide made for use with the cap or K-Y Jelly or some other water-based lubricants. (See also "Diaphragm.")

CERVIX

Imagine the interior of the vagina as a sort of long, narrow lobby or waiting room. At the far end of this room there's a sort of doorway, sealing off the noise and confusion of the reception area from the quiet inner sanctum of the uterus, or womb. That door is called the cervix—a bulging, fleshy plug about the diameter of a quarter. (Actually, strictly speaking, the cervix is the lower end of the uterus itself.) In its center is an opening (called the os) that's normally about the size of a drinking straw—a tiny passageway through which the voyaging sperm cell must slip before it can reach its goal of conception. (Just before childbirth, this same opening dilates to about 10 centimeters, or the width of five fingers, in order to make way for the descending baby's head. It's through this wondrous secret portal that life passes twice—both coming, as a sperm cell, and going, as a baby.)

Various contraceptive devices, such as the cervical cap and the diaphragm, do their job by blocking off this cervical opening and thus preventing the egg-hunting sperm cell from entering the uterus.

Unpleasant Signs of Infection

Infections of the cervix, known as cervicitis, are fairly common—but fortunately they can usually be taken care of in short order with antibiotics or fungicides. The first sign of cervicitis is usually a vaginal discharge that increases just after menstruation, or sometimes bleeding, pain on intercourse, a burning sensation during urination or even low back pain. All of these symptoms should be brought to the attention of a gynecologist.

That's because similar symptoms may also be a signal of cervical cancer, the second leading cause of cancer deaths (after breast cancer) in women over 40. One of the first warning signs is vaginal bleeding between periods, after intercourse or after menopause; sometimes there's also increased vaginal discharge. The best defense against cervical cancer is the Pap test. It's a simple, painless procedure in which a tiny scraping of cervical tissue is taken and examined under a microscope in order to catch any cell abnormalities at an early stage, when they're still fairly easy to treat and before they have a chance to become malignant.

The American Cancer Society recommends an annual Pap test and pelvic examination for all women under 18 who are or have been sexually active and for all women over 18. After a woman has had at least three consecutive satisfactory, normal annual examinations, the Pap test may be performed less frequently at the discretion of her physician.

CHLAMYDIA

The people most likely to get it probably have never even heard of it. But *Chlamydia trachomitis,* a kind of shrewd and persistent bacterium, is responsible for what is now the most common sexually transmitted disease

(STD) among young adults. Something like four million new cases of chlamydial infection are now reported every year; sexually active adolescent women are its favorite targets.

"It's so pervasive in the young adult population that I think everybody needs to be screened," says Sandra Samuels, M.D., director of Student Health Services at Rutgers University in New Brunswick, New Jersey. "We've seen it in people who are promiscuous and in people who have been monogamous for five years. People can be carriers for a long time without even knowing it."

We're Talking Subtle

Chlamydial infections are sometimes called the "silent STD" for that reason: The symptoms can be so mild that many people don't even know they've been tagged until they've passed the infection on to their partners or it's progressed to a more serious phase. About 80 percent of infected women have no symptoms at all. Once an infected woman does develop symptoms, though, they usually include genital itching and burning, an odorless, thick, yellow-white vaginal discharge, dull pain in the abdomen or bleeding between periods. Men are much more likely to have noticeable symptoms, which usually include pain on urination or a watery discharge from the penis.

The real problem with chlamydia is that its primary target is the reproductive system, and once it gets in there it sets about causing as much trouble as possible. The danger is greatest in women: In them, untreated chlamydial infections can lead to infertility, pelvic inflammatory disease, ectopic (tubal) pregnancy or infections of the cervix. Pregnant women who have chlamydial infections can also transmit the disease to their babies, who may pick up conjunctivitis (eye infections) or pneumonia.

The Leapfrog Effect

The good news is that chlamydia is usually pretty easily treated with antibiotics, usually doxycycline or tetracycline. But Dr. Samuels points out that it's very important that both you *and* your sex partner get the full course of treatment before resuming sex, because the little buggers are exceedingly persistent and may simply leapfrog to the untreated partner. Also, she says, after you've taken the full course of antibiotics, you should go back to the doctor for a follow-up test to make sure the chlamydia colony is completely wiped out.

In a two-year study she conducted among the student population at Rutgers, Dr. Samuels was distressed to find a "persistently high incidence of positive posttreatment chlamydia cultures" among women who'd come into the student health center for treatment. The reason? "We invariably learned, on further questioning, that their sexual partners either were not treated at all or did not take the full course of treatment."

In theory, at least, condoms are "the only thing that offers any protection whatsoever" from chlamydia (except, of course, abstinence), Dr. Samuels says. Even so, in her survey, condoms didn't seem to help much at all: Chlamydia infection rates among students using condoms or diaphragms were about the same as those among students using the Pill or nothing at all. Her theory: The students weren't using condoms and/or contraceptive foam *consistently,* which is the only way they'll do you any good.

Practically speaking, what else can you do to protect yourself from a potentially dangerous disease that you can carry for years without even knowing it? Well, there's no completely satisfying answer. But "periodic screening for chlamydia would be a wise idea, especially if you're in a high-risk group," Dr. Samuels suggests. The highest-risk group: Sexually active women under the age of 24 who don't use condoms, a diaphragm or any other form of barrier contraception. Also, if you've got some other STD, especially gonorrhea, you're much more likely to have chlamydia as well.

Some doctors recommend that all women who've changed sex partners within the past year have a chlamydia test every time they have a Pap test. The chlamydia test is cheap, painless and quick—new in-office test kits allow doctors to give you a fairly accurate yes-or-no answer within 15 minutes.

CHOLESTEROL

Consider for a moment the rather wondrous spectacle of the male erection. Stirred to life by some passing fancy, this humble coil of flesh is suddenly and utterly transformed. What was, a moment before, an undistinguished and disorderly heap is within a matter of seconds transfigured into a rigid, towering tool. What was a cloud becomes a sword. What was a field of hay becomes a tree. It's amazing!

Even urologic specialists still do not fully understand how it works. The basic principle, though, is fairly simple: Once a man is aroused, arteries supplying the penis dilate dramatically, and eight times the normal amount of blood rushes in and fills its spongy tissues, causing them to swell to the point of rigidity. After orgasm, tiny valves release the blood, which rushes away through the veins. Blood flow, in other words, is at the very heart of the mystery of erection. Which brings us to cholesterol. If the small arteries that supply inrushing blood to the penis become clogged with fatty debris and plaque (just as the coronary arteries to the heart become clogged in heart disease), the penis cannot fully inflate. The worse the blockage, the limper the erection.

The "Canary in the Mineshaft"

That, in brief, is the depressing explanation for many cases of impotence, according to information coming out of sexual research centers around the country in recent years. It is, of course, not the only physical cause of impotence, but it is worth considering. It's also why you're reading about cholesterol in a book about sex. Blockage of blood vessels due to high-fat, high-cholesterol diets is not restricted to the heart's coronaries (they're just the most famous of the arteries affected). The arteries that supply blood to the penis clog up, too—and often do so *sooner* than the coronary arteries. In fact, specialists in male impotence now believe that over half the men who are about to have a heart attack or stroke experience impotence during the months before the attack. Impotence in older men, in effect, may be a "canary in the mineshaft," a warning of a much more serious crisis in the offing.

"Our research suggests that impotence is no longer something that endangers only your sex life—it's a warning that your life itself may be in danger," says John Morley, M.D., director of geriatric research, medicine and education at the St. Louis Veterans Administration Medical Center and the man who's done some of the most interesting recent work on vascular disease and impotence.

Millions of Men at Risk

It's widely acknowledged that perhaps as many as one-quarter of all men over 50 will at some point in their lives have problems getting an erection and that many of these men will be impotent due to arterial blockage. That means that something like one-eighth of all men over 50—millions of husbands, fathers, uncles—are having erection problems caused by clogged arteries. And they could well be at risk for something much worse.

This alarming finding was clarified and underscored by a study conducted by Dr. Morley's research group a few years ago. First, 130 impotent men had their penile blood pressure readings taken by means of a kind of ultrasound imaging process. Roughly half of them (46 percent) turned out to have measurably reduced blood flow to the penis. But the follow-up was the real kicker: The researchers continued to monitor these men for the next two to three years, during which time 26 percent of the men with low penile blood pressure had heart attacks or strokes. By contrast, only 4.5 percent of the men whose penile blood pressure was normal had strokes or heart attacks.

"Penile Angina"

Can this kind of impotence actually be used to *predict* an impending heart attack or stroke? Dr. Morley's group has found that low penile pressure readings are as reliable a predictor of heart disease as the exercise stress test—long considered the gold standard of such tests. In fact, he's taken to calling low penile blood pressure readings "penile angina," since it predicts heart disease risk just as severe chest pain does.

"There is no question that if you develop impotence due to arterial blockage, you are at high risk for developing vascular disease in other parts of your body," he concludes.

The bottom line in all this: If you're a man over 50 who's having troubles with impotence, it might be wise to see a cardiologist as well as a sex therapist. (Don't forget, though: Not *all* impotence is caused by vascular disease—you might discover your arteries are as clean as a baby's.) If vascular disease turns out to be the problem, it's time for a full court press against dietary fat and cholesterol, time to step up your exercise program, quit smoking (if you do) and concentrate on destressing your life. If the damage has progressed beyond the point of no return, there are a variety of new surgeries available, including a sort of "penis bypass," which can help restore blood flow to the regions in question. And of course, there is a bewildering array of other promising new impotence treatments available. (For more, see "Erection Problems.")

CIRCUMCISION

Is the circumcised penis—shorn of its shroud of skin, unsheltered and bare as a mushroom cap in the rain—a fairer thing than the uncircumcised one? Women who've had close encounters with both kinds are

60

divided on the question, according to Alex Comfort, M.D., Ph.D., author of *The Joy of Sex*.

Does circumcision have any effect on sexual pleasure or performance? Well, when William Masters, M.D., and Virginia Johnson, of the Masters and Johnson Institute in St. Louis, posed this question to the men they were studying back in the 1960s, virtually all of them replied that uncircumcised men have better ejaculatory control than men who've been relieved of their foreskins. Their reasoning was simple: In uncircumcised men, the exquisitely sensitive glans (head) of the penis is wrapped in the foreskin, shielding it from direct stimulation and thus slowing the ascent to orgasm and ejaculation.

But Masters and Johnson, unsatisfied with commonsense explanations, put this conjecture to the test. They matched 35 circumcised men with 35 uncircumcised men of about the same age and ran some routine neurological tests on the sensitivity of their penis and glans. Their conclusion: "No clinically significant difference could be established between the circumcised and uncircumcised glans during these examinations." They also pointed out something else: In 29 out of the 35 uncircumcised men, the foreskin fully retracted during intercourse, exposing the glans to direct stimulation. Practically speaking, for most of these men, it really made no difference whether they had a foreskin or not.

On the question of aesthetics, it seems, circumcision is a subjective thing, but when it comes to sensitivity, it seems to make no difference at all.

The 40-Year Debate

It's other kinds of questions about circumcision—particularly those concerning its long-term health effects—that have everybody so steamed. Although this simple, 15-minute operation is the most common surgery performed in the United States, the debate over whether it should be routinely performed on baby boys has been raging for 40 years or more. Its opponents call the operation "child abuse"—unwarranted, unnecessary and just a horrific thing to inflict on a baby. Nature laid this mantle of skin over the head of the penis in order to protect it, they say; who are we to hack it off, whether our reasons be cosmetic or religious? Circumcision proponents, on the other hand, claim that recent medical evidence shows the operation can reduce the risk of urinary tract infections, cancer of the penis and many sexually transmitted diseases.

But first: What is circumcision? This is not an unreasonable question, since one rather startling study showed that 48 percent of a group of mothers did not even know whether the father of their child was circumcised or not.

How It's Done

Boy babies are born with a shaft of skin, called the foreskin, or prepuce, covering the head of the penis. The uncircumcised baby penis looks kind of like a tiny sausage that's not been tied up at the end. At birth, in almost all baby boys, the foreskin is attached to the penis in such a way that it cannot be pulled back all the way; it's designed to cover up the glans, and that's the way it stays. But as the child grows older, the foreskin gradually begins to unhitch from its moorings so that by age three almost all boys can fully unsheathe the glans.

Modern circumcision, generally performed on infants who are about a week old, involves fitting a bell-like device over the head of the foreskin-covered penis and then, with a scalpel, gently cutting the foreskin away, leaving the glans completely exposed. The circumcised penis looks more like a mushroom than a sausage.

The short-term effects of circumcision are minimal—even though there's no question that it hurts, as anybody who's watched the operation can testify. (Even today, it's often performed without anesthesia.)

The rate of postoperative complications is somewhere between 0.2 and 0.6 percent (less than 1 in 100), usually minor local infections or a bit of excess bleeding. The risk of death is practically nil: It's usually given as 1 per 500,000 procedures, but one careful student of circumcision says he knows of only 1 death in more than 2 million operations.

Pros and Cons

It's the long-term effects that are controversial.

Urinary tract infections. In a series of celebrated studies of over 400,000 baby boys circumcised at U.S. Army hospitals, Thomas Wiswell, M.D., a neonatologist at Walter Reed Army Medical Center in Washington, D.C., has shown that circumcised boys are more than ten times less likely than uncircumcised boys to have urinary tract infections (UTIs) during infancy. Apparently the warm, often wet inner surface of the foreskin tends to harbor bacteria like *Escherichia coli,* which can invade the urethra and cause infections. UTIs can be serious, leading to kidney infections, hospitalization and even death.

On the other hand, opponents point out that girl babies get even more UTIs than boys, and nobody is suggesting all girl babies have surgery. Operating on a hundred babies to save one from infection is the sort of reasoning that led to the practice of routine tonsillectomy—something almost nobody advocates anymore.

Cancer of the penis. Circumcision practically eliminates the risk of penile cancer. Although cancer of the penis is really quite rare (a little over 1,000 cases are reported each year), it's also terrifying—a quarter of these men die, and the rest may lose most or all of their penises to surgery, followed by radiation or chemotherapy. Penile cancer occurs almost exclusively in men who haven't been circumcised. Of the more than 60,000 cases of penile cancer that have occurred in the United States since 1930, fewer than 10 have involved circumcised men, Dr. Wiswell reports.

On the other hand, penile cancer is almost never found in anyone except men whose standards of personal hygiene are revolting. In Sweden, where circumcision is rare but people tend to keep frightfully clean, the incidence of penile cancer is almost precisely the same as it is in the United States. All of which seems to support the basic contention of the anticircumcision camp: Keeping yourself clean works just as well as circumcision, and it doesn't involve mutilating your genitals.

Sexually transmitted diseases. Although this evidence is the shakiest, a variety of studies seem to suggest that circumcised men are less likely to pick up sexually transmitted diseases, including gonorrhea, syphilis and perhaps even AIDS. One study showed that uncircumcised men are twice as likely as circumcised men to have gonorrhea or genital herpes and five times as likely to have candidiasis or syphilis.

The New Policymakers: Parents

The upshot of all this is that some pediatric policymakers have recently tempered their positions on the subject of neonatal circumcision. Back in 1975, the official policy statement of the American Academy of Pediatrics (AAP) was that "there is no absolute indication for the routine circumcision of the newborn." The AAP still does not recommend *routine* circumcision. But in a much more guarded statement issued by an AAP task force in 1989, the group noted that "newborn circumcision has potential medical benefits and advantages, as well as disadvantages and risks." Parents should be presented with all the evidence, pro and con, and be allowed to make their *own* choice, the AAP now says.

One thing to remember, though: Because of the host of woes caused by poor genital hygiene, especially cancer of the penis, uncircumcised men need to make a lifelong habit of thoroughly washing the foreskin. The foreskin should be gently pulled back—but only as far as it will go without resistance—and swabbed with soap and water daily.

CLITORIS

It's an anatomical irony that perhaps only God could explain: The most sexually sensitive spot on most women's bodies—the clitoris—is positioned in such a way that it's often not directly stimulated during normal intercourse. It sits, snug and secret, concealed by the multiple lips of the labia and a hood of skin, on a mound high above the opening of the vagina. In most women, it can be found at the peak of the inverted V formed by the inner lips of the labia.

The late Dr. Alfred Kinsey called the clitoris "the phallus of the female," but you could just as easily call the penis the clitoris of the male. Anyway, a baby girl's clitoris is formed from the very same embryonic tissue that becomes the head of the penis in a baby boy. Both penis and clitoris are richly endowed with nerve endings, so they're exquisitely sensitive to the touch. They even look the same: The clitoris is a shaft, an inch long and a little skinnier than a pencil, with a glans (head) and a foreskin. The comparison really isn't so obvious, because most of the clitoris is tucked away in the soft tissue forming the wall above the vagina and is covered by a veil of skin called the clitoral hood. In some women, the head of the clitoris protrudes, like a tiny bud; in others, it is completely hidden. Its size can vary, too, but whether it's large or small has nothing to do with how sensitive it is.

Clitoral Erection

During arousal, the clitoris becomes engorged with blood just as the penis does, swelling in diameter and (in some women, at least) also in length. Strangely enough, though, during the height of arousal the clitoris retreats demurely beneath its veil of skin rather than rearing up for the world to see, like a penis. It may even seem to disappear altogether, so that an ardent lover, eager to find it just when he wants it most, may search in vain.

What is the physiological *purpose* of the clitoris? The penis, its male equivalent, has a couple of purposes: to provide a channel for the discharge of urine and ejaculate and also to provide sexual pleasure. But the clitoris seems to have only one purpose: to give pleasure. When he speaks to women's church groups, Jude Cotter, Ph.D., a psychologist and sex therapist in private practice in Farmington Hills, Michigan, likes to tell them: "God wanted you to have an orgasm. How do I know? Because He gave you a clitoris, and the only known purpose of the clitoris is to give sexual pleasure. It has no other function."

Hogwash from Dr. Freud

Yet for much of this century, the clitoris was regarded as much less important to a woman's sexual fulfillment than the vagina, largely because of the misbegotten notions of Sigmund Freud, turn-of-the century founder of psychoanalysis, and his followers. In Freud's view, the clitoris is a sort of vestigial, inferior penis, considered the centerpiece of sexual delight only by girls who discover it during masturbation and by immature, neurotic or frigid adult women who cannot break this fixation as they get older. What a woman *should* do as she matured, Freud taught, was learn to transfer the source of her sexual pleasure from the clitoris to the vagina. The only right and proper way for a mature adult woman to experience sexual pleasure was through vaginal orgasm—penetration of the vagina by a penis, without any additional stimulation of the clitoris.

This notion came to be known as the clitoral/vaginal transfer theory, and it drove lots of women crazy. Distressed that they still seemed fixated on the clitoris, legions of women sought the help of marriage counselors and therapists, who valiantly sought to transform their immature "clitoral responses" into grown-up "vaginal responses." But nothing worked, because the whole business, it turns out, is pure Freudian hogwash—a biological impossibility. A bed of nerve endings just doesn't jump from one place to another like that. For most women, the centerpiece of sexual delight *is* the clitoris, and it doesn't change no matter how old you get.

The Search for the "Magic Spot"

Still, in recent decades, there has been a continuing debate—often quite heated and usually tinged with one sort of ideological fervor or another—about the precise location of the "magic spot," the focus of female sexual arousal. Freud insisted it was the vagina. Dr. Kinsey, Masters and Johnson and others insisted it was the clitoris. (In fact, in an odd turnabout, it's the clitoris instead of the vagina that tends to get overpromoted today, particularly by feminist writers and therapists.) More recently, other researchers have suggested that in many women, the most sensitive area is the "G-spot"—a dime-sized spot on the roof of the vagina, several inches inside the opening. (See "G-Spot.")

But the latest round of research suggests something even more interesting: that there's a wonderful diversity of sexual responses among women, and no single theory holds true for everyone. Shere Hite reports that 70 percent of the thousands of women who answered her questionnaires said they required some clitoral stimulation to reach orgasm—meaning, of course, that 30 percent of the women achieved orgasm some other way. Some women, it appears, are more clitorally sensitive, others are more vaginally sensitive, and neither one is right or wrong.

Finding the "Love Button"

Even though devotees of Freud have dwindled, many women still feel uncomfortable or embarrassed about touching their clitoris during lovemaking, says Lonnie Barbach, Ph.D., assistant clinical professor of medical psychology at the University of California, San Francisco, School of Medicine. And many men feel they're somehow inadequate if their partner feels the need to stimulate her clitoris during intercourse. "There is a myth that it is somehow wrong to touch yourself while making love with someone else. An unspoken rule dictates that you only touch me and I only touch you, but we never touch ourselves," Dr. Barbach says.

But it's worth overcoming these preconceptions, because there are lots of women who simply can't reach peak arousal unless their clitoris is sufficiently stimulated. Take some time to help your partner locate your "love button" precisely—preferably in a gentle, playful way. If it doesn't embarrass you, turn on a light to allow for a better look. Dr. Barbach even suggests that—if you can get over your modesty about it—a great way to show your partner precisely where you like to be touched is to allow him to watch you masturbate. That way, he can tell exactly where your clitoris is and in the future know how to pleasure you more precisely.

Probably the best way to stimulate the clitoris is go straight to the point and do it by hand (his or hers), or with a roving tongue. But there are also many ways to do it during intercourse as well. Dr. Barbach suggests trying the position that most closely resembles the position the woman uses when she is masturbating alone. Or a couple can try something described in old marriage manuals as "riding high"—any position in which the man rides up on the woman, so that his pubic bone rocks away against her clitoral region. Although this may not be sufficient in itself to trigger orgasm, it can get her partway there. Or he can penetrate her as deeply as possible and then, rather than thrusting in and out, rock from side to side or gently churn round and round. This stimulates the clitoris but allows him to last, since it doesn't cause an excess of ecstasy by rubbing too hard against the head of the penis. (For more, see "Sexual Positions.")

Coitus Interruptus

Coitus interruptus—withdrawal of the penis from the vagina just before ejaculation—is a very ancient, very crude and quite ineffective form of birth control. Out of 100 women whose partners use (or try to use) the withdrawal method, about 18 will become pregnant during the first year of typical use. By contrast, only 3 out of 100 women who use the Pill can be expected to get pregnant, based on typical use.

Coitus interruptus has its advantages: It's free, requires no equipment and thus is available for use at the spur of the moment. However, it tends to have one unsettling side effect: pregnancy. It just doesn't work very well, for a variety reasons. Withdrawing just before the moment of ejaculation requires the will-power of Hercules, and most men simply can't muster it every time. It's a terribly unsettling interruption of lovemaking, likely to leave the woman as unsatisfied as the man is unnerved. It loads all the responsibility on the man and all the consequences on the woman; thus, it's a terrific setup for future arguments if she gets pregnant.

And finally, even if he does succeed in pulling out before he reaches orgasm, she may still get pregnant. That's because during sexual arousal and long before full-blown ejaculation occurs, a tiny droplet of clear, sperm-loaded liquid some-times escapes from the tip of the penis—in a sort of reproductive warm-up routine—which is enough to cause conception.

Communication

Sex therapists like to say that good communication between partners is as essential to good sex as any other single thing. But the fact is that very few people really do know how to talk to their partners about sex.

"One of the most amazing things to us about sexual behavior is how reticent most people are to talk with their lovers about sex. . . . We see plenty of couples whose well-intentioned caresses fall short of the mark because they're too much, too soon, too little, too late," William Masters, M.D., and Virginia Johnson, of the Masters and Johnson Institute in St. Louis, have observed.

You shouldn't beat yourself up too badly if you still feel a little sheepish and embarrassed about discussing your sexual needs. For one thing, we're simply unused to hearing people talk, with love and specifics, about sex. There are few role models whom we can emulate—there is no Jane Fonda of sexual communication. For another thing, it's hard to talk to your lover about sex without sounding like you're judging or criticizing. And then, of course, there's the enormous cultural chasm that separates men from women, which makes sexual conversations sometimes seem like a fireside chat with E.T. Add to that the fact that both men and women, for different reasons, have difficulty talking to each other about sex, and you've got a surefire setup for communications failure.

Why Men—and Women—Don't Ask

"Men are supposed to know everything about sex, so they feel foolish if they have to ask about what pleases their mate," says Lonnie Barbach, Ph.D., assistant clinical professor of medical psychology at the University of California, San Francisco, School of Medicine. Just having to ask shows that they're not a macho superhero. Many men also would simply prefer to communicate non-verbally, because they're not really comfortable verbalizing *anything.* They argue that talking about sex spoils the spontaneity.

Women, on the other hand, were brought up to believe that it's not "nice" to talk about sex, or even to act as if you're interested in it. ("If he really loved me, he'd know what I want.") Sex becomes an ESP guessing game. It happens, says Dr. Barbach, that one partner will persist for years in some habit (like ear kissing) that he or she thinks turns the other on but that in fact causes only repulsion or irritation.

There are times when it really isn't necessary to talk to your lover about sex—like when things are going great. It's not unheard-of for couples to have a satisfying, long-standing sexual relationship and never feel the need to say a word about it. But when one of you begins to feel used or unloved or unsatisfied, it's time to talk.

Take a Little Time

Sometimes the best way to deal with sexual dissatisfaction is to face it head-on. Set aside a "safe" block of time, free from the intrusions of children, ringing phones and work, advises Dr. Barbach. It doesn't have to be long—15 minutes is probably plenty. It's probably best to choose a time other than during or after sex and a place other than bed, because that way it doesn't seem so much as if you're criticizing or judging your partner.

Think of what you're going to say beforehand and try to make it simple, concise and unambiguous. Ask for your partner's full attention. Begin on a positive note by telling your lover what you like and appreciate and how much you want the relationship to work. Then go on to add that "there is a problem with our sex life that I'd like us to work on." Try to use "I" statements (what I really need; what I'd like; what I wish) rather than "you" statements (you never do this; you always do that), because it's less judgmental.

Since talking about sex can be so emotionally loaded and emotions can so wildly distort what you're trying to say, it's important that you make sure you're being understood. Bernie Zilbergeld, Ph.D., a clinical psychologist in the Human Sexuality Program at the University of California, San Francisco, suggests using the "talk and listen" approach. That simply means that you ask your lover to listen and say nothing while you're talking. Try to communicate your message as clearly as possible, and stick to one main point. Then, when you're done, ask your lover to tell you (in just a sentence or two) what he or she thinks you meant. If there's some misunderstanding, explain yourself again and ask for your lover's new understanding of what you're trying to say. Proceed in this way until you both feel you've understood one another.

"It's truly amazing how often we aren't understood and how often we don't understand others," says Dr. Zilbergeld. "The feeling of being understood is a powerful one and in itself can bring people closer together."

Keep It Simple

Remember to keep your message short and sweet—a sexual telegram, not an opus.

"The concept of communication sounds very serious and frightening to many people," says Dr. Zilbergeld, but "no one is suggesting that Shakespearean odes are necessary." Most of the time, what works best is just to keep it short and simple. If you fear that your partner may reject your suggestions utterly, relax.

"Most women are very open to the idea of trying to make your love life better," says Dr. Zilbergeld. "If you just approach her in a nice, loving way—say, 'I love our sex life, but I'd like for us to try some new ways to keep it interesting'—I think you'll find she may well have some ideas of her own." (Men might, too.)

Be Specific; Make a List

"Very often, I'll discover that the guy has desires he's never brought up," says Dr. Zilbergeld. "And the woman says, 'I try to please him, but when I ask him what he wants, he says, "Everything you do is great." ' Women hate that. Men need to learn how to ask." (So do women.) And be specific about it.

For couples who really need to broach the subject of sex with each other but are having trouble breaking the ice, therapists sometimes have them do a simple list-making exercise, says Dr. Barbach. Both partners just make a written list of everything they think sets the stage for good sex and then share their lists with each other. "We're both relaxed . . . no interruptions . . . we've spent some time talking or just being together beforehand . . . candlelight . . . " Doing this exercise can be an innocuous way of easing into the subject of sex and perhaps raising issues that need to be raised.

CONDOM

Not so long ago, condoms were unspeakable things dispensed from machines in unspeakable truck-stop bathrooms. Now they seem almost as respectable as the Pledge of Allegiance.

It's fear of AIDS, of course, that has brought about this national change of heart.

Several studies have shown that latex condoms—especially if they're coupled with a spermicide—can dramatically reduce the chances that somebody who is infected with the AIDS virus will pass on that potential death sentence to a sex partner. In one study of the heterosexual spouses of AIDS patients, 82 percent wound up developing antibodies to the AIDS virus (suggesting that they themselves had become infected)—if the couple did not use condoms. But among spouses of AIDS patients who *did* use condoms, only 17 percent became infected (even though sometimes the condoms broke or were used improperly). In other words, consistent use of condoms can dramatically reduce—although not completely eliminate—the risk of contracting the twentieth century's scariest plague.

The Condom as Shield

That in itself is probably enough reason to consider using condoms. But they can also reduce the risk of a host of other sexually transmitted diseases (STDs), including gonorrhea, chlamydia, herpes and a few others you've probably never heard of. "Used consistently and correctly, condoms are highly effective in preventing acquisition and transmission of most STDs," say the authors of *Contraceptive Technology 1990–1992,* the bible of contraception.

Condoms are much more effective in killing microbes that cause STDs (not to mention sperm) if they're used in combination with a spermicidal foam, jelly or cream. But of course, double the effectiveness usually means double the trouble, and lots of people just don't bother to do both. So in 1982, a uniquely American solution came on the market: the spermicidal condom, a condom precoated, inside and out, with sperm-killing nonoxynol-9. These products, now widely available, save you some bother, and they really work. In one study, the percentage of sperm still moving inside a spermicidal condom after 30 seconds was 10.35; at 60 seconds, 4.3 percent; and at 2 minutes, 1.5 percent. By contrast, in a regular, untreated condom, 55.9 percent of sperm were still moving at 30 seconds, and 50.2 percent were still moving after 2 minutes.

The Rubber of Choice

It's also been found that latex condoms offer better protection against STDs than natural membrane or "skin" rubbers. Natural membranes are perforated with microscopic holes, too tiny to be seen but big enough to allow wee viruses (like HIV—human immunodeficiency virus, the one that causes AIDS) to pass through. In short, particularly if you're using condoms specifically to avoid STDs, a *spermicidal latex condom* is the rubber of choice.

Actually, the use of condoms as STD shields has a long and venerable history. One of the condom's earliest promoters, the sixteenth-century Italian anatomist Fallopius, peddled the things not so much for their ability to prevent pregnancy as for their ability to prevent syphilis. In a pamphlet he published in 1564, he described how a small linen sheath could be fitted over the head of the penis, thus protecting the user from the dread disease. (Fallopius also falsely claimed to have invented the device, although it had already been used for centuries. However, he gets credit for naming it. He derived that odd little word, *condom,* from the Latin *condus,* meaning "receptacle.")

How Effective Are They?

But what if you're worried only about such mundane, nineteenth-century problems as pregnancy? Casanova, that famous rake, once remarked that the condom would "put the fair sex under shelter from all fear," but that's not exactly so. Condoms are considered only a moderately effective form of birth control. Typical-use failure rates are generally given as about 12 percent—meaning that during one year of use, about 12 out of 100 women whose partners used condoms would get pregnant, if they used them in the usual slipshod, inconsistent, impatient human way they're normally used. (By comparison, the typical-use failure rate for the Pill is about 3 during one year; for the diaphragm, about 18; and for nothing at all, 85.)

But this failure rate is mostly the fault of the user. The esteemed authors of *Contraceptive Technology* estimate that if condoms were used perfectly—every time, and without any slipup—the failure rate would be more like 2 percent.

Unfortunately, condom use in the real world bears almost no resemblance to the sort of meticulous precision that doctors like to imagine. "The only way condoms can be counted upon to work even reasonably well is if they're used *consistently, every time* you have sex—and most of the students I see, unfortunately, simply don't use them that way," says Sandra Samuels, M.D., director of Student Health Services at Rutgers University in New Brunswick, New Jersey. "Even students who know people who've died of AIDS are not using them properly."

Students, she says, tend to use condoms only if they've got them handy or only during the woman's fertile period (which, of course, is difficult to define precisely). Or they'll use them for the first two or three months of a new relationship, then stop. Deciding to have sex without using a condom becomes a symbol of trust, a sign that the relationship has entered a new stage of commitment. But the heart is fickle, and most relationships don't last. And perhaps even worse, "people can be carriers of almost all the STDs—herpes, AIDS, chlamydia, gonorrhea—without showing any overt symptoms," says Dr. Samuels. "Dropping the condom, even if you know and trust your partner, is foolhardy."

What about Breakage?

In comparison with the risk of human foolishness, the risk of condom breakage is relatively small. (Of course, almost anything seems small next to human foolishness.) One recent survey of 282 couples who regularly used condoms found that a condom broke about once every 161 times they had intercourse. If these folks had intercourse twice a week, or around 100 times a year, that means about two-thirds of these couples could expect to break one condom in a year.

A couple of cautions: Avoid using a condom that's more than two years old (generally considered its safe shelf life). Store them in a dry place away from heat and light. A glove compartment or a wallet—the condoms' most famous storage places—are bad places to keep them.

And don't use petroleum-based lubricants like Vaseline or Crisco or certain vaginal medications, including Monistat, Premarin, Estrace, Femstat or Vagisil, which can cause latex condoms to deteriorate with amazing rapidity. Studies have shown that within an hour of contact with latex, these substances will cause a 20 to 50 percent loss in latex's ability to provide a barrier to microscopic organisms. Instead, use a water-based lubricant like K-Y Jelly, saliva or a dollop of spermicide cream.

How to Use Them

To use a condom properly, remember the first rule: It should be put on *before* the penis makes contact with the vagina. (The penis, by nature overeager, will exude small amounts of sperm-loaded ejaculate well before full-fledged ejaculation takes place.) Place the correct side of the condom against the head of the penis (you can tell you've got it on backward if it won't unroll) and then unroll it all the way down to the base of the penis. Pinch the tip as you roll it on, so that a half inch of empty space is left at the end. Don't leave a bubble of air at the tip, because this may cause the little devil to burst.

It's best to wait until the woman is well lubricated before entering, because an unlubricated vagina is more likely to tear the condom. (For this reason, a condom is also more likely to tear during anal intercourse.) After ejaculation, remove the condom and avoid spillage of its contents. Check for leaks and discard it. If you discover a leak, have your partner apply spermicide to her vagina without delay. If you're really worried, you might also want to check with your doctor about a "morning-after pill" like Ovral, which can greatly reduce her chances of getting pregnant if taken within 72 hours after intercourse.

Ladies' Choice

Male condoms have been around for hundreds of years, but in 1992, an advisory panel to the Food and Drug Administration (FDA) recommended approval of the first *female* condom. The product, also known as a vaginal pouch, is manufactured by Wisconsin Pharmaceutical Company and marketed under the brand name Reality. The condoms should be available soon in drugstores, without a prescription, for about $2 apiece.

The device looks like a larger version of a male condom, except that it has a ring at each end. One ring, at the closed end of the condom, is slipped over the cervix like a diaphragm. The second ring, at the open end, lies over the vaginal opening, with the sheath between the rings completely covering the interior walls of the vagina. The condom is made of polyurethane rather than latex; the manufacturer says it is stronger and more resistant to penetration by viruses and bacteria than latex.

Some have hailed the device as a medical breakthrough, but members of the FDA panel were a little less enthusiastic. Even while recommending its approval during public hearings on the matter, they repeatedly noted that the device doesn't actually work that well. For one thing, pregnancy rates for women using the condoms are slightly higher than rates for women using diaphragms, cervical caps or contraceptive sponges. That's partly because during intercourse, the device tends to get pushed down into the vagina, slip out of place or get removed prematurely. Also, even though company data showed that the condom can provide 100 percent protection against trichomoniasis (a common STD), more than 60 percent of women didn't use it correctly—so they were no better protected against trichomoniasis than if they had used nothing at all.

Even so, despite all its shortcomings, panel members repeatedly cited the "moral imperative" of giving women a device of their own to protect themselves against AIDS. "Until now, a heterosexual woman's best protection against AIDS depended entirely on the cooperation of her partner," Cynthia Pearson, of the National Women's Health Network, told the panel. Now women have a choice that doesn't involve convincing anyone except themselves.

CONTRACEPTIVES

To find out more about a specific form of contraception, look up "Condom," "Intrauterine Device (IUD)" or whatever you'd like to know more about elsewhere in this book. To get a better idea of how all the major forms of birth control compare with one another in terms of effectiveness, consult the table below. The figures given are the number of pregnancies that can be expected per 100 women during one year of use. "Perfect Use" is what would be expected when the method is used as intended. "Typical Use" takes into account the all-too-human qualities of forgetfulness and inaccurate use—especially in the heat of the moment. (See also "Cervical Cap," "Coitus Interruptus," "Diaphragm," "Norplant," "The Pill," "Rhythm Method," "Spermicides," "Tubal Steriliza-tion" and "Vasectomy.")

Method	Typical Use	Perfect Use
Voluntary sterilization		
Men	0.15	0.1
Women	0.4	0.2
Norplant	0.2	0.2
The Pill	3.0	
Combination		0.1
Progestin only		0.5
IUD	3.0	
ParaGard (copper T380A)		0.8
Progestasert		2.0
Condom	12.0	2.0
Diaphragm/cervical cap	18.0	6.0
Contraceptive sponge		
Women who have not		
had a child	18.0	6.0
Women who have had a child	28.0	9.0
Withdrawal	18.0	4.0
Fertility awareness methods	20.0	
Postovulation method		1.0
Basal body temperature method		2.0
Vaginal mucus method		3.0
Calendar method		9.0
Contraceptive foams		
and suppositories	21.0	3.0
No method	85.0	85.0

CREMASTERIC REFLEX

When a skinny-dipping man jumps into a freezing lake, something odd happens to his testicles. Normally, they hang free of his body in a pendulous sac of flesh called the scrotum. But after contact with the cold, suddenly they lift, clinging to his body like a pair of balloons magnetized by static electricity.

This little genital oddity is no accident. It's caused by a reflex of the cremaster muscle, which controls the elevation of the testes. When it's hot outside, the cremaster muscle allows them to hang loose; when it's cold, it reels them in. Why? Because the testicles must be kept at precisely 94°F (4° lower than the rest of the body) in order to maintain optimal sperm production. This reflex is part of an ingenious heating and cooling system that helps a man's body maintain an unwavering testicular temperature, no matter how cold (or hot) it may be outside. (For more, see "Testicles.")

CRYPTORCHIDISM

(undescended testes). *See* Testicles

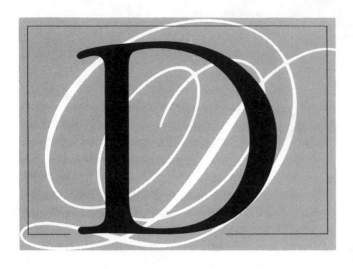

DEPRESSION

Sexual desire is the fullest flower of good health. When you feel good—aglow with happiness, full of physical zest—you tend to feel sexy. But when you're blue, sex is the farthest thing from your mind. Loss of sexual desire, in fact, is one of the most common symptoms of depression.

"As a cause of sexual dysfunction, depression is as real as diabetes," says C. Norman Shealy, M.D., Ph.D., of the Shealy Institute for Comprehensive Health Care in Springfield, Missouri.

Body or Mind?

It's not exactly clear which comes first—the psychological *feeling* of depression or the sexually dispiriting physiological changes that go along with it. Not that it really matters. All that really matters is that depression can alter the body's sexual functioning so profoundly that physical changes (at least in men) can be measured even during sleep.

This was discovered fairly recently during studies of the nocturnal penile tumescence test. The test is a way of measuring whether a man is having normal erections while he's asleep (a healthy man will have a series of them during the dream or REM—rapid eye movement—phase of sleep). The test is used by therapists as a screening device to determine whether an impotent man's erectile problems are caused by some underlying physical impairment or by psychological difficulties. Until recently it was believed that no psychological condition could interfere with nighttime erections. If the guy was having poor erections while he was asleep, so the reasoning went, there must be something physically wrong with him. If not, the problem was probably "all in his head."

But now it's known that depression is perhaps the only exception to that rule. Studies have shown that depressed men who are physically healthy in every other way tend to have fewer nighttime erections, or erections that are softer or more short-lived, than men who aren't depressed. And once the clouds of depression clear, their erections usually return to normal.

Desire Phase Disorders

What do you *do* if you have sexual problems due to depression? Unfortunately, there's no completely satisfying answer. "Sexual problems like retarded ejaculation are the easy stuff to treat—it's the *desire phase* disorders (like depression) that are tough," says Robert Birch, Ph.D., director of the Arlington Center for Marital and Sexual Concerns in Columbus, Ohio.

If you go to see a psychiatrist, it's very likely that he or she will prescribe an antidepressant medication, typically something from one of two classes of drugs— the tricyclics (such as Elavil or Tofranil) or the monoamine oxidase inhibitors (such as Nardil or Parnate). The trouble is, many of these drugs have sexual side effects—including, ironically, loss of sexual desire. Even the alleged wonder drug for depression, Prozac, can have sexual side effects in some people.

A good sex therapist or psychologist (who, not being an M.D., can't prescribe drugs) may be just as capable of helping you as a psychiatrist. Recent studies comparing the effectiveness of drug therapies for depression with drug-free "talking therapies" have shown that they're both about equally effective, observes psychologist and sex therapist Jude Cotter, Ph.D., who has a private practice in Farmington Hills, Michigan.

"The only time I'd refer a patient to a psychiatrist for medication is if there was really extreme depression—somebody who almost needed a jump-start to get out of the hole they're in," says Dr. Cotter. "These drugs are very expensive and have so many side effects that I think they should be used only with extreme caution."

Who Loves You?

In Dr. Cotter's view: "A good sex life comes out of a good love relationship. When a person is having a problem, whether it's depression or anything else, the first thing I do is look at that person's relationship. One of the things I always ask myself is, Who does this person have to hug them and kiss them and love them?"

By working to help patients find a loving partner or to reactivate the love in their current relationship, he feels he can help lead them out of the gloom. (For more information, see "Sex Therapy.")

One thing you could do to help *yourself* climb out of depression: Start working out more often. At least one recent large-scale study showed that people who are physically inactive are about twice as likely to be depressed as those who are moderately active. If you can force yourself to start moving again—walk, play tennis, swim—it may help restore your self-esteem, and then who knows what may follow? (See "Exercise.")

DESIRE

She wants to make love three times a week and smooch and cuddle the other nights. He is satisfied coming to her sexually once a month. And therein lies one of the most common problems involving sexual desire: a mismatch of appetites.

"We see this all the time, and it only stands to reason: We don't usually screen our potential partners for their level of sexual desire, especially over the long term," says Stephen B. Levine, M.D., medical director of the Center for Human Sexuality at University Hospitals in Cleveland, Ohio. "In the early stages of a sexual relationship, you just make love a lot, and both of you are happy. The problem tends not to emerge until later."

Adds Robert Birch, Ph.D., director of the Arlington Center for Marital and Sexual Concerns in Columbus, Ohio: "If two married people want to make love only once every six months, that's perfectly fine—there *is* no problem. It's only when there's a discrepancy in desire that there's a problem."

There are some simple ways for two people to accommodate each other sexually without forcing themselves to have intercourse more often (or less often) than they'd really like to, Dr. Levine says.

"One easy solution is masturbation, just to relieve the tension," he says. "If you don't feel you can impose on your partner as often as you'd really like to, you may have to learn to substitute high-quality lovemaking for frequent lovemaking, and masturbate just for relief." Some people may have a little trouble accepting masturbation as a part of the repertoire of marital sex, but the truth is, experts say, it's common, and nobody should feel guilty about it, especially if it helps you stay sexually satisfied—and married.

Low Sexual Desire

Another common problem is low sexual desire—either failing to initiate sex or failing to respond when your partner initiates. People tend to think of this as a female problem, but actually, says Dr. Birch, it's equally common, and perhaps even more common, among men. In the popular mind, men are supposed to be ready to have sex anywhere, anytime. It's no wonder that when their desire begins to diminish, they panic.

Occasionally, inhibited sexual desire can be caused by some physical problem, such as side effects of medication (high blood pressure drugs, for instance), hormone imbalances or chronic diseases such as alcoholism. But the truth is that this kind of problem is a relatively uncommon cause of low desire.

"We can spend a lot of money working a patient up to make sure they're physically okay, but usually the problem is partner-specific, meaning that it's something in the relationship," says Dr. Birch.

Sex, after all, is a physical expression of what's going on in a relationship. If you're seething with repressed anger, or you feel manipulated or pressured to have sex when you don't feel like it, or you feel distaste for your partner, or you're just bored—your lack of desire is not an illness, it's an eloquent expression of your feelings.

Dissecting Desire

To get at the bottom of lack of desire between long-term sexual partners is often a difficult, time-consuming therapeutic task, partly because low sexual desire can be caused by so many different things, says Dr. Levine. But it's helpful to realize that sexual desire is not merely a base biological need, a carnal appetite, like hunger. Actually, he says, it's not one single force but three different forces—a biological *drive,* a mental *wish* and a more complex *motivation*—all cunningly intertwined. Learning to distinguish the difference can help pinpoint the problem.

Sexual *drive* is the biological urge to have sex, the carnal appetite. In men (and, surprisingly, in women as well) sex drive is triggered by the hormone testosterone. For a variety of reasons, some people seem to have a greater sex drive than others. Those with a sex drive that is set on "high" begin having sex earlier in life and want it more frequently than those with a low sex drive. It's almost as if we're born with sexual thermostats with the dial set to one temperature or another (the trouble is, nobody has yet figured out how to reset it). But "sex drive is only one element of desire—and not the most important one, either," says Dr. Levine.

Sexual *wishes* are the social aspect of sex. Why do older people continue to have sex, even after their biological drive has greatly diminished? Because it makes them feel good. It makes them feel loved and valued. It makes them feel energetic, or masculine, or feminine, or less alone, or any of a number of other things that have little or nothing to do with bodily appetites. Sex drive is physical; a sex wish is a thought.

Sexual *motive* is the most complex aspect of desire—and, in Dr. Levine's view, the most important part. Some people have sex very frequently, but it's not because their bodies are turbocharged with testosterone. It's because they simply value the experience and build their lives around it, for any number of reasons. To them, life without frequent sex is unthinkable. Their *motive* for having sex is deeply rooted in their whole personalities, in their past sexual experiences, in their sexual identity.

"A man may be able and ready to have sex and find his mate physically appealing, but somehow still not want to bring his body to her," Dr. Levine says. "The ideas and thoughts that either inhibit or allow you to bring your body to your spouse are what I call motivation, and these things can hold incredible power."

When sex is like skyrockets in flight, wish, desire and motivation are all pulling in the same direction, and we don't waste time trying to tell the difference. We just call it love. But more commonly, our sexual experiences are more complex and conflicted, with one or another of these powerful forces pulling in different directions.

A man, for example, may avoid making love to his wife, although he claims he'd like to do so more often (wish). At the same time, he occasionally masturbates in response to fleeting excitation or flirting (drive). But the plain fact is, he has no desire for her (motive). Could be time for therapy.

DIABETES

Approximately half of all diabetic men will eventually develop erectile dysfunction [the inability to get or maintain an erection firm enough for intercourse]." That flat proclamation, from a doctor writing in a medical journal, is widely accepted by doctors and diabetics alike. But what many of the two million diabetic men who have erection problems *don't* know is that a significant number of them, particularly those under the age of 50, may be able to restore their sex lives simply by bringing their blood sugar back under control or by dealing with underlying psychological stresses.

Test My Sugar, Sugar

Before seeking treatment for diabetes-related impotence, a man needs to do everything he can to get his blood sugar under control with diet and medication, says E. Douglas Whitehead, M.D., associate clinical professor of urology at Mount Sinai School of Medicine and a director of the Association for Male Sexual Dysfunction in New York City. Dr. Whitehead is an authority on diabetic impotence. If you're under the care of an internist who regularly monitors your blood sugar, you should know if it's out of control—and if you're not monitoring it yourself, you probably should be. "For some of these men—perhaps as many as 20 percent—their impotence will resolve spontaneously once the blood sugar is stabilized," Dr. Whitehead says.

Another 10 percent of diabetic men with erection problems may be experiencing difficulties because some other medical problem—such as pneumonia or any significant infection in the body—is throwing their carefully controlled blood sugar out of whack. Once *that* problem is dealt with, sexual potency may return, Dr. Whitehead says.

Oh, Noooo . . . Not Diabetes

For another large group of these men, their erection problems are primarily psychogenic—medicalese for "it's all in your head." For some, it seems, simply being diagnosed as a diabetic is enough to wilt their ardor, due to the prevailing belief that the disease *always* causes impotence and therefore their sex lives are over. For others, the psychological stress of coping with a chronic disease takes the bloom off the rose. Or depression and guilt can come into play, as when a man comes to believe that he's having sex problems because he's neglected his diet or medication and that the impotence is entirely his own fault.

If you doubt the mind's power to affect a man's sexual prowess, consider this: One six-year follow-up of a group of diabetic men showed that 36 percent of them had a "spontaneous remission" of their sexual problems when they started a new relationship or when old problems in their current one were cleared up. Another five-year study of 466 men with diabetes also reported the same sort of amazing turnarounds, although in only 9 percent of the men.

"Diabetic men are no different from nondiabetic men in the sense that they're subjected to the same environmental stresses and interpersonal problems that nondiabetic men have" — and any of these things can cause difficulties in bed, observes Dr. Whitehead.

Only Your Doctor Can Tell

On the other hand, diabetes is a complex disease (a group of diseases, actually), and it could very well be that the erection problems are caused by physical damage due to the diabetes itself. The problems might also be the result of *both* physical and psychogenic problems. The key thing to remember, says Dr. Whitehead, is that for many patients it's wrong to reach *any* conclusion until a complete medical workup has been done. Yet in his experience, only about 25 percent of the diabetic men who are concerned about their erection problems actually get the right sort of evaluation and treatment.

A huge number of men don't seek professional advice for their problems at all, or they opt for quack mail-order remedies. And even among those who do see a doctor, fully half are given advice that is inadequate or ill-informed, according to Dr. Whitehead. Either they're sent to a psychotherapist without first undergoing a physical exam to rule out organic problems or they're given testosterone pills or injections without first establishing whether they've got a hormone deficiency (which is unlikely). Sometimes they're simply given a pat on the back and told that they've "had enough sex already." Or they may even be handed that old line so familiar to women — "it's all in your head" — whether this has been conclusively established or not.

Ideally, Dr. Whitehead advises, diabetic men with erection problems should seek help from a urologist with a special interest in male sexual dysfunction. If your family physician doesn't know of one, you may wish to seek more information from a major medical center with a department of urology or a residency training program in urology. These institutions should have a urologist on staff with the training and expertise to evaluate and treat your condition. Alternately, a man with diabetes might seek treatment from a sexual medicine center. Again, your family physician might be able to point you in the right direction.

Some Important Clues

Still, there are a few seat-of-the-pants generalities that may help you determine whether your problem may be caused primarily by mental or physical problems. In general, Dr. Whitehead says, the erection problem is *probably* psychogenic if:

- It appears suddenly, rather than gradually (shortly after the diabetes is diagnosed, for instance).
- It occurs only with certain partners or in certain situations.
- You also feel decreased desire.
- You have problems ejaculating or reaching orgasm.
- You have other bad feelings, like shame, guilt, hostility or depression.

By contrast, the impotence is *probably* caused by organic or physical problems if:

- The onset is gradual, with a progressive decrease in hardness and frequency of erections.
- It occurs in all situations—in the morning, during intercourse and during masturbation.
- You can get an erection, but you can't seem to maintain it.
- Your sexual desire is undiminished.

Cause Unknown

What, precisely, is the connection between out-of-control blood sugar metabolism and erection problems? Well, researchers aren't really sure, but there are three prime suspects: damage to peripheral nerves, blood flow problems and damage to the internal structure of the erectile tissue itself. Diabetes, over the long haul, often damages the tiny nerves that serve the body's far-flung regions, especially the fect and legs, and may also ravage the nerves that operate male erections. People with diabetes are also highly prone to developing atherosclerosis, and it could be that this deadly buildup clogs the vessels that supply blood to the penis. (Some studies have shown that diabetic men with impotence do have blood flow problems in the penis, but so do diabetic men *without* sexual problems. And yes, that does make the whole thing a little confusing.)

There are, of course, two main varieties of diabetes—Type I (a rarer, more severe form that tends to show up in childhood and requires insulin injections) and Type II (which usually appears in adulthood). Both types are characterized by problems in the metabolism of glucose—the sugar that supplies the body's energy. Both types have a dispiriting effect on sexuality, although so far it's not clear whether one type has a worse effect than the other.

New Tricks for Impotence

Unfortunately, for many diabetic men, simply keeping the blood sugar under control or developing a positive mental attitude is not enough to restore the sexual potency of youth. Action of a bolder sort is called for. The good news is that there are many medical treatments and products for impotence now available. (For more on these treatments, see "Erection Problems.")

Effects in Women

In women, the sexual side effects of diabetes seem to be much less severe than they are in men. Several studies have suggested that about a third of diabetic women have trouble producing vaginal lubrication. One anatomical study of these women showed degeneration of nerve beds in the clitoris, although that didn't seem to affect their ability to reach orgasm. As a practical matter, one of the most troublesome sexual problems for diabetic women is an increased susceptibility to vaginal infections, since disturbances in blood sugar metabolism encourage bacteria to move in and make themselves at home. (See "Urinary Tract Infections.")

DIAPHRAGM

The diaphragm is one of the tried-and-true barrier contraceptives. A dome-shaped rubber cup with a flexible rim, it is liberally smeared with up to a tablespoon of spermicidal cream or jelly and inserted into the vagina. The diaphragm fits snugly over the rounded bulge of the cervix, holding the spermicide in place and covering up the tiny cervical opening through which sperm must pass to cause pregnancy. It can be inserted either just before inter-course or up to 6 hours beforehand, and it should be kept in place for 6 to 8 hours afterward but for no longer than 24 hours.

Diaphragms have to be prescribed and fitted by a doctor. Because proper fit is so crucial, doctors often advise women to return for refitting annually, after weight gain (or loss) of 10 pounds or more and after pregnancy.

When it's correctly fitted, a diaphragm blocks the upper vagina and cervix, but it may not fit tightly all the time during lovemaking or in all coital positions. That's why most manufacturers (and doctors) recommend that these devices be used with spermicidal jelly or cream.

How Well Do They Work?

If the diaphragm is used correctly and used *every time* you make love, it can be an effective form of birth control, with very few side effects. So-called perfect-use failure rates for the diaphragm are generally given as about 6 percent—meaning that for every 100 women who used a diaphragm for a year, there would be about 6 pregnancies. But people aren't perfect (most of us don't even come close), and when diaphragms are used in the forgetful, haphazard, sometimes frenzied way they usually are, the rate of failure is more like 18. These typical-use failure rates are about the same as those for the cervical cap (really just a smaller version of the diaphragm) and the vaginal sponge, known collectively as *vaginal barrier methods* because they work in essentially the same way.

By way of comparison, typical-use failure rates for the Pill or the IUD would produce around 3 pregnancies among 100 women over the course of a year, sterilization would produce considerably less than 1, and using no birth control method at all would produce around 85.

How to Decrease Your Risk

Of course, all these numbers are just averages—actual pregnancy rates vary dramatically. As with all birth control methods, experienced, older, regular users of diaphragms tend to have much lower pregnancy rates than inexperienced users. What can you do to make sure your risk of getting pregnant is *lower* than average? Well, don't be afraid to use more than one kind of birth control, like condoms or the Pill, in addition to the diaphragm.

There are a few risk factors that *increase* your chances of getting pregnant while using a diaphragm, say the authors of *Contraceptive Technology 1990-1992,* the reigning authority on all aspects of birth control.

- Frequent intercourse (more than four times a week)
- Being less than 30 years old (younger women are more fertile)
- A personal sexual style that makes it difficult to use the diaphragm consistently
- Having previously gotten pregnant while using birth control (of any type)
- Some ambivalent feelings about whether getting pregnant is a good idea

What all this adds up to is that a woman's risk of getting pregnant is *roughly doubled* if she's less than 30 or likes to make love more than four times a week. If you fall into this category, it doesn't mean that you *can't* use the diaphragm. It *does* mean that you must be all the more meticulous about using it correctly and consistently.

One other cautionary note: Studies strongly suggest that it's a lousy idea to use oil-based sexual lubricants with a diaphragm. Oil-based lubricants, such as mineral oil, baby oil, suntan oil, vegetable oil or butter, cause significant deterioration of latex condoms after only an hour's exposure. (Obviously, a diaphragm is not a condom, but they're made from similar materials.) Some kinds of vaginal medications—including hormones and infection-fighting creams such as Femstat, Monistat and Vagisil—also caused a rapid breakdown of the latex. If you need more lubrication during intercourse, try saliva, a commercial lubricant or even a little extra squirt of spermicide.

STD Protection: The Big Bonus

Both women and men complain that diaphragms can be a pain to use. They're about as romantic as a wet sock. They're messy. They can destroy the spontaneity of lovemaking. You have to either anticipate sex or interrupt it in order to use them. And they require a whole routine every time you make love (unlike, say, the Pill, which can be blissfully ignored).

But diaphragms (and all other barrier methods, including the cervical cap and condoms) offer one big advantage, too: They are the only kind of birth control available that seems to offer significant protection against sexually transmitted diseases (STDs). In one study, for example, the relative risk of contracting gonorrhea was more than 50 percent lower among women who used diaphragms and/or spermicides compared with those who used the Pill or were sterilized. Studies have also shown that diaphragm users are significantly less likely to contract pelvic inflammatory disease or tubal infertility, two unpleasant consequences of STDs.

In effect, diaphragms appear to give the cervix (and, by extension, the upper reproductive tract) a temporary suit of armor, protecting it against invasion by voyaging viruses, bacteria and infected semen. This seems to be why diaphragms also protect women against *cervical neoplasia* (a term referring to cancerous or noncancerous tumors on the cervix). Since it's thought that one important cause of cervical neoplasia is contact with semen infected by a virus called human papillomavirus, researchers think the diaphragm may help by shielding the surface cells of the cervix from viral infection. Various studies have shown that using a diaphragm, cervical cap or sponge *plus* spermicide is more effective in preventing cervical neoplasia than a diaphragm alone.

The Downside

For most women, using a diaphragm plus spermicide has no serious side effects. A few women develop a little bit of skin irritation, from either the latex or the spermicide (which often goes away if you just switch to a different spermicide). Urinary tract infections (UTIs) are more common among diaphragm users than among women using other methods, apparently because diaphragm users tend to develop significantly more bacterial colonization in the vagina. Doctors suggest that women plagued with recurrent UTIs be refitted with a smaller diaphragm, and if that doesn't help, try switching to a different kind of birth control.

Some women who are particularly sensitive in the area known as the "G-spot" (a dime-sized area on the roof of the vagina, usually several inches inside the opening) complain that using a diaphragm interferes with the pleasure they get from direct stimulation of this area. For them, getting fitted with a cervical cap often restores them to their former glory. (For more, see "G-Spot.")

But the most serious potential side effect, though by far the rarest, is toxic shock syndrome. This potentially fatal disorder is caused by toxins released by certain strains of a nasty little bacterium called *Staphylococcus aureus*. Just remember the warning signs of toxic shock syndrome, and if any of them develop, take out the diaphragm and contact your doctor.

- Sudden high fever
- Vomiting and diarrhea
- Dizziness, faintness, weakness
- Sore throat, aching joints and muscles
- A sunburnlike rash

One other important precaution: Women who use diaphragms should be careful to clean and disinfect them after each use, because dirty diaphragms can harbor a rogue's gallery of microorganisms that cause STDs. Doctors recommend washing the diaphragm with soap and water and soaking it in alcohol for at least 20 minutes after each use. After cleaning, the diaphragm should be dried, dusted with cornstarch (not scented talcs) and stored in a cool, dry, dark place.

DOUCHING

Douching is a practice that may seem as feminine and proper as a lilac-scented thank-you note: Millions of women have been taught that as part of their routine hygiene, they should regularly flush the vagina with either water and vinegar or a commercial preparation. And many women do: In one survey of nearly 7,000 American women, 32 percent reported they'd douched at least once within the previous week.

Most women who douche do so for general cleanliness, others do it because they are bothered by vaginal odors or secretions, and a few do it because they believe douching will protect them against sexually transmitted diseases. Some (heaven help them) even think it will prevent pregnancy if they do it after lovemaking.

But the truth is that the douche has been oversold. For one thing, the fairly common myth that it can be used as a form of contraception is a cruel joke, because by the time a woman is able to douche, it's too late. Studies have shown that within 15 seconds after ejaculation, some sperm have already entered the cervical canal and are furiously paddling toward the uterus, bound for glory. But even douching for cleanliness is problematic. Too-frequent douching can increase the risk of a variety of feminine ills, including ectopic (tubal) pregnancy (in which an egg is fertilized outside the uterus, usually during its descent down the fallopian tube), pelvic inflammatory disease (or PID, a general term referring to any genital infection that passes into the reproductive organs, causing inflammation and possibly infertility) and even cervical cancer.

"There are bacteria in the vagina, and they're *supposed* to be there—if you irrigate those bacteria out, you're more likely to have vaginal infections as a result," explains nurse-midwife Katy Head, director of the Allentown-Bethlehem Birth Midwifery Center in Allentown, Pennsylvania.

A Douche a Day Means Trouble

In one major study, a group of women with PID was compared with a group of women who were free of the disease. The researchers found that "those who douched three or more times per month were 3.6 times more likely than those who douched less than once per month to have confirmed pelvic inflammatory disease."

PID, in turn, increases a woman's risk of tubal pregnancy, because these reproductive infections often leave scars on the interior lining of the fallopian tubes, blocking the egg's passage through them.

Also, in another study, medical researchers studied the douching habits of a large group of women in Utah, some of whom had cervical cancer and some of whom did not. Their finding: "Essentially no association was found in women who douched once per week or less, but in those who douched more than once per week, a consistent relation was demonstrated. . . . Frequent douching (more than once per week) may be a biologic risk factor for cervical carcinoma." In this study, at least, the *kind* of douching preparation the women used didn't seem to matter much; what mattered was how frequently they used it.

On the other hand, says Head, "some women have fairly heavy vaginal secretions, which tend to develop a musty odor, and are prone to yeast infections, especially during the summer. For them, it's a matter of self-image: They just feel cleaner and better if they douche. I have no problem with that at all, so long as they don't do it too often."

Usually, though, a healthy vagina really has no need of human efforts to sanitize it. The mucous membranes that line its interior surface produce secretions that continuously cleanse it, even during menstruation. As one gynecologist likes to say, only half joking, "the vagina is the world's greatest self-cleaning oven."

DREAMS

If you dream that you're having sex with the butcher's wife, or the butcher, or even the butcher's dog—forgive yourself. Sex dreams, including those that may seem disturbingly perverse by daylight, are an almost universal human experience. The late Dr. Alfred Kinsey found that about 70 percent of women, and nearly all men, had sex dreams—often so torrid they resulted in orgasm. In fact, a few women in his study (about 5 percent) actually reached orgasm for the first time in their lives during sleep.

Interestingly enough, Dr. Kinsey also found that the better educated his subjects were, the more often they had sexy dreams. For instance, adolescent boys who later went on to college had nocturnal emissions triggered by sex dreams *seven times* more frequently than boys who never made it beyond grade school. Dr. Kinsey attributed this difference to the greater imaginative capacities of the brighter boys. Feel free, in other words, to consider your next steamy dream as proof of your superior intelligence. Don't forget, though, that even animals appear to have sex dreams. There have been some reports of sex dreams in a cat (with ejaculation), a shrew (with a teeny erection) and dogs. When they're in heat, some female dogs will moan and groan during sleep, and their vaginas will swell and grow wet.

Women's Dreams Differ

In general, sex dreams aren't as universal, or as frequent, in women as they are in men. Still, more than two-thirds of the 8,000 women in Dr. Kinsey's sample reported having "overtly sexual" dreams, and 37 percent reported having had orgasms during sleep at least once. The women who did dream to orgasm had such dreams roughly three or four times a year, although a handful of his subjects (no doubt the ones with the biggest smiles) reported having dream-induced orgasms more often than once a week.

The content of women's dreams differs from that of men's dreams: In one study of 100 male and 100 female college students, women were more likely to dream about kissing and petting, men were more likely to dream of intercourse. The women's dream lovers were more likely to be someone they actually knew, but for men, the dream partner was more likely to be a stranger. Also, oddly enough, women often considered pregnancy and childbirth dreams to be associated with sex, and one out of seven of these dreams involved orgasm.

The Older You Get, the Better It Gets

While many things about sex seem to diminish with age, women's sex dreams actually seem to increase in frequency as they get older. In Dr. Kinsey's sample, only 2 percent of girls from adolescence to 15 had sex dreams—but among women in their forties (the peak period for sexual dreams), 22 to 38 percent of women reported having erotic dreams. It's a little sad to note that men reach their peak frequency for sexual dreams in their late teens or twenties—20 to 30 years before women reach *their* peak. The well-known sexual mismatch between men and women, whose responses and life cycles seem forever out of synch, is reflected even in sleep.

The Male Experience

Men, of course, are very often left with physical evidence that they've had a sex dream: sticky sheets. Wet dreams, or nocturnal emissions, tend to begin a year or so after a young boy reaches adolescence and reach their greatest frequency during the teens and early twenties. Still, Dr. Kinsey found a huge variation: About 17 percent of boys never have wet dreams at all, while others have them so frequently it becomes a laundry problem—some have orgasms almost every time they wake up, although they may wake up two or three times a night.

For men and women both, it's a distressingly common experience to wake up moments before the climax of orgasm—even though (in the case of a man) the dreamer may actually be ejaculating when he awakes. Dream lovers, like the rainbow's end, seem ever out of reach.

Homosexual Dreams

Sex dreams are a way of discharging physical urges in a safe, harmless way. And experts say that if some of these nocturnal fantasies are disturbing to our waking sense of propriety—like homosexual or incestuous dreams—it's best not to get too worked up about it.

"It's really not that unusual for a heterosexual man or woman to have an occasional homosexual dream," says Robert L. Van de Castle, Ph.D., a behavioral psychologist and dream expert at the University of Virginia. "Besides, a homosexual dream may not be about homosexuality at all. It may simply be about learning to love or appreciate oneself."

It's important to pay attention to the *feelings* associated with sexual dreams to get a better idea about your subconscious attitude toward their content, Dr. Van de Castle says. Do they make you feel alarmed, guilty, aroused? Even if the dreams depict things you might find objectionable in real life, there may be a comforting message about your own sexuality in them.

" 'Normal' human sexuality is not just a simple missionary position–only sort of thing—it's much more varied and diverse, and that's reflected in dreams," says Dr. Van de Castle. "To the degree that we find sexual diversity within ourselves, hopefully it can help us appreciate the sexual diversity in other people."

Everything Is a Penis

To hear Freud tell it, of course, almost *everything* in a dream (and in life) is sexual. In Freud's view, dreams are the fulfillment of some repressed infantile wish—nearly always a sexual one. Since these wishes are usually unacceptable to the conscious mind, the theory goes, the unconscious mind expresses them in dreams in disguised, symbolic form. The psychoanalyst's task becomes one of deciphering the *latent content* of a dream (its true, hidden meaning) from its *manifest content* (its overt imagery).

In Freudian dream interpretation, every image that's a receptacle (boxes, bowls, houses) or enclosing (rooms, tunnels) is taken to be a symbol representing the vagina. So are mouths, ears and eyes. Everything that's oblong or suggests penetration (sticks, knives, umbrellas, pencils or nail files, which suggest rubbing up and down), along with hands, feet and the number three, represents the penis. (One penis plus two testicles equals three.) Walking up and down stairs or ladders suggests intercourse (bouncing up and down—get it?).

The trouble is, not all sex dreams are about boxes or umbrellas—sometimes they're as blatantly, unashamedly sexual as a naked breast. They're not disguised at all. This poses a real problem for Freudians, who are forced to argue that this sort of dream conceals a still deeper, more taboo sexual urge. But "this argument that nothing is ever what it appears to be is very unconvincing to me," says Dr. Van de Castle. "If, according to Freud, all weapons and tools are symbols standing for the penis, then what does it mean when one dreams about a penis? Does it mean that the person is really dreaming about a gun or a hammer?"

Anyway, all their arcane arguments aside, psychologists and dream experts are generally agreed on one thing: If you have a dream that produces an orgasm, it's a sex dream. And *anybody* can understand that.

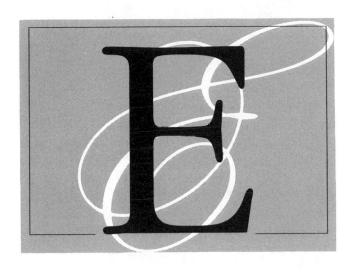

EJACULATION

Because it is drenched in such exquisitely distracting sensations, few men realize that ejaculation is actually a two-part process—and that ejaculation and orgasm are not the same.

The first phase of ejaculation is what sex therapist and psychiatrist Helen Singer Kaplan, M.D., Ph.D., founder of the Human Sexuality Program at New York Hospital–Cornell Medical Center, calls *emission*. During this phase—the last step on the highway to heaven, so to speak—muscular contractions squeeze milky, protein-rich ejaculatory fluids out of the prostate and the seminal vesicles and mix them with sperm. The resulting brew (semen) is squeezed into a little chamber at the base of the urethra (the pipe through which semen and urine exit the body), where it lies ready for the launch.

William Masters, M.D., and Virginia Johnson, of the Masters and Johnson Institute in St. Louis, called the sensations produced by this process "ejaculatory inevitability"—the feeling that, as Dr. Kaplan has described it, the gun is loaded, the trigger is pulled, and there's no turning back. You get that feeling because ejaculation has already begun.

The final phase, *ejaculation* itself, normally follows a fraction of a second later. Respiration, blood pressure and heartbeat, already rising rapidly, reach their peak. So does vasocongestion (the process by which various key body parts become engorged with blood). Rhythmic contractions of muscles near the base of the penis drive the semen up and out the urethra, usually in from one to five spurts. (It's not possible to ejaculate and urinate at the same time, because of a valve system that shuts off the bladder just before orgasm.)

A Teaspoon for Two

The actual volume of ejaculate varies quite a bit from man to man—it tends to decrease with age and increase with the length of time since the last ejaculation. It usually amounts to about a teaspoonful, although in one study of 46 Swedish men, the volume of the men's ejaculate ranged from a few drops to up to 8.8 milliliters (nearly 2 teaspoons). (Tip for the weight-conscious: There are at least 5 calories in the amount of semen ejaculated by the average man.)

Ejaculation usually produces such a tremendous sensation of release because, after it occurs, vasocongestion (the damming-up of blood) becomes its opposite (the letting-go of blood). Suddenly, all that trapped, shivering blood is unleashed, and the engorged parts gradually return to their former relaxed condition. At the same time, there's a tremendous release of muscular tension.

Here's something else it's important to remember: Well before a man feels the great spasm of ejaculation, a dewy drop or two of *preejaculate* may emerge from the tip of his penis with so little fanfare that he probably won't even notice it. Even a drop of this lubricating fluid, produced by the Cowper's glands, can contain millions of sperm—more than enough to impregnate a woman. That's why the withdrawal method doesn't work very well as birth control and why condoms should be put on before the penis ever makes contact with the vagina.

Go Rest, Young Man

Many men don't realize their bodies have what's known as a *refractory period* between ejaculations. In other words, the body simply cannot repeat the amazing physiological performance of erection and orgasm without a little rest first. The refractory period gets longer as you get older. In an 18-year-old, it may last as little as 5 to 15 minutes, but by the time you reach 60, the R&R required between ejaculations is more likely to be 18 to 24 hours. The period varies from man to man—the more frequently a man usually ejaculates, the shorter the in-between period is likely to be.

Orgasm or Ejaculation?

Actually, although it may feel like it, and although they usually occur simultaneously, ejaculation is not quite the same thing as orgasm. It's possible to have one without the other. Men who've had prostate operations, for instance, often have what are known as *dry ejaculations*—they experience orgasm, but they don't ejaculate. (The semen backs up into the bladder and is harmlessly voided during urination, a process known as *retrograde ejaculation.*)

What's the difference between ejaculation and orgasm? In his book *Male Sexuality,* Bernie Zilbergeld, Ph.D., a clinical psychologist in the Human Sexuality Program at the University of California, San Francisco, describes orgasm simply as "what you feel" and ejaculation as, well, ejaculation. Some men, he says, have trained themselves to have orgasms without ejaculating and may even be able to have multiple orgasms, like women. Other men complain that they ejaculate, but they miss the big payoff—they just don't feel very much at all. One way for these men to increase their orgasmic pleasure, Dr. Zilbergeld suggests, is to practice Kegel exercises, which strengthen the muscles of the pelvic floor and improve blood flow to the penis. (See "Kegel Exercises.")

Learning Ejaculatory Control

One of the most common problems with ejaculation, of course, is that it comes too soon—or at least, the man has little voluntary control about when it occurs. One survey showed that a third of all adult men think they suffer from what's come to be known as *premature ejaculation*—even though there's no real agreement on the meaning of that term. Masters and Johnson, for instance, have said that a man should be diagnosed as having premature ejaculation if he reaches climax before his partner more than 50 percent of the time. But Dr. Zilbergeld's view of the matter seems more sensible and does away with the term completely. To him, *ejaculatory control* just means the man is able to control, at least fairly well, when he will ejaculate. He can pleasure himself and his partner for a luxuriously long time, or he can finish up quickly—it's up to him. To be able to do so contributes so much to satisfying sex—and to be unable to do so is so unsatisfying—that it deserves a special entry of its own. (For more, see "Premature Ejaculation.")

EPIDIDYMIS

The epididymis is a structure mounted on the back side of each testicle and containing a tiny, tightly coiled tube. Fully unwound, that tube would stretch a full 20 feet. After being formed in the testicle, immature sperm cells enter this dark maze, where they gradually mature to the point where they are able to move forward with their familiar lashing movement. The epididymis, in effect, is a sort of elementary school for sperm. Once they leave it, they pass into the vas deferens, a 20-inch tube that coils back into the body, around the bladder and back down to the urethra, through which they pass during ejaculation.

Although you can readily feel the epididymis as a soft swelling on the back of each testicle, usually a man is completely unaware of this humble duct work until it gets infected. This fairly common condition—known as epididymitis—can be caused by bacteria of various kinds (such as those that cause chlamydia or gonorrhea infections), urinary tract infections, infections of the prostate and sometimes tuberculosis. Symptoms often include sudden severe pain in the testicles, swelling and tenderness in the scrotum (usually on just one side, although both sides can sometimes become infected at once). These symptoms call for a trip to the doctor. The infection is generally treated with antibiotics, prescribed to knock out the organism responsible for infection. Treatment also calls for avoiding sex and alcohol and for bed rest with the testicles elevated—all in all, a rather miserable but effective combination.

ERECTION

In many ways, erections sum up the whole male way of doing things: They appear with dramatic and swashbuckling suddenness (at least in younger men), they look like tools or weapons, their use involves aggressive action rather than passive acceptance—and underlying the whole performance is the constant fear that they won't work.

Men's worries often take the form of concern that their erections are too small. But such fears are highly overrated, because no matter how much penises may differ in the flaccid (nonerect) state, studies have shown that they are amazingly similar when they're erect. A penis that's relatively small when flaccid will swell proportionally more than one that's a little more impressive in its unaroused state. Erection, you might say, is the great equalizer of penis size. Just for the record, the average size of the erect human penis is about 6 inches, although it can vary from 4 to 8 inches.

But more to the point—at least if you're concerned mainly about pleasuring your partner, not about outshining your male competitors—an additional inch or two makes almost no difference at all.

"The part of the vagina where a woman experiences sexual pleasure is still an area of controversy—but at the very least, it's fairly well agreed that for most women, the greatest pleasure comes when the first [outer] third of the vagina is stimulated," says Ted McIlvenna, Ph.D., president of the Institute for the Advanced Study of Human Sexuality in San Francisco. "Going in deeper doesn't give most women any extra pleasure."

The Body's Erector Set

Actually, male erections are the most dramatic manifestation of one of the most basic processes of sexual arousal—vasocongestion (the concentration of blood in the genitals and the female breasts). Vasocongestion causes the clitoris to become erect, too (as well as the multiple lips that surround it), and although clitoral erections are equally pleasurable, they're not nearly as noticeable as the male variety.

There are still some mysteries surrounding the actual mechanics of a man's erection, but basically it goes like this. Due to the nature of the nerves that supply the penis, the whole show can be touched off in only one of two different ways: by physical touch (so-called reflexogenic erections) or by erotic thoughts (psychogenic erections). Just as you cannot control what arouses you, you also cannot get an erection just because you want one, no matter how hard you try. This is not a personal failure. It's just the way your motor and sensory nerve pathways work.

The penis itself is composed mainly of three cylinders that lie side by side along the length of the shaft—two big ones lying on top (the corpora cavernosa) and a smaller one underneath (the corpus spongiosum), which contains the urethra, or urinary drainpipe. These cylinders are wrapped in a sheath of tight-fitting though stretchable skin. Once stimulated by thought or touch, the nerves respond by opening up millions of tiny sphincters along the walls of these cylinders, and fantastic amounts of blood pour in, filling up the millions of tiny sinuses, or balloonlike sacs. Once these sacs are filled and distended, the cylinders squeeze off the veins that normally drain blood out of the penis. The result is that eight times the normal amount of blood is trapped inside the penis, creating (ideally, at least) a rigid, towering erection.

Stabilizing the Tower

Rigid as it may be, how come a man's erection doesn't wobble all over the place, or even buckle, during intercourse? Because the rigid corpora cavernosa extend all the way down to the bone that you sit on, giving the erection a rocklike foundation, explains urologist and microsurgeon Sherman J. Silber, M.D., in his book *The Male*. Whales, bears, walruses and other creatures have solved the "wobble" problem by means of a bone that runs right up inside the penis, giving their amorous intentions some support. But the human erection, says Dr. Silber, "is more exquisitely refined than that of any other animal."

The late Dr. Alfred Kinsey, who never seemed to tire of studying even the smallest details related to sexuality, found a great variety in the angle of men's erections. Most men of all ages reported they usually had erections very slightly above the horizontal, but some (15 or 20 percent) said theirs were fully 45 degrees above horizontal, and a few (8 or 10 percent) reported their erections were practically vertical, almost flat against their bellies. Dr. Kinsey also found that with increasing age, the angle of a man's erection tends to gradually droop.

It's also been known since 1945 that most men will have three to five good, unused erections during the night. These nocturnal salutes usually correspond to the dream or REM (rapid eye movement) phase of sleep and generally last 20 or 30 minutes apiece. Interestingly enough, they're usually not triggered by sexy dreams. Instead, it's now believed that dreaming itself causes erections because it induces a state of heightened physiological arousal.

Dr. Kinsey found that most men averaged a little more than one morning erection a week, with the greatest frequency (twice a week) reported by men between 31 and 35. Some guys ascribe this morning surprise to having a full bladder (morning erections are sometimes called "piss-hards"), but a full bladder has nothing whatsoever to do with having an erection. More likely, they're a last hurrah left over from your final dream of the night.

Quite a few drugs, both illegal and medicinal, can hinder a man's ability to get erections. (See "Illegal Drugs" and "Medications.") And occasionally, a man's erections will be painful or noticeably crooked, a condition that is sometimes caused by Peyronie's disease. (See "Peyronie's Disease.")

Effects of Aging

As a man ages, it usually begins to take more time, and more physical stimulation, for him to become erect. As a teenager, he could get a substantial erection in 10 seconds flat, but at 60 it may take 10 minutes of special attention before he comes to attention.

This was demonstrated by two researchers at the University of Southern California who showed the same erotic movie to two groups of men while monitoring their responses. The younger men (19 to 30) got erections almost six times faster than their elders (48 to 65).

A man's erections also tend to become a little less firm as he gets older, and after orgasm, he tends to lose his erection more quickly. Dr. Kinsey found that teenage boys could maintain an erection (before ejaculation) for nearly an hour, but men between 66 and 70 could keep it up for only 7 minutes.

The last and perhaps most noticeable erectile change brought on by age is an increase in the amount of "downtime" that must occur between erections. This refractory period may be as little as 5 to 15 minutes in an 18-year-old, but by the time you reach 60, it may take as long as 18 to 24 hours before the body can repeat the performance.

All of these changes are quite predictable, but they're not necessarily a curse. They're completely normal and natural, for one thing. And for another, sloweddown sexual responses can open up a whole new world of lovemaking that's all the sweeter because it lasts longer. For men who, in their younger days, tended to pop off so quickly that it was all over before it began, getting older can be a genuine blessing.

The Penis/Heart Connection

With all this talk of hydraulics and refractory periods, it's easy to begin thinking of erections as some kind of remarkable machine, completely disconnected from the body. But it's important not to forget that "the penis is connected to the heart," says Stephen B. Levine, M.D., medical director of the Center for Human Sexuality at University Hospitals in Cleveland, Ohio.

"Men believe that they're supposed to be able to have intercourse with anybody, at any time, even somebody they don't particularly care for—but it's a sign of our own alienation from ourselves that we believe this," Dr. Levine says. We're not robots, and our bodies are not machines. "If you occasionally have trouble getting an erection, that doesn't mean you're a wimp or a homosexual," he says. "That means you're just like everybody else."

Some therapists even argue that when it comes to male sexual performance, entirely too much attention has been focused on the erection. Bernie Zilbergeld, Ph.D., a clinical psychologist in the Human Sexuality Program at the University of California, San Francisco, has written that "the erection is considered by almost all men as the star performer in the drama of sex, and we all know what happens to the show when the star performer doesn't make an appearance."

But by focusing so much attention on that little fellow who's supposed to snap to attention at the slightest provocation, we put an almost unbearable burden on men. After all, there's no way he can fake an erection, and it's virtually guaranteed that there will be times when he can't get one. The penis is not the only sexual part of the body, says Dr. Zilbergeld. And besides, it's possible to have a delicious sexual encounter without an erection—and even without intercourse.

There are times, however, when happy talk from therapists is just not enough. The man wants an erection, and he can't get one. Thankfully, there are an amazing number of treatments now available. (For more, see "Erection Problems.")

ERECTION PROBLEMS

If this were a medical textbook, you'd find the following discussion under the heading "impotence"—an unpleasant medical term for men who have trouble getting an erection or keeping it long enough to make love. But *impotence* is such a terrible word, implying that a man is feeble, powerless, washed up, over the hill (it actually derives from the Latin *impotentia,* meaning "lack of strength"), that we'll try to refrain from using it too much here.

A man having trouble getting an erection is just that: a man having trouble getting an erection. In most other ways, he's probably every bit the man he ever was—in fact, since erectile difficulties tend to crop up after the age of 40 or so, it's likely his worldly career and earning power are peaking at the same time this loneliest of problems makes its first appearance.

Just to clarify: Virtually every man has trouble getting an erection from time to time, and although this can be extraordinarily distressing, it's only natural. What's *unnatural* is the idea that a man should be able to produce a towering erection at the slightest provocation, with any partner, at a moment's notice. Unrealistic expectations only set the stage for disappointment.

"In any other part of a person's life—running a race, hitting a ball—you'll have some days when you can just perform better than other days. But men rarely realize that this is equally true of their sexual lives," says Richard E. Berger, M.D., professor of urology at the University of Washington and coauthor of *BioPotency: A Guide to Sexual Success.* "If you lose an erection, or can't get one, the best thing to do is try to understand *why* it happened. Often there's something else going on, like chronic tiredness, stress, alcohol, nicotine or drug use—things you can do something about."

The worst thing you can do, he says, is worry about it too much. Men often begin thinking of their erection as the key part of what amounts to a sexual performance, a kind of Super Bowl of Sex—in other words, something at which it's possible to fail. They begin to worry that they *will* fail, especially if it's happened a few times already. That initial worry leads to the downward spiral of anxiety, self-doubt and self-observation that William Masters, M.D., and Virginia Johnson, of the Masters and Johnson Institute in St. Louis, called "performance anxiety"— one of the most common psychological causes of erection problems and one that's sometimes difficult to overcome. (See "Performance Anxiety.")

A Curable Epidemic

But for a huge number of men, the trouble is more intractable than that. For them, erectile difficulties have become a chronic, long-term problem, and that's the subject of the rest of this chapter. *Chronic impotence* (if you'll pardon the phrase) is sometimes defined as the inability to achieve and maintain an erection long enough for sexual intercourse in at least 25 percent of attempts. Other doctors say the term simply means that difficulties crop up often enough to be recognized as a problem by a man or his partner. However you define it, such a distressing situation is extraordinarily common: It's estimated that one in every nine or ten American males is chronically impotent—that's ten million men, and perhaps many more. Studies have shown that nearly 20 percent of men are chronically impotent by the time they reach age 55; 30 percent by age 65; and over half by age 75.

These huge numbers are no particular comfort to a man suffering from such humiliation—or to the woman who loves him. The man, afraid to "fail" if he attempts sex, often pulls back from his partner, fearful, anxious and ashamed. The woman, for her part, often blames herself, fearing that she is no longer attractive to him, that she no longer turns him on or perhaps even that he's taken another lover. What is in many cases a relatively minor mechanical problem can sometimes become a marital catastrophe.

Even so, there's plenty of good news to spread around. In fact, over the past decade, there's been a virtual revolution in treatments for male impotence, and many men who once would have had to resign themselves to a life without sex now have an almost bewildering array of options.

"The real tragedy, though, is that as many as 90 percent of these men may be suffering needlessly," says E. Douglas Whitehead, M.D., a director of the Association for Male Sexual Dysfunction in New York City and an associate clinical professor of urology at Mount Sinai School of Medicine. "Impotence is primarily an epidemic with a cure. Great strides have been made in recent years, not just in diagnosing the causes of impotence but in doing something about them."

How to Head Off Problems

Before we get into a discussion of all the treatments now available, though, let's pause a moment to consider a few ways to prevent the problem in the first place. Chief among the ways men can maintain a "potent lifestyle" are eating a low-fat, low-cholesterol, high-fiber diet and doing regular aerobic exercise. Yes, it's boring, and you've heard it before, but it's true. The reason is simple: A lifetime of eating fatty foods and not exercising leads to clogged arteries. And clogged arteries mean that blood flow is impeded to the penis as well as the heart. And since erections depend on robust blood flow, "anything that keeps those vessels clean will reduce your chances of developing erection problems," Dr. Berger says. In fact, in one study, researchers found that more than 75 percent of impotent men had at least some problems with arterial blood flow to the penis.

Even though it's usually older men who have heart attacks, heart disease is slow and insidious, and it begins early in life—which is why you're never too young to start protecting yourself. The same is true of sexual potency. In his book *BioPotency* (coauthored with Deborah Berger), Dr. Berger reports on a Czechoslovakian study in which doctors examined the penile arteries of a group of deceased men whose ages ranged from 19 to 85. The results showed that all the men 38 years old and older had at least some blockage in these arteries. The message: The time to begin preserving your sexual longevity is *now*.

Dr. Berger makes these general recommendations.

- Generally, cut back on your intake of fatty meats and eggs, whole milk, ice cream, cheese and butter. Trim the fat off meat and broil or roast instead of frying. Rarely, if ever, eat organ meats like liver or sweetbreads.

- Increase your intake of fish and poultry.
- Keep salty, processed foods to a minimum.
- Eat plenty of fresh, whole fruits and vegetables and whole grains.
- Work out regularly—ideally, for 20 to 30 minutes at least three times a week.

Is It the Body or the Mind?

Once you do decide to seek help at a clinic or with a qualified urologist, it's nice to know that your odds of success are extremely high. "Almost everybody can be treated successfully," says Dr. Berger, "because even if we can't fix the underlying problem, we now have ways to go around it."

This is a dramatic turnabout from 20 years ago, when most sex specialists believed that for the vast majority of men, their sex problems were "all in their heads"—and hence very difficult to treat. Today, though, most specialists think precisely the opposite is true: that 50 to 75 percent of men with erection problems have some physical (and usually treatable) trouble that's to blame. In one 1986 study of 1,500 men who visited sex clinics for erection problems, more than 70 percent were diagnosed as having erection problems caused by some physical, rather than psychological, disorder.

Even so, there's no clear line that separates the body from the mind, and both are almost always involved.

"There's seldom such a thing as purely physical impotence, because if a man can't get an erection once, he starts to worry about it, and when it happens again, he worries even more, until he begins to expect to fail," says Dr. Berger. "Even after the initial, physical cause of erectile difficulty has been treated, it's not uncommon for men to still need a little therapy to overcome those fears and negative expectations."

Expect a Few Questions

At the clinic, the first thing a specialist will attempt to determine is the *primary* cause of your problem. The most basic question is, Is it mainly physical, or is it mainly psychological? (Again, these things are often devilishly intertwined, but one or the other undoubtedly came first.)

Experts say your erection problems probably have some *psychological* cause if:

- They appeared suddenly, rather than gradually.

- They occur only with certain partners or in certain situations (for instance, if you can get a rigid erection while masturbating, but not with your wife).
- You also feel decreased desire for your partner.
- You have problems ejaculating or reaching orgasm.
- You have other bad feelings, like shame, guilt, hostility or depression.

By contrast, the impotence is *probably* caused by organic or physical problems if:

- The onset is gradual, with a progressive decrease in hardness and frequency of erections.
- It occurs in all situations—in the morning, during intercourse and during masturbation.
- You can get an erection, but you can't seem to maintain it.
- Your sexual desire is undiminished.

Expect to be asked about all these areas as the doctor tries to determine whether your problem has a mental or physical basis.

The doctor may ask a few other questions about your life and health, too.

Could a prescription drug you're taking be the problem? It's now believed that as many as a quarter of all cases of impotence are caused or made worse by medications, according to Paul Church, M.D., a urologist at the New England Deaconess Hospital in Boston. (See "Medications.")

Could it be alcohol? A drink or two can have a mildly aphrodisiac effect, but heavy drinking is one of the most common causes of impotence. Long-term drinking can be disastrous, reducing the blood levels of male hormones and sapping sex drive. (See "Alcohol.")

Could it be smoking? Good erections require robust blood flow, but smoking constricts blood vessels, squeezing off circulation. That's probably why a very high percentage of impotent men are heavy smokers. (Quitting may not lead to a sexual renaissance, but it certainly can't hurt.)

Old Reliable: The NPT Test

You could very well ask yourself all those questions without going to a sex clinic at all, of course. But you *couldn't* move on to the next stage: high-tech medical testing to determine whether the cause (if physical) is centered in the nerves, blood vessels, hormones or somewhere else. Just a few years ago, doctors were only able to distinguish between physical and psychological impotence. Today, armed with a space-age array of testing devices, it's often possible to precisely pinpoint the problem and then target the treatment.

Actually, the test you're most likely to get is one of the oldest and simplest — the venerable nocturnal penile tumescence (NPT) test. Although it's not as reliable as it was once believed to be, many specialists still consider the NPT test to be the gold standard of impotence tests. Its basic premise is simple: Normally while he's sleeping, a healthy man will have erections that last 20 to 30 minutes every 90 minutes or so. The NPT test is just a way of determining whether this is occurring or not. If a man is not having normal erections while he's sleeping, there's probably some underlying physical problem to blame. If he is, the problem is likely psychological. The NPT test can be done in a sleep lab, under carefully monitored conditions, in which both the frequency and rigidity of nighttime erections are measured. It can also be done more cheaply, but with slightly less accurate results, at home.

The Most Common Problems

These and other tests can be used to narrow the search to the primary, underlying problem. A fair percentage of cases turn out to be caused by chronic diseases of one kind or another. The most common cause of organic impotence, it's now believed, is vascular disease, which interferes with the lusty blood flow that's so critical to producing a rigid erection.

The next most common cause is diabetes, affecting an estimated two million men in the United States. (For more, see "Diabetes.") People with diabetes often suffer from neuropathy (tingling and numbness in the hands and feet due to damaged nerves), which is the most common cause of neurological impotence. Quite a few other men have impotence due to bladder, rectal or prostate surgery or spinal cord injuries.

Sometimes, hormonal problems may turn out to be the cause, but this is really fairly rare (perhaps 5 percent of all cases). Some men believe that their erection problems are due to a gradual decline in testosterone levels caused by aging and that testosterone pills or shots will restore their sexual youth. In the relatively rare instances in which this is actually true (often due to a condition called hypogonadism, or malfunctioning testicles), the treatment is testosterone replacement, which generally restores both sexual desire and erections. But if your testosterone levels are normal, shots are almost universally ineffective, Dr. Whitehead says. (For more, see "Testosterone.")

Consider Counseling

If the battery of hormonal, neurological and vascular tests comes up with nothing, consider yourself a lucky man. And consider seeing a sex therapist. In general, sex therapy does not last terribly long, and it is not a matter of delving into your deepest childhood traumas. Instead, its goal is much simpler: to enable you to have a satisfying sexual relationship. It's possible the problem can be resolved in relatively short order. If you're unsure where to find someone to help you, write to the American Association of Sex Educators, Counselors and Therapists, and they'll supply you with a list of therapists in your area. Send a self-addressed stamped envelope, and $1, to AASECT, 435 North Michigan Avenue, Suite 1717, Chicago, IL 60611-4067. (See "Sex Therapy.")

An Amazing Array of Treatments

Of course, correct diagnosis does you no particular good unless there's a treatment available to match the problem. Fortunately, there are so many that sometimes *choosing* is the challenge. Just remember, though, that "the bottom line is vaginal penetration," Dr. Whitehead says. That may sound a bit cold and mechanical, but it underscores a point: The key to success is realistic expectations. None of these treatments will make you a teenager again, or solve a preexisting problem in your marriage, or give you a sexual appetite that's noticeably different from the one you have now. All have drawbacks of one kind or another.

But the right solution, coupled with the right attitude, could go a long way toward restoring the sexual sweetness in your life.

Love Potions and Vacuum Devices

Some doctors, faced with an impotent man who is reluctant to take more drastic measures to solve the problem (such as surgery, shots or an implant), may suggest that he try a drug called yohimbine (Yocon or Yohimex) for two or three months. It's kind of a "first try" approach, which seems to induce erections in something less than a third of a third of the impotent men who try it. Yohimbine, in fact, is now the most commonly used nonhormonal drug for the treatment of impotence. (For more, see "Yohimbine.")

In recent years, vacuum constriction or negative pressure devices have gained popularity because they, too, are fairly cheap and noninvasive, and if they don't work, at least they probably won't hurt you. They're often prescribed for older patients who aren't candidates for surgery and don't want to learn self-injection. Vacuum devices also require a prescription.

Basically, this the way they work: You fit a clear plastic cylinder over your limp penis, get a good air seal, then pump all the air out of the cylinder with a hand or electric pump. The vacuum that's created engorges the penis with blood, producing an erection that is frequently rigid enough for intercourse. Then you slip a rubber band–like constriction ring off the end of the cylinder and over the base of your erection, trapping the blood there long enough to do your honorable duty. It's unwise to wear the ring any longer than 30 minutes, however, because you've basically applied a tourniquet to something you'd rather not lose. (Men with severe vascular problems may have to limit its use to 15 minutes.)

The erection is a little fatter, and feels a little cooler, than a normal erection. It's not rock-hard, either; instead, the devices produce something that's ingloriously referred to as "an erection–like state" — firm enough to insert, but not much more. Also, because it goes no farther south than the constriction ring, the erection tends to wobble about rather than standing straight up.

One 1990 study looked at the experience of 29 men who used the Osbon ErecAid vacuum device (one of the most common models) for six months. These men reported significant improvements in the quality of their erections, the frequency with which they attempted intercourse, the frequency of orgasm and their overall sexual satisfaction. After six months, only 7 of the men (19 percent) had dropped out. (In self-injection programs, which we'll discuss next, dropout rates run as high as 40 percent or more.)

"Vacuum devices appear to provide a safe, effective, inexpensive, noninvasive treatment for erectile failure that enjoys high patient and partner acceptance," reported the researchers, a team of urologists and psychiatrists from Case Western Reserve School of Medicine in Cincinnati. Other studies have shown that after anywhere from 3 to 22 months of use, 80 to 85 percent of couples use the device at least twice a month and are satisfied with the results.

Vacuum devices are not without their shortcomings, of course. Many men complain that they're a little painful to use and that they produce speckling or spotting on the penis, caused by minor bruising (this goes away by itself, however). Also, because the urethra is squeezed off, the device usually blocks ejaculation — so they're not a good choice for couples trying to conceive. (It doesn't *always* work like this, though, so you can't use them like a contraceptive.) And of course, the erection itself lacks rigidity. These are all relatively minor problems, though. No serious medical complications have been reported with vacuum devices.

Self-Injection Therapy

In recent years, some of the biggest news in impotence treatment has been the development of shots that produce long-lasting erections within minutes. In properly selected patients, in proper doses, the injections produce good erections in 3 to 5 minutes and last 30 minutes to an hour or more, nearly every time they're used. The kicker: The shots must be injected directly into the penis itself. And yes, that alone has been enough to scare lots of men away from even trying *intracavernosal self-injection therapy.* (Actually, the needles are exceedingly tiny, and pain—usually very minor—is really not the most significant worry about this kind of treatment.)

After almost a decade of use, self-injection therapy is considered a "safe and effective treatment for organic impotence," according to a panel of specialists convened by the *Journal of the American Medical Association.* Studies have shown that the treatments also have a positive effect on marital satisfaction and psychological well-being.

One unexpected bonus: "Some patients we start on self-injection therapy get better spontaneously—we don't know why," Dr. Whitehead says, with an air of mystification. "But if we had given them surgical implants before we tried the shots, it would have been a shame."

This self-injection treatment was discovered accidentally in 1982, when an injection of the drug papaverine produced a rigid, long-lasting erection in a male patient. Papaverine, it turns out, had accomplished this feat due to its action as a potent muscle relaxant. Normally, a pair of long, narrow erectile chambers inside the penis (the corpora cavernosa) hang limp and empty. When the muscles that control the flow of blood into the penis come in contact with papaverine, they relax, allowing incoming arteries to dilate. Blood pours into the waiting chambers, the penis awakes, and a firm erection is the result.

Since the discovery of papaverine, at least two other drugs have been added to the arsenal of impotence injections: phentolamine mesylate and prostaglandin E1, a synthetic form of a naturally occurring body chemical. These three drugs (and others) are sometimes used together and sometimes separately; sometimes two are used together.

The Drawbacks of Self-Injection

Still, like every other form of impotence treatment, injections have their drawbacks. The most worrisome ones:

- Frequent injections in or around the same area may begin to cause scarring, or small, hard nodules, on the shaft of the penis. In one study, 57 percent of patients using the injections for a year developed small fibrous nodules on their penises.
- Sometimes the longed-for erection doesn't go away (a condition called

priapism). If a drug-induced erection lasts more than 4 hours, it can cause irreparable damage to the spongy tissue within the penis, leaving you with no real option but an implant. If you find yourself in this unforgettable situation, you have to find your urologist, or a hospital emergency room, to drain off the blood that's trapped in the penis and then get a shot of epinephrine (or some other drug) to deflate your ardor.

• Some men develop facial flushing, dizziness or low blood pressure or may have difficulty ejaculating.

• Sometimes abnormal liver function develops. The condition seems to go away when the treatment is discontinued.

Why Do Men Drop Out?

Injection therapy has its advantages. But over the few years that it's been in use, something rather revealing has emerged: A very high percentage of men eventually give up on it, even if it's working.

"If the patient is a young guy, 30 or 40 years of self-injection just doesn't seem reasonable," Dr. Whitehead explains. "Patients are concerned about long-term effects, and frankly, so are we—after all, this therapy has only been used for about 7 years. Its long-term effects are unknown. Others get tired of injecting themselves; it's certainly not spontaneous. And sometimes, of course, there are complications."

(Because the long-term effects of the shots are unknown, in fact, some doctors suggest that the therapy shouldn't be continued for longer than 18 months.)

Facing the Knife

In some cases, the problem turns out to be feeble or impeded blood flow to the penis caused by a problem in the arteries or veins in the neighborhood. Although this problem has long been understood, it wasn't until recently that surgeons could actually repair the blood vessels themselves. Today, surgeons with super-naturally steady hands are able to perform a variety of operations that either increase blood flow to the penis or block its escape through the veins, thus restoring a man to sexual wholeness.

Perhaps 5 percent of impotent men, or less, are candidates for this kind of microvascular surgery.

In one such operation—a kind of "penis bypass surgery"—an abdominal artery is rerouted around a clogged or damaged penile artery and connected to one or both of the other main arteries leading into the penis. Five-year follow-up studies have shown that 80 percent of the men who undergo this procedure achieve sexual success, according to Harin Padma-Nathan, M.D., codirector of the Research Center for Sexual Function at the University of Southern California.

In another type of operation, called *penile venous ligation,* surgical repairs are done to leaky veins. In order to produce a firm erection, incoming blood must be trapped inside the erectile chambers of the penis. Normally to do this, the veins squeeze shut, trapping blood inside the penis in the same way a stopper traps water in a filling bathtub. But men whose veins don't close off properly, and who thus can't retain an erection, can now have them surgically repaired.

Unfortunately, the success rate for this kind of operation is disappointingly low—less than 50 percent. At some centers, the initial success rates were promising—over 75 percent in some cases. But as time went by, the repairs began to leak again, like faucets that stubbornly insist on dripping, no matter what you do. Venous outflow problems seem to be one of the most difficult impotence problems to correct, urological surgeons say, and some centers have stopped performing the operation because of its disappointing long-term results.

There is a fallback position, though: If the surgery fails, the man is still a candidate for an implant, Dr. Whitehead says.

Implants: The Last, Best Hope

The most drastic option available to you—a surgical implant—also has the highest success rate of any impotence treatment we've discussed so far. According to recent studies, more than 90 percent of the men who have the surgery, and their partners, are satisfied with the results. And a 90 percent success rate, after all, is better than your chances of having a successful marriage.

Still, it's important to emphasize that this is the *last* option you should consider, and only after everything else has failed. Having a stiff or semistiff rod permanently implanted into your penis is about as invasive as you can get. And once it's done, there's no turning back: The surgery frequently alters normal blood flow, so that without the implant, you may get no erection at all.

Implants are increasingly common—about 30,000 of these operations are performed annually, on men mostly between the ages of 50 and 70. They've been used for the treatment of impotence caused by diabetes, heart disease, spinal cord injuries, Peyronie's disease (bent penis), pelvic surgery for prostate cancer, chronic alcoholism and a host of other problems. There are over a dozen different kinds of implants, but basically they break down into two categories.

Noninflatable implants. These are the simplest, least expensive devices, which can sometimes be implanted with only a local anesthetic. A pair of bendable rods are implanted, side by side, into the two long, narrow erectile chambers that lie inside the penis. Sometimes the rods are made of silicone rubber with a bendable or hinged metallic core. You bend them outward for sex, then back for the rest of the time. The downside is that they remain permanently stiff. Although they're fairly well concealed under clothes, there may be times (like in public restrooms or locker rooms) when the implant is uncomfortably obvious.

Inflatable implants. These types can be inflated and deflated, more closely simulating a "real" erection. This is done by means of a tiny pump, a storage reservoir and a pair of rodlike inflatable cylinders that are implanted in the shaft of the penis. When the spirit moves, you activate the pump with a finger, which passes fluid from the reservoir into the implants, producing an erection. After the erection has done its honorable duty, pressing the deflate valve returns fluid to the reservoir, and the penis grows limp again.

Inflatable implants have gone through several generations of improvement. The first models, introduced in the 1970s, came in three parts. Inflatable cylinders were implanted in the penis itself, the pump was implanted in the scrotum, and the reservoir was tucked into the lower abdomen. Everything was connected

HOW TO FIND PROFESSIONAL HELP

The vast majority of men having erection problems never seek professional help—even when sexual difficulties have brought a marriage to the brink. By some estimates, fewer than 10 percent of impotent men ever see a doctor about the problem or get a checkup at a sex clinic. In other words, seeking medical help doesn't mean you are weak or in some way a failure: It means that you have more courage, and more willingness to confront your problems, than the vast majority of your peers.

Whom should you see when you decide to take the big step? It's possible you're lucky enough to have a knowledgeable internist or family doctor to turn to, although "unfortunately, many are uninterested or not sensitive to the needs of patients with sex problems," says E. Douglas Whitehead, a director of the Association for Male Sexual Dysfunction in New York City and associate clinical professor of urology at Mount Sinai School of Medicine. It would be better to find a urologist who has some special interest in male sexual dysfunction (although only about a third of urologists do). To find out whether a particular urologist in your area is qualified, try looking in *The Directory of Medical Specialists,* which lists the background and specialties of doctors and is available in most public libraries. Or if there's a medical school near you, the urology department may have a sex clinic. Or just look in the Yellow Pages, where local sex clinics are probably listed.

by tubing. However, all that plumbing, no matter how ingenious, meant that malfunctions and infections were fairly common. Later, in the 1980s, two-piece devices were introduced (both pump and reservoir were implanted in the scrotum), eliminating the need for abdominal surgery. In the latest generation of devices, pump and reservoir are built into the implant itself, making the surgery even simpler. (One drawback is that these new devices can't hold as much fluid, so the erection tends to be less firm.)

In some centers, patients are hospitalized for two or three days to give them intensive antibiotic therapy before, during and after the operation. Intercourse is usually prohibited for a month after the surgery. Implants are usually covered by most major medical insurance programs and by Medicare, if the impotence has a physical cause.

How Safe Are They?

In the early days, as many as 60 percent of implants malfunctioned or became infected over the first five years. Today, though, the rate of malfunction after the first five years has been reduced to something less than 5 percent, and infection rates are about 2 or 3 percent, according to recent studies. One other positive note: Even when the implant malfunctions and has to be removed for one reason or another, many men request that it be replaced. Dr. Whitehead says virtually all his patients who develop such problems ask to have a new device implanted.

The ideal implant candidate, most urologists say, is a man who is otherwise in reasonably good health, has a healthy sex drive, has normal ejaculation, orgasm and sensation in his penis and has a partner who is comfortable with the idea.

For many men—especially compared to a life without sex—a little bit of hydraulic assistance may seem like a small price to pay.

EROGENOUS ZONES

An erogenous zone is a sexual hot spot—a place that's especially erotic when kissed, touched or fondled. There are many of them, some better known than others, but they've all got one thing in common: They're covered with skin. Skin, in fact, is the body's largest erogenous zone—the only one, really. All of the delicious body messages of sex come to you through the nerve endings that are nestled within your skin.

Some parts of the body, like the clitoris, the tongue and the nipples, have come to be known as erogenous zones because they're more richly endowed with nerve endings and thus more exquisitely responsive to the touch than other body neighborhoods. But the truth is that there's not a nook or cranny of the flesh, from the soles of the feet to the nape of the neck, that can't produce an erotic sigh.

"There is no part of the human body that is not sufficiently sensitive to effect erotic arousal and even orgasm for at least some individuals in the population," the late Dr. Alfred Kinsey observed. No kidding! Among the more than 12,000 people he interviewed for his books, Dr. Kinsey found a handful of women who could reach orgasm merely by the kissing or fondling of their earlobes, a few men who could reach orgasm if a lover kissed their nipples and several women who could actually climax through the stroking of their eyebrows!

But it's wrong to think of erogenous zones as rigid, unchanging things, like the switches on a VCR. They may vary considerably from person to person and even vary from one day to the next.

"Women complain, 'He never varies in what he does!' And the man says, 'But you said that's where you like to be touched!' What's often ignored is that a person may like to be touched one way one day and somewhere else, differently, the next," says sex therapist Shirley Zussman, Ed.D., a director of the Association for Male Sexual Dysfunction in New York City and former president of the American Association of Sex Educators, Counselors and Therapists. "The key thing is to be sensitive to your partner, so that you know not only where they like to be touched but how."

Women's Hot Spots

Generally, all the evidence seems to suggest that compared with men, women tend to be less focused on the genitals and more sensitive to the entire body's potential for sensuous pleasure.

"For most women, being touched and stroked all over is an essential prelude to arousal, perhaps because it takes them longer to become aroused than men," says Dr. Zussman. Still, once you've gotten beyond the tactile generalities, there are certain areas that most women find highly arousing.

The *clitoris* is an unmistakable erogenous zone in most women. Both the glans (head) and the shaft of the clitoris are highly responsive to the touch— sometimes so much so that it hurts if they're touched too roughly or without lubrication. In a series of now-famous experiments, Dr. Kinsey had five gynecologists using glass, metal or cotton-tipped probes explore the genitals of almost 900 women to find out which areas were most sensitive. Ninety-eight percent of the women could feel the probe touching their clitoris, often evoking erotic feelings of "considerable intensity." The clitoris, in other words, is the hot spot of hot spots.

The *labia minora,* the inner lips of the genitals, are richly supplied with nerves, especially on their secret, inner sides. In Dr. Kinsey's studies, 98 percent of the women could feel a touch on either the inner or the outer side of the lips. "As sources of erotic arousal," he observed, "the labia minora seem to be fully as important as the clitoris." The labia majora—the fleshy outer lips—seem to be considerably less sensually sensitive.

The *entrance of the vagina* is a definite pleasure zone. Most women find the so-called vestibule of the vagina (the funnel-shaped area between the inner lips, just above and outside the vaginal opening), as well as the first inch and a half of its interior, to be the sweetest of spots. That's because these areas are richly supplied with nerve endings. Interestingly enough, the deep inner walls of the vagina seem numb by comparison—only 14 percent of the women in Dr. Kinsey's sample could even feel it when the probe gently stroked them there, and relatively few of them said they masturbated by means of deep vaginal penetration. Modern researchers point out, though, that some women are wildly responsive to deep pressure (not light strokes) applied to the roof of the vagina, several inches inside the opening—an area that's come to be called the "G-spot." (For more, see "G-Spot.")

The *breasts and nipples* receive mixed reviews. Many women respond to erotic attentions to the breast and nipples—but an equal number find that being stimulated in these areas either does not lead to arousal or even makes them uncomfortable. Studies have shown that although 90 percent of women say their partners like to kiss or stroke their breasts during sex, only about 50 percent actually enjoy it. Some women find it painful, especially just before or during menstruation, when the breasts may become tender.

What Arouses Men

It's often said that men are more focused on the erotic potential of their genitals, to the exclusion of other body parts, than women are. But even if that generalization is true, it's also true that there's a good deal of variation in the sensitivity of the male genitals from one place to another. For most men, in descending order of pleasure, it goes something like this.

The *frenulum* (the area underneath and just behind the glans, or head of the penis) is usually the most sensitive spot.

The *rim of the glans,* sometimes called the coronal ridge, is also highly sensitive all the way around.

The *urethral meatus,* the tiny slit through which urine passes, is worth investigation.

The *shaft* of the penis, relative to these other spots, is much less sensitive, and so is the skin of the scrotum.

Also, don't forget the *breasts and nipples.* Most men (and women) feel a little funny about the man's nipples being stimulated during sex play—but lots of men are sensitive there. In fact, Dr. Kinsey reported that "there may be as many males as there are females whose breasts are distinctly sensitive."

In Search of the Less Obvious

The *mouth, lips and tongue* are, of course, one of the body's premiere erogenous zones—something that's known to almost all the higher animals. During sex play, fish, lizards and most mammals will put their mouths on their partners' bodies, sometimes for hours at a time. A stallion mounting a mare will nibble, lick and snuffle her with his mouth and nose almost continuously. (Is it any wonder that in both humans and animals, the two most erotically sensitive places—mouth and genitals—have a habit of coming together during sexual encounters?)

In many men and women, the *perineum*—the skin between the anus and genitals, the place you'd make contact with if you straddled a fence post—is highly sensitive to touch. Dr. Kinsey found that "many males are quickly brought to erection when pressure is applied on the perineal surface at a point which is about midway between the anus and the scrotum." This rather secretive spot can be reached by direct pressure with a finger, through the rectum or (in women) by deep penetration of the vagina.

Earlobes become engorged with blood during sex, swelling and becoming increasingly sensitive to touch.

The thin skin on the inner surface of the *thigh* is richly endowed with nerves, and in some people stimulation of this area makes for an especially arousing adventure. Other erogenous zones—all arousing to *some* people—include the throat, the armpits, the anus, the navel, the abdomen, the toes and who knows what else?

There may be others known only to your partner (or as yet unknown to him or her)—but you'll never find them until you set out on a Lewis and Clark expedition over the frontiers of your lover's flesh.

ESTROGEN REPLACEMENT THERAPY.

See Hormone Replacement Therapy

EXERCISE

What's the effect of regular exercise on sex? For most people, it acts as a mild, and quite legal, aphrodisiac. A variety of studies have shown that men and women who keep themselves trim and toned tend to have lustier sex lives, and remain sexually active later in life, compared with people who are relatively inactive. There is an outer limit to this cheerful news, however: Driven, compulsive exercisers actually have *lower* sex drives than people who understand the meaning of moderation.

Women's Sexual Second Wind

The libidinous effects of exercise have been demonstrated in both men and women. Linda DeVillers, Ph.D., an adjunct professor of psychology at Pepperdine University in Los Angeles, was intrigued when she noticed that after a day of swimming or skiing, she felt sexually stirred up. She wondered if other women might experience a similar "sexual second wind" after exercise and polled 8,000 female readers of a fitness magazine to find out. A quarter of these women reported that they, too, felt sexually aroused immediately after working out; only 3 percent said their libidos seemed to flag.

The long–term effects of exercise were even more pronounced. Almost a third of the women reported they had sex more often after beginning their exercise program, 40 percent said they'd noticed an increase in their ability to be aroused, and 89 percent said exercise had given their sexual self-confidence a boost.

Sexual Aerobics for Men

Another study showed similar effects in a group of 78 sedentary middle-aged men. Researchers at the University of California, San Diego, rounded up these healthy but inactive men, whose mean age was 48, and put them on a vigorous, nine-month-long exercise program. Although they worked into it gradually, by the sixth month the men were doing sustained aerobic exercise (pushing their hearts up to 75 to 80 percent of their maximum aerobic capacity) for a full hour at least three times a week. A similar group of 17 middle-aged, sedentary men was put on a program of moderate walking for an hour about four times a week. Both groups kept detailed diaries about all sorts of things, including their sex lives, during the first and last months of the program.

After nine months, predictably enough, the men on the no-nonsense exercise program had increased their overall fitness levels by 30 percent. At the same time, by a variety of different measures, their night lives had also gotten considerably more entertaining. Their frequency of intercourse increased by 30 percent (to three times a week), the frequency of orgasms increased by 26 percent, and the frequency of masturbation increased by 50 percent (to roughly once every ten days). At the same time, their sexual dissatisfaction or dysfunction (such as trouble achieving or maintaining an erection) noticeably decreased. In short, these newly fit middle-aged men underwent a kind of renaissance of randiness.

Walkers increased their fitness levels by only 3 percent during the study, compared with a 30 percent increase among the more strenuous exercisers. (Obviously, the walkers weren't breaking any speed records.) Even so, walkers reduced their anxiety as much as the exercisers, bumped up their levels of good cholesterol and reported more sexual fantasies and more desire for intercourse than before the study started. Walking may not qualify as Olympic-level training, but don't overlook its mild-mannered benefits.

Exercise, Sex and Aging

Studies of a different sort have shown that people who keep themselves in fighting trim also tend to stay sexually active far later in life than more pedestrian mortals. In one small-scale study, a behavioral scientist at Bentley College in Waltham, Massachusetts, looked at the sex lives of 160 Masters swimmers, one group in their forties and another in their sixties. These people were not just moderately fit, they were superfit, training an average of an hour a day, four or five days a week—a few of them even more.

"The men and women in our study reported sex lives more like those of people in their twenties and thirties than those of their contemporaries," reported Phillip Whitten, Ph.D., and his research associate Elizabeth J. Whiteside. "Not only that, the people in their sixties reported sex lives comparable to those in their forties," making love an average of about seven times a month.

Why Fit Equals Sexy

What, precisely, is the connection between staying fit and staying sexy? Well, there are a few obvious things, like enhanced self-esteem. When you look good, you feel good — and your partner feels good about you. Eighty percent of the Masters swimmers rated themselves as attractive or very attractive, but they were just being humble — their spouses or lovers rated them as even more attractive than they rated themselves. But there is a physiological explanation as well. Cardiovascular fitness seems to have a direct effect on men's sexual performance, because attaining and maintaining a serviceable erection requires good circulation. One of the body's responses to regular exercise is increased blood volume throughout the entire body, including the genitals.

Exercise also has an effect on circulating levels of testosterone — the hormonal trigger of sex drive in both men and women. Although the physiology is complex and the studies don't all agree, quite a few have shown that testosterone levels rise after short-term, moderately vigorous exercise. One study showed significantly elevated serum testosterone levels after men ran on a treadmill for 30 minutes — although in women, these levels rose only after 120 minutes of exertion.

The Outer Limit

Like almost everything else, exercise is best if it's seasoned with reason. If a little jogging is great for your love life, a whole lot of jogging is not necessarily better. It's well known, for instance, that female athletes who train too ferociously or get too lean develop athletic amenorrhea — in effect, their bodies turn off the menstrual cycle. Their bodies are saying, in essence, "I'm under terrific stress — now is a lousy time to get pregnant!"

Quite a few studies have also shown that continuous, exhausting exercise drives down testosterone levels and takes the steam out of the libido. Rather dramatic declines in testosterone have been shown in male ultramarathon runners after a 100-mile race, for instance. And one study of fanatical, driven male athletes, who tended to be as obsessed with leanness as anorexics and took up running with an almost religious zeal, found that their marriages were also "often impersonal and asexual."

How much exercise does it take to drive down testosterone levels—what, in effect, is the outer limit? Well, fortunately, it's *way* out there. A researcher at the University of Michigan, Ann Arbor, Ariel Barkan, M.D., has estimated that you'd have to run around 200 miles a week to seriously disrupt your hormones. By contrast, "there appears to be something magical about running 30 miles per week," says Jay Schinfeld, M.D., a triathlete who is also chief of endocrinology at the Temple University School of Medicine in Philadelphia. You don't have to exercise *that* hard to experience the positive effects of exercise on sexuality, but once you start going above it, you increase your risk of injury—as well as of losing interest in old Frank Sinatra records.

EXPERTS

When it comes to the complex and mysterious realm of sex, what, exactly, is an expert? There are plenty of sex therapists and psychologists who are perfectly willing to go on TV talk shows and dispense free advice about how to conduct your sex life. But the fact is that there are only two experts who *really* matter: you and your partner.

No one knows what is pleasurable to you better than you do. No one can say with more certainty what turns you on more than you can. And no amount of expert advice can tell you—precisely—what sends your mate to Cloud Nine except your own loving, exploring touch and the response that it elicits.

As a culture, we are inundated with the advice of experts, newspaper pundits, syndicated sages and self-help books like this one. There's lots to be learned from all these sources of information, but it's dangerous to take them too seriously. It's best to learn what you can, take what you need and throw the rest away. Don't sanctify *anybody's* notion of what's "true" about sex, because it may not be true for you. (And what could be deadlier than to have the grim, judging visage of Sigmund Freud hanging in the darkness over your bed?)

Besides, every "sex expert" of this century—including Freud, Kinsey, Masters and Johnson—has been at least partly wrong, and the current crop of experts no doubt will also turn out to be at least partly wrong. When Freud declared that the vaginal orgasm was the only right and proper way for women to experience

120

sexual pleasure, millions of women were left wondering what was the matter with them. *They* didn't experience the greatest pleasure that way. When certain modern-day experts began insisting that the clitoral orgasm was the only possible way to go, millions of other women couldn't figure out why they enjoyed vaginal penetration so much. In these instances, people felt they were "wrong" only because the experts were wrong.

The fact is that human sexuality is a wonderfully diverse, wonderfully individual thing. It's yours. As long as you do it with love and mutual consent, there is no right way or wrong way to do anything. Just have faith in your body and your own experience. *That's* the thing to trust—not the advice of experts.

Consult a psychologist, a sex therapist, your family doctor, a urologist interested in sexual problems or a gynecologist if you're experiencing a problem. Just don't feel that you have to rely on them for advice about what's supposed to feel good for you.

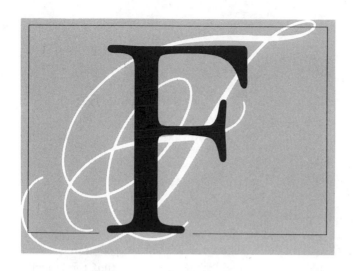

FANTASY

First of all, don't worry. Almost everybody—male and female, young and old, prudish and promiscuous—has sexual fantasies. And surprisingly often these fantasies involve things that (in real life) would be considered unusual, unnatural and maybe even illegal. "Although once regarded as symptoms of emotional, sexual and psychological disturbance . . . sexual fantasies now are widely recognized as positive forms of erotic expression," one team of sex researchers recently observed.

The mind, after all, is the body's most fertile erogenous zone. Without sexual fantasies, sex itself may seem sterile, mechanical and uninteresting. In fact, it's been discovered that sexually dysfunctional men and women rarely have erotic fantasies during foreplay, sexual intercourse or masturbation. And people who suffer from what are known as *hypoactive desire disorders* (lack of interest in sex) also seldom unreel torrid movies in their minds. These people may consciously squelch such thoughts because they feel guilty or embarrassed about them, or they may simply not have them at all. As part of their cure, many sex therapists actually help these self-censored folks unleash the erotic potential of their minds by teaching them how to fantasize. Some women who've never had an orgasm, in fact, are able to become orgasmic simply by allowing themselves to indulge in their erotic fantasies during sex.

Fantasy as Reality

Sexual fantasies are without doubt the most common kind of human sexual experience—and sometimes they're so vivid, and so steamy, that they hardly qualify as "fantasies" at all. It's now believed that about 1 percent of women can actually bring themselves to orgasm through fantasy alone—without touching themselves, or being touched, at all. At a recent conference of sex educators and therapists, Beverly Whipple, R.N., Ph.D., a sex researcher at Rutgers University in New Brunswick, New Jersey, presented a study of ten such women. Under laboratory conditions—despite the extraordinary unsexiness of being wired up and monitored by a crowd of researchers—seven out of ten of these women had a bona fide climax, solely through the erotic use of their minds.

Functions of Fancy

Sexual fantasies can serve a variety of purposes. One of the most common, reported by 71 percent of men and 72 percent of women in one recent study, is to heighten sexual arousal. "One of the most frequent patterns we have encountered is the use of a particularly treasured fantasy to move from the plateau phase of arousal," say William Masters, M.D., and Virginia Johnson, of the Masters and Johnson Institute in St. Louis. "Some men and women report that they are unable to be orgasmic unless they use fantasy this way."

Sex fantasies, because they're completely safe and completely private, also allow you a way to let your sexual feelings out for an uninhibited romp. You can explore all sorts of sexual situations—and have all sorts of sex partners—without being held personally accountable. (In one study of college students, over 30 percent of the men admitted that in a lifetime of erotic fantasizing, they'd had sexual "encounters" with over a thousand partners.) You can release pent-up sexual pressures and tensions harmlessly. And you can "preview" an anticipated sexual activity, partly as a way to diffuse your fears, partly to rehearse the scene in advance and troubleshoot potential problems. Adolescents often use fantasy this way.

Far-Out Fantasies

One thing that's important to remember, though: Just because you fantasize about something doesn't mean you'd actually want to do it, even if you could. Fantasizing about, say, a homosexual encounter, or bondage, may be a way of discharging your fears, or perhaps just your curiosity, about such practices. And it's fairly well known that some women fantasize about being raped—but that doesn't mean they are actually longing to be forced into having sex. (Nancy Friday, a writer who spent nearly a decade investigating men's and women's sex fantasies, suggests in her book *Forbidden Flowers* that often women who have rape fantasies grew up in sexually repressed households and that, for them, the fantasy of being "taken" by an overpowering male is often the only acceptable way to allow themselves to be sexual.)

Studies at the Masters and Johnson Institute have shown that women who have "unusual" fantasies (of being raped, of having sex with animals, of sadomasochistic sex) have no interest in actually doing these things. But interestingly enough, about two-thirds of the men who were interviewed for these studies said they might want to try out their fantasies, if given the chance.

Sometimes, of course, bizarre sex fantasies *do* get out of control. People may become compelled to act out strange fantasies or become so obsessed with a fantasy that their flesh-and-blood partners fade into unimportance. Experts say one hallmark of real trouble (what's now known as a *paraphilia*, or perversion) is when a person finds himself compelled to bring a specific, aberrant fantasy to mind, every time, in order to become sexually aroused or have orgasm.

How Men and Women Differ

How do men's erotic fantasies differ from women's? A variety of studies have shown that our sexual imaginations are almost as different as our bodies. For one thing, men have sex fantasies far more frequently than women do—about twice as often, according to most studies. (There's interesting evidence that all sex fantasies are tied to androgens, or male sex hormones, which trigger the libido in both men and women but are far more prevalent in men.) According to one review of the literature on sex fantasy, other generalizations can also be made. Men's fantasies tend to be dominated by visual images, especially genital images, are more likely to involve multiple, often anonymous partners, are more active and aggressive and move more quickly to explicitly sexual acts. Women's fantasies, by contrast, are more personal, often focusing specifically on someone they actually know, emphasize touching, feeling and emotions, unfold more slowly and tend to include more caressing and nongenital touching.

Sound suspiciously familiar? Well, it doesn't end there. Bruce J. Ellis of the University of Michigan and Donald Symons, Ph.D., of the University of California, Santa Barbara, note that men's and women's erotic fantasies are also mirrored almost perfectly in the literature of erotic fantasy: male-oriented pornography and female-oriented romance novels. Pornography is highly visual, highly explicit and focuses on "sheer lust and physical gratification, devoid of encumbering relationships." Romance novels, by contrast, are primarily love stories—a woman's personal, emotional search to "identify and marry the one right man who will remain hers for the rest of her life." There is very little overlap in the fantasy worlds depicted by these two genres, just as there is almost no market for male-oriented romance novels or hard-core pornography for women.

Ah, sex and the sexes! Will we ever understand each other?

Should You Share?

Should you share your sex fantasies with your partner? Well, it all depends. Masters and Johnson report that many people find that when they share their spiciest fantasy with a partner, somehow the whole thing just fizzles. Actually acting out fantasies can be disappointing, too; sometimes the thrill lies in its secrecy and the fact that reality doesn't intrude. You never get cold or uncomfortable or sticky, and you can stop it any time you like. Says Nancy Friday: "I think that for every person who has written to me about the joys of performing their sexual dreams in reality, there have been three or four who knew in advance that it wouldn't work or who tried it and were disappointed."

Still, what if you're one of the people who love it? You never know until you try. Sex therapist Lonnie Barbach, Ph.D., assistant clinical professor of medical psychology at the University of California, San Francisco, School of Medicine, suggests that the two of you try spinning out a fantasy *together.* Or imagine this—one of you could spin out the story while the other provided the physical stimulation. Or you could try acting out a fantasy, such as going to a motel bar and pretending you've just met, having a little getting-to-know-you chitchat, then going upstairs and making love as if for the first time.

Or you might want to try a sort of modified acting-out. One woman had fantasies of wild, passionate sex, so she and her husband would wear old T-shirts and rip them off each other during sex. What better proof could you get of the reality of fantasy than shreds of T-shirt scattered all over the bedroom floor?

FATIGUE

Fatigue plays an enormous role in almost everybody's sex life these days. I see couples who work 12-hour days who have no sexual dysfunctions at all but who simply never get around to it because they're so exhausted," says sex therapist Shirley Zussman, Ed.D., a director of the Association for Male Sexual Dysfunction in New York City and former president of the American Association of Sex Educators, Counselors and Therapists.

Other sex therapists across the country are hearing the same thing. "Among working women, especially women with kids, chronic fatigue is the most common obstacle to a good sex life, the number one complaint," says Jude Cotter, Ph.D., a psychologist and sex therapist in private practice in Farmington Hills, Michigan.

In fact, about one out of every five Americans who walk into a doctor's office complains of fatigue. Chronic fatigue can have an impact on every area of your life, including sex. When all you long for is sleep, it's hard to get interested in sex (or stay interested) once your head hits the pillow. Doctors say that's because chronic fatigue can interfere with sexual functioning in at least two different ways. It can inhibit your interest in sex (a desire problem), or it can dampen your ability to become aroused once things start getting physical (an arousal problem). Either way, chronic fatigue throws a wet sheet over everything.

If your fatigue is simply a scheduling problem (too much to do, not enough time), consider these modest suggestions.

Plan ahead. We all have blue-movie fantasies of wild, reckless, spontaneous sex—sex that "just happens." And sometimes it really does. Other times, though, life gets so overscheduled you may have to put "spontaneous sex" on your calendar for Thursday at 7. Yeah, it does seem awfully unromantic. But if learning to schedule time for sex means you have sex more often, what's so bad about that? Says Dr. Cotter: "A good sex life doesn't fall out of heaven. Sometimes you've got to work to make it happen."

Have a morning glory. It's easy to fall into the routine of having sex just before falling asleep at night, but for many people that's the worst possible time. Your love life gets what little energy is left after the day is done, and sometimes there's almost nothing left. But if you think about it, among all the priorities in your life, do you *really* think love should be last in line? Try reversing your priorities for a change, beginning the day with lovemaking instead of ending it that way. If Saturday morning is the only time it's feasible to linger abed, and you've got kids, try having a sitter come early Saturday morning, lock the bedroom door, and don't come out till you're through.

Get back in sync. Sometimes a couple's schedules get so out of sync with each other that they're never in bed, awake and feeling ready for sex at the same time. By the time she's ready for bed at 11, he's already asleep, or vice versa. The only way to stoke up the smoldering fires is to get up earlier, or go to bed later, or in some other way synchronize your watches. (Sometimes out-of-sync schedules are deliberately arranged that way, to avoid sex or intimacy, Dr. Cotter observes. If that's the case, this could be a very difficult pattern to break. If not, it may be a simpler problem to solve than you think.)

Try a mini-vacation. If you find that your interest in sex returns while you're on vacation, it could very well be that fatigue and stress are at the root of the problem. Obviously, you can't jet off to Barbados every time you feel like making love. But consider the concept of the mini-vacation—little 18- to 24-hour chunks of paradise slipped into your schedule throughout the year. Just checking into a local hotel overnight (especially one with lavish room service) can give your sex life a real boost.

Unexplained Fatigue

We're all stretched a little thin these days, but for some people, no amount of sleep will ever be enough. It's *not* just a scheduling problem. Chronic, unexplained fatigue that doesn't go away even when you've had plenty of sleep may be due to some other kind of trouble. Here are several likely possibilities.

Anemia. Oxygen is the stuff of life, and it's delivered to every far-flung cell in your body by red blood cells. But when red blood cell counts drop below normal (anemia), the result, almost always, is chronic fatigue. Women who bleed heavily during their periods may deplete their body's stores of iron, which is necessary for oxygen transport. Insufficient iron can also result in chronic tiredness, according to James D. Cook, M.D., head of the Division of Hematology at the University of Kansas Medical Center. Occasionally men also develop an iron deficiency due to gastrointestinal bleeding (which is often virtually symptomless).

A thin, pale diet (especially one lacking iron, protein and vitamin B_{12}) may also cause anemia. Among the best food sources of iron are beef liver, dark turkey meat, lean ground beef, lima beans, sunflower seeds, prunes, broccoli and spinach.

Drug side effects. Fatigue can be a side effect of quite a few different drugs, including antihistamines, pain relievers, diuretics, high blood pressure medications, antibiotics and birth control pills. Sometimes it's a *combination* of drugs that puts you to sleep. If you suspect a nonprescription medication is making you drowsy, try switching to another brand, or stop taking it altogether. (Check the product insert to see if fatigue is listed as a side effect.) If you suspect a prescription medication is the problem, *don't* stop taking it without checking with your doctor first. There are so many medications on the market, it's very likely the physician will be able to substitute another drug that won't take the starch out of your sex life.

Chronic fatigue syndrome. A few people who come into a doctor's office complaining of fatigue—less than 5 percent, doctors say—suffer from a complex and baffling disorder that's come to be known as *chronic fatigue syndrome.* So far, it's not at all clear what the cause may be, although the Centers for Disease Control (CDC) in Atlanta is currently conducting a massive study to examine every possibility, from pesticides and fertilizers to Epstein-Barr virus. According to an expert panel convened by the CDC, people who truly have chronic fatigue syndrome have a flulike illness that has produced debilitating fatigue for at least six months and that doctors have concluded is not due to any other physical or psychiatric illness. (Psychological stresses, especially depression, can also cause chronic fatigue.) Classic symptoms of chronic fatigue syndrome include chills or low fever, a sore throat, swollen lymph glands, muscle weakness or discomfort, headaches, joint pain without swelling, insomnia or forgetfulness. If that description sounds like you, it may be time to begin your search for relief—beginning with your family doctor.

Other possibilities. In some cases, doctors say, fatigue may be one of the first signs of a serious disorder like hepatitis, a thyroid problem, mononucleosis, tuberculosis, an infection or something else. It could be an early warning sign from a body in distress. So if that washed-out feeling doesn't go away even when you're on vacation, see your doctor. A correct diagnosis could bring back your zest for sex and might even save your life.

FEMININE HYGIENE DEODORANT SPRAYS

Whole industries are built on the insecurities of women, and feminine hygiene deodorant sprays are a classic example. Not only are they entirely unnecessary, doctors say, but many women have allergic reactions to the chemicals they contain. They can irritate the vagina and the vulva (as can deodorized or scented tampons and some commercial douches), producing redness and inflammation of sensitive inner skin. In fact, the Food and Drug Administration has suggested, and may soon require, that all these sprays carry a warning to this effect on the label.

An unusually strong-smelling vaginal discharge is generally a sign of vaginal infection, and it should be treated by a doctor, not covered up with chemicals. As a general rule, washing your genitals daily with mild soap and water, making sure to dry yourself thoroughly, is a much better way to keep yourself smelling fresh. (For more information about preventing infections, see "Pelvic Inflammatory Disease" and "Yeast Infections.")

But there's something more fundamental about "intimate deodorants" that's objectionable. Where did we ever get the idea we were supposed to smell like corsages, instead of human beings? We're here in the flesh, and our bodies produce odors—rank, musty, briny—especially when we get sexual. That's normal, natural, completely wholesome. That's how we were made.

The French, of course, look at the question of female odor quite differently than we do. To them, it's not something to be covered up but to be celebrated. *Cassolete* is a lovely word of theirs, meaning, literally, "perfume box" but referring more poetically to the animal smell of a clean woman—her hair, her skin, her sweat, her whole physical being. They consider all of it to be seductive, arousing, sexual and uniquely *her own*. To spray away those musky private vapors and replace them with the scent of fake lilacs, mass-produced in a factory, should be some sort of a crime.

If you insist upon using deodorant sprays anyway, doctors recommend that you never spray them directly into the vagina, because they can be especially irritating to mucous membranes. And if you notice redness or itching, stop using the spray immediately.

FOREPLAY

If intercourse is the entrée, foreplay is the appetizer—which, as anybody knows, can be the tastiest part of the meal. On the other hand, sometimes it's also nice to have an entire banquet consisting of nothing but hors d'oeuvres, with no main course at all.

This, in fact, is the way some sex experts (including William Masters, M.D., and Virginia Johnson of the Masters and Johnson Institute in St. Louis) prefer to look at foreplay. To them, even the word *foreplay* is mildly objectionable, because it implies that all sexual touching is just a prelude to intercourse, which may or may not be the case. To them, *noncoital sex play* is a better term, because it includes everything, takes the pressure off everybody and doesn't seem quite so desperately goal-oriented.

Well, whatever you call the delectable rites of arousal, and wherever they lead, they're still wonderful—and terribly important—especially to the woman.

The Light Bulb and the Iron

In one study, a group of 709 female nurses were asked to rank the importance of 15 different things (such as fatigue, stress and lack of tenderness) that interfered with their ability to reach orgasm. The women's most common complaint, outranking all the others by a good margin, was that their partners did not spend enough time in foreplay. Men, overly focused on the "goal" (intercourse), tend to hurry through it all. They tend not to slow down and take enough time to linger, to be playful, to explore—and to help their partners be satisfied.

How long is long enough? Well, only you and your partner can really tell for sure. But when these sexually experienced adult women were asked how long they'd *prefer* that their lovers indulge in foreplay, they replied (on average) about 17 minutes. That may seem like a long time, but the rewards of patience are rich. When Paul Gebhard, a collaborator of the late Dr. Alfred Kinsey, went back and reexamined the Kinsey group's data, he found that only 7.7 percent of the women whose lovers spent 21 minutes or longer on foreplay *failed* to reach orgasm.

"A man's sexual responses are like a light bulb: You turn it on, and it goes from cold to hot almost instantly. When you turn it off, it cools down right away. But a woman's responses are more like an iron: You turn it on, then wait and wait and wait until it heats up; and after you turn it off, you wait and wait and wait until it cools off," explains Jude Cotter, Ph.D., a psychologist and sex therapist in private practice in Farmington Hills, Michigan.

Foreplay is the way we smooth out the differences—slowing down the man a little, speeding up the woman a little, and meeting (let's hope) somewhere in the middle. Technically speaking, there's some interesting evidence that it's not so much that women's sexual responses are innately slower than men's but that they require more foreplay because it's harder for them to reach orgasm *through* *intercourse*. Dr. Kinsey felt that masturbation is a truer measure of women's actual sexual capacity than intercourse—and discovered that, even though many women are slow to respond during coitus, they could often masturbate to orgasm within a minute or two. To him, this showed that women's innate sexual capacities are really quite similar to men's.

All-Day Foreplay

The pleasure and utility of extended foreplay is not some great secret, and it's certainly not strange or unnatural—a huge variety of animals, including most mammals, will bite, scratch, nuzzle, smell, urinate upon, mount and otherwise make intimate contact with their partners for minutes, hours or even days before intercourse is attempted. "The student of mammalian mating behavior, interested in observing coitus in his animal stocks, sometimes may have to wait through hours and days of sex play before he has an opportunity to observe actual coitus," Dr. Kinsey wrote, with his usual air of professorial dispassion.

We're not animals, of course, but we, too, do better when we work up to sex slowly. In fact, if you think of foreplay as anything that gets you aroused about your partner, the whole dance begins long before you take off your clothes.

"One of the things that men don't understand is that if a guy spends the afternoon with his partner, and they stop and get a sandwich, they joke and kid around, they laugh, they hug—to the woman, that's foreplay," says Dr. Cotter. "Men want to know, What's the right technique for foreplay? Well, part of it is to go for a walk with her, spend some time with her, do things that are sensitive and kind.

"If he stops and buys a single long-stemmed rose on Tuesday, for no particular reason at all, he will probably have fantastic sex on Wednesday."

Sweet Sexual Signals

One way to make this sweet, lingering sort of foreplay a little bit more sexually explicit, he says, is to develop a sexual signal. Whenever she touches her ear in public, say, or yawns, or runs her finger along her throat, that means: "I can't wait to get you home in bed." Or, if you've got a slightly oddball sense of humor, you can give his penis a name. Call it "your friend," let's say. She calls him at work and says, "I sure will be glad to see you and your friend when you get home." Or, "Do you think your friend will still remember me when he sees me?" Or, "Why don't you introduce me to your friend when you get home?"

Says Dr. Cotter: "Women are usually very sensitive to a man's sexual cycle; they usually know when he's going to want to make love that night. Using these little signals can help enhance this sense of sexual anticipation tremendously."

Mistakes We Make

When it comes to actually getting physical, men and women often make similar mistakes. From their own intimate observations, Masters and Johnson say that during foreplay both men and women tend to do things that they think would turn *them* on. For instance, many men stroke the shaft of the clitoris vigorously and rapidly, in imitation of the way men masturbate, or they plunge a finger deep into the vagina—even though many women find this unarousing or even uncomfortable. By contrast, one of the men's most common complaints is that women don't grab the penis firmly enough; they treat the man's genitals as gingerly as they do their own.

(Interestingly enough, homosexual couples—who know from personal experience what a certain kind of erotic touch feels like—tend to be much more sensitive to their partner's needs, Masters and Johnson have found. Lesbians, for instance, know that the breasts are often tender just before a period and so treat them gently—something men often don't understand.)

The answer? Communication. It doesn't necessarily have to be verbal, but it's important to let your partner know, in one way or another, what feels good and what doesn't. (For more, see "Erogenous Zones.")

Aging Adds Awareness

As a man gets older, his sexual responses slow down a bit. The instant, unstoppable erections of his teenage years now rouse themselves more slowly, more reluctantly, and usually require more manual help in order to become fully rigid. In other words, the aging male begins to need more foreplay. In many ways, this is a blessing, because his sexual arousal cycle falls into closer sync with a woman's—the light bulb begins turning into an iron.

For the older male, foreplay doesn't only mean touching. It may also take the form of visual stimulation, like watching X-rated videos, because older men are more quickly aroused by the visual than they are even by manual stimulation of the genitals, Dr. Cotter has observed. Women, who may feel uncomfortable or even offended by steamy movies, should perhaps bear with their male partners on this, he says.

Enjoy the Afterglow

Even if intercourse is the entrée of sex, there's no reason to skip dessert. Yet many people, men in particular, tend to fall asleep or jump up and go watch the late show shortly after intercourse.

"Very often, when the guy is finished, he's finished, and he wants his report card—he wants to know how it was," says Dr. Cotter. "But for many women, the wind-down part after intercourse—the hugging and kissing, the feeling of closeness—is the nicest part. Often there are times when she has intercourse just because of the aftermath."

Men need to be more sensitive to women's fondness for this sweet, intimate afterglow, Dr. Cotter says. But women also need to be more up-front about communicating their love of this special time to men.

FREQUENCY

The right frequency for sex is as often as you both enjoy it," says Alex Comfort, M.D., Ph.D., in *The Joy of Sex.* "Don't be compulsive about frequency (or worried if friends say theirs is lower than yours). You aren't being scored." All of which seems like eminently sane advice in a culture obsessed with scoring everything, from bowling championships to orgasms per week.

Still—let's face it—everybody is interested. It's normal to wonder if you're normal.

A 1991 study by the National Opinion Research Center at the University of Chicago found that American adults reported having sexual intercourse an average of 57 times in the preceding year (about once a week). Married people were more active than singles, reporting having intercourse 67 times in the preceding year. And as in all other sex surveys, there was a steady decline with age, dropping from 78 times a year (three times every two weeks) for those under 40 to eight times a year (once every six weeks or so) for those over 70.

But this is only the frequency with which people have *intercourse.* When you include all varieties and permutations of human sexual behavior (including masturbation, wet dreams, mutual sex play that includes orgasm but not inter-course and everything else), the numbers are considerably higher. The late Dr. Alfred Kinsey found that the average white American man under age 30 had an orgasm (by whatever means) a little more than three times a week. When you consider the total male population of all ages, he found, the rate is closer to twice a week. (Oddly enough, the frequency with which married women have sex is often reported to be a little lower than that of married men. How is that possible? The University of Chicago researchers concluded that both men and women lie, at least a little, about sex—men inflating, women deflating, their sexual activities.)

So, What's Normal?

Still, all these numbers are just averages—a lumping together of vastly diverse individuals with wildly differing appetites. They tend to hide one of the most fascinating things about human sexuality: that the range of behavior that could be considered "normal," including sexual frequency, is astoundingly vast. The range is so great, Dr. Kinsey marveled, that it "raises a question as to whether the terms 'normal' and 'abnormal' belong in a scientific vocabulary." For example, among the 12,000 men interviewed by Dr. Kinsey and his colleagues, they found one man—apparently healthy and well-adjusted—who had ejaculated only once in the previous 30 years. At the opposite extreme, there were 12 men who were accustomed to averaging more than 29 ejaculations per week (over four times a day). One distinguished and accomplished lawyer had apparently found enough time between trying cases to average over 30 ejaculations a week for 30 years (or so he said). The difference between those two extremes, Dr. Kinsey calculated, is 45,000 times! As a biologist, he couldn't help but note that variations in behavior of that magnitude would be absolutely unheard of in the animal kingdom.

And these men were not just freaks at the lunatic fringes of human sexuality. Even in a relatively small group, Dr. Kinsey found, it would be reasonable to expect some people to be having orgasms only once or twice a year and others to be having them 10 or even 20 times a week. In the average person's circle of friends, in fact, there's probably at least one who is in the habit of reaching orgasm every day, or even more often than that, Dr. Kinsey noted.

His statistics bear this out: While three-quarters of the men he studied reported having between 1 and 6.5 ejaculations a week, a quarter of the men fell outside even that broad range of behavior—having sex even more, or even less, frequently. And among women, the range of variation is even greater, he found.

All of which should be at least a little comforting to almost everybody. When it comes to sexual frequency, "normal" covers just about everything.

The Incompatibility of the Sexes

All those averages also disguise another important fact about sexual frequency: In some ways, men and women are fundamentally incompatible.

If you chart the lifelong sexual frequency of the average man, as Dr. Kinsey did, you get a steep, sudden uphill climb during early adolescence, which peaks at around age 16 or 17. For most males, this is the time of greatest sexual activity, usually averaging more than three orgasms a week. But as they pass into their twenties, men's sexual activity begins to gradually decline in frequency, and it continues to decline, gently and steadily, on into old age. In fact, Dr. Kinsey wrote: "There are no calculations in all of the material on human sexuality which give straighter slopes than the data showing the decline with age." That steady decline in sexual frequency holds for both married and unmarried men.

This typical male sexual history stands in dramatic contrast to what seems to be the natural pattern of a woman's sexual life. If you look at the sexual history of single women, you don't find this dramatic early peak followed by a long decline. Instead, a woman's level of sexual activity tends to remain steady throughout her life, from adolescence on through to old age. Unmarried women, Dr. Kinsey found, averaged between 0.3 and 0.5 orgasms per week (a little less than once every two weeks) between adolescence and the age of 60.

On the other hand, not everybody has less sex as they get older. In fact, one recent study found that 15 percent of people over 65 said they were having more sex than ever before. If you're in this salty group, why should you care about what everybody else is doing (or not doing)?

Discrepancies of Desire

There's one more reason all these sexual averages shouldn't be taken too seriously: They aren't worth a hoot if there's a discrepancy between what you and your partner consider the ideal frequency for having sex. If you want to make love three times a week, and your mate only feels the urge once a month, you've got a problem. (The myth is that it's the man who wants sex more often than the woman, but most sex therapists say it's just as often the other way around.)

"Differences in sexual desire are a very common problem, but most couples manage to negotiate a compromise," says Domeena C. Renshaw, M.D., psychiatry professor and director of the Sexual Dysfunction Clinic at Loyola University School of Medicine in Chicago. "You have to be willing to negotiate."

Negotiate? Like two lawyers haggling over a contract? Well, sort of. If you value your relationship, and if the issue is important enough, experts say that both of you will have to give a little—just as in a fairly negotiated contract.

When you're trying to work out sexual differences, advises Bernie Zilbergeld, Ph.D., a clinical psychologist in the Human Sexuality Program at the University of California, San Francisco, you'd do well to ask yourself two questions: What, *precisely,* do you (or your partner) want more of—intercourse, oral sex, physical intimacy or what? "The partner less inclined to have more sex may be willing to increase the amount of physical contact or sexual activity other than intercourse, but may not be willing to have intercourse more often," he notes. This can be an opening for compromise.

The second question: Is the issue here the physical act of sex or only its symbolic meaning? Sometimes a woman (or a man) may want sex because it's the only time she or he feels loved, but there are other ways to make someone feel loved. If there was more physical affection in the relationship, there might not be such a great need for sex.

Adds Dr. Renshaw: "Sometimes women complain, 'You don't show me any acceptance or love, you just want intercourse.' At the same time, there are also men who feel she gives him sex, but she doesn't give him any feeling of intimacy. The emotional satisfaction is not there."

In both cases, the issue is not sex at all, but the feeling of being loved. In working out disagreements over sexual frequency, it may be helpful to distinguish the difference.

Still, notes Dr. Zilbergeld, "if a disagreement assumes major proportions and can be neither resolved nor dropped and is causing real problems in the relationship, the chances are excellent that sex is not what you are disagreeing about. Get some help before it wrecks the relationship."

FRIGIDITY

When a man complains that his wife is frigid, you can almost picture her lying there in bed, frosty and unresponsive as a statuette of ice. She may even imagine herself that way, too.

The trouble is, the term *frigid* is both too vivid and too vague. It creates an indelible mental image not only of iciness and unarousability but also of deliberate cruelty, conscious withholding and perhaps some deep and terrible psychological disturbance. Maybe she's a man-hater, a latent lesbian. Maybe she was sexually abused as a child. Maybe she really *does* have a heart made of snow.

It also suggests that her mate has nothing whatever to do with it. He's blameless; she's frigid. As we all know, though, relationships (and sex troubles) are always far knottier than that. It could very well be that he simply cannot acknowledge how much his behavior is contributing to the problem. (One old saying—equally unfairly—completely reverses the blame: "There are no frigid women, only clumsy men.")

At the same time, it's not at all clear what the word *frigid* really means—which is one reason sex therapists hardly ever use it anymore. Does it mean that she has little desire for or interest in sex? If so, it's not a problem unique to women—despite all the myths, men are just as prone to low sexual desire as women are, many sex therapists now report. Does it mean she has trouble getting aroused? That she can't seem to reach orgasm? This problem is now usually, and more accurately, referred to as being *preorgasmic.*

In other words, from the point of view of a therapist seeking to understand what's going on in a troubled relationship, "She's frigid" can mean so many different things it's practically useless as a descriptive term.

On the other hand, the word may be overused at least partly because it really does describe *something.* Alex Comfort, M.D., Ph.D., in *The Joy of Sex,* describes it nicely: "Real frigidity is when a woman who loves her man and isn't consciously scared of any part of sex still fails to enjoy it when they've both taken the trouble to see that she should."

In that case, it may be time to consider therapy. (See "Sex Therapy.")

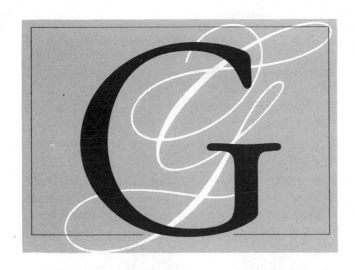

GINSENG.

See Aphrodisiacs

GONORRHEA

The AIDS epidemic has upstaged all the rest of the old-fashioned sexually transmitted diseases (STDs), but that doesn't mean they've gone away. Gonorrhea ("the clap")—one of the oldest known diseases—is still flourishing, and it's still just as ugly as it ever was. In fact, it is the most frequently reported infectious disease in the United States, according to the Centers for Disease Control in Atlanta. Something like a million cases of gonorrhea are reported in the United States every year, and another million (mostly among teenagers and young adults) are thought to go unreported.

The key things to remember about gonorrhea are these: It's highly contagious and potentially dangerous—and it may cause no symptoms at all.

That Tingling Sensation

Gonorrhea is named after *Neisseria gonorrhoeae,* or gonococcus, a nasty and tenacious bacterium that thrives in warm, damp places such as the urinary tract, the cervix (the most common site of infection in women), the mouth and the rectum. Like gossip and wildfire, it spreads. In addition to spreading from contact between the genitals during intercourse, it can spread from a man's penis to his partner's throat during oral sex (pharyngeal gonorrhea), from the penis to the rectum during anal sex and from the genitals to the mouth via the fingers.

Even so, people who are infected may have only mild symptoms or none at all, at least during the early stages—which is one of the reasons gonorrhea so readily makes the rounds.

Men who do develop symptoms usually notice them fairly quickly—one day to two weeks after having sex with an infected partner. The first sign is often a tingling sensation in the urethra (urinary exit pipe), followed by pain and burning during urination and a discharge of milky white pus. If left untreated, the discharge continues to increase for two or three months. For men, the real danger is that the infection will ascend into the seminal vesicles, the epididymis or the prostate, potentially causing sterility. It can also cause narrowing of the urethra, making urination permanently more difficult. The bacteria also can sometimes get loose elsewhere inside the body, infecting the joints, heart valves, brain or bloodstream.

The Danger to Women

In women, the incubation period is generally longer—7 to 21 days. The early symptoms, if they show up, usually include a painful burning sensation during urination or a yellowish or whitish vaginal discharge. Left untreated, these symptoms may degenerate into abdominal pain, bleeding between periods, vomiting and fever.

But the real danger to women is that the bacteria will invade the reproductive system, usually the ovaries and fallopian tubes, causing pelvic inflammatory disease, which can result in infertility and a host of other serious complications including an increased risk of ectopic (tubal) pregnancies.

Pregnant women carrying gonorrheal infections may also pass the disease on to their babies during childbirth. Because of the danger of gonorrheal eye infections that can lead to blindness in infants, most states require that the baby's eyes be treated with eyedrops (silver nitrate or penicillin) just after birth. And many doctors recommend that pregnant women have at least one gonorrhea test during pregnancy.

Gonorrhea-Safe Sex

The best way to protect yourself from gonorrhea is to become a monk or a nun or to practice monogamy. If that's unrealistic, use condoms, which have been shown to be highly effective in preventing the spread of gonorrhea (and many other STDs as well). Barrier contraceptives like the diaphragm or the cervical cap, plus spermicidal creams, foams and jellies containing nonoxynol-9, will also help protect you (although not as well as condoms).

The Good News

About the only good news on this dismal subject is that effective treatment is available, if the disease is quickly and correctly diagnosed. Diagnosis is made with the help of a Gram stain test, usually available in a clinic or doctor's office. It is accurate more than 90 percent of the time. A culture test (which takes a couple of days) is considered even more reliable, especially for women.

Although treatment regimens vary, doctors usually use the antibiotics ampicillin, amoxicillin or some type of penicillin to treat gonorrhea. These drugs are often given along with a tablet of probenecid, which slows down the rate at which the body excretes antibiotics and in this way increases their effectiveness. You may also be given a second antibiotic (such as tetracycline) to take at the same time. That's because many gonorrhea carriers are also infected with *Chlamydia trachomatis,* another noxious bacterial STD.

In recent years, there has been increasing concern about new antibiotic-resistant strains of gonorrhea, which were apparently introduced from the Far East in the 1970s. Even ordinary gonorrhea is so clever at adapting to antibiotics that increasing resistance was noticed almost as soon as penicillin was introduced back in the 1940s. Today, the dosage of penicillin used to treat it is a hundred times stronger than it was 50 years ago. Fortunately, new, improved antibiotics (such as spectinomycin or ceftriaxone) can usually knock out these new strains of supergonorrhea.

No matter what the doctor prescribes for you, it's important that you go back for a follow-up test once you're through taking the medicine, usually in a week or ten days. You're not cured until you've had a repeat test showing that you're disease-free.

And—this may be the most difficult part—you should also inform your sex partner (or partners) and suggest they get treatment, too, even if they have no symptoms at all. Not only could the disease be as harmful to them as it is to you, but if you're continuing your sexual relationship, you could be reinfected. The human body doesn't build up enough antibodies to gonorrhea to prevent reinfection, so even after the bacteria have been blasted out of your body, they could come right back if you're not careful. (James Boswell, the celebrated biographer of Samuel Johnson, was also famous for something else: The poor devil got gonorrhea 12 different times.)

G-SPOT

For something no bigger than a bean, the "G-spot" has caused a furor all out of proportion to its size. Its proponents claim it's a breakthrough discovery in female sexuality, a secret erotic hot spot largely unknown until the 1980s. Its detractors (including, to be honest, virtually all medically trained sex researchers) counter that it doesn't exist at all. Meanwhile, throngs of women have either discovered its sensuous pleasures or have given up trying to find it and concluded that the whole thing is a hoax.

What touched off the ruckus was a 1982 book called *The G-Spot and Other Recent Discoveries about Human Sexuality,* by Alice Ladas, Ed.D., a Manhattan psychologist, Beverly Whipple, R.N., Ph.D., a sex researcher at Rutgers University in New Brunswick, New Jersey, and John Perry, Ph.D., a psychologist and sexologist. These researchers had rediscovered a long-forgotten article, published in 1950, by the German obstetrician and gynecologist Ernst Grafenberg, M.D., in which he described a small area on the upper wall of the vagina that—in some women, at least—was so erotically charged that it could produce orgasms completely independent of clitoral stimulation. The tissue in this area, Dr. Grafenberg wrote, seems to be surrounded by erectile tissue like part of the penis and during sexual stimulation swells to the size of a dime.

The Grafenberg spot, or G-spot, as Dr. Ladas, Dr. Perry and Dr. Whipple called it, could be found directly behind the pubic bone, in the upper front wall of the vagina, about 2 inches inside the opening. Although its exact size and location varied, it could usually be found about halfway between the back of the pubic bone and the front of the cervix, near the neck of the bladder. If you imagine a clock inside the vagina with 12 o'clock aimed at the navel, they explained, the G-spot could usually be found somewhere between 11 o'clock and 1 o'clock.

Female Ejaculation

The three authors reported that many of the women who were sensitive to stimulation of the G-spot often ejaculated a clear fluid during orgasm—sometimes a few demure droplets, sometimes a gush of it. Although many of these women also felt the powerful urge to urinate just before orgasm, and some were convinced they *were* urinating during sex (much to their chagrin), these authors argued that this mysterious fluid was not urine at all.

Early chemical analysis of samples of this ejaculate showed it to be markedly different from urine and to apparently have components like that secreted by a man's prostate gland. These authors and others postulated that the fluid was produced by a group of ducts called the Skene's glands, located near the urethra, which evolve in the embryo from the same tissues that form the prostate in men and are sometimes referred to as the "female prostate." This theory, however, is still highly controversial (along with almost everything else about the G-spot). In fact, subsequent studies have found the fluid to be suspiciously urinelike, after all.

Where Was It Hiding?

So where does this "yes, it exists; no, it doesn't" controversy leave us? How could something so central to women's sexual response have escaped the attention of clinicians, gynecologists and ordinary lovers for so many centuries? Well, proponents claim that it *didn't*. Female ejaculation, they point out, was described by Aristotle and Galen as long ago as the second century A.D., and the seventeenth-century Dutch anatomist Regnier De Graaf described the "female prostate" in detail, noting that " . . . during the sexual act it discharges to lubricate the tract so copiously that it even flows outside the pudenda [external genitals]. This is the matter which may have been taken to be actual female semen." Some primitive peoples, not knowing any better, were so familiar with female ejaculation that they named it. The Bataro tribe of Uganda, for instance, had a custom called *kachapati,* or "spray the wall," in which older women taught young ones how to ejaculate.

Proponents also argued that the G-spot had remained largely undiscovered because (unlike the clitoris, which is a distinct, protruding organ) it lay deep within the vaginal wall and usually only responded to deep, firm pressure. (This

142

may be part of the reason women sometimes feel orgasmic sensations during childbirth, they suggested, since the baby's head is applying deep pressure on the vaginal walls.) Even the late Dr. Alfred Kinsey missed it, they claimed, because during a series of famous experiments he had five gynecologists examine the genitals of over 800 women by *gently stroking* the vagina, clitoris and other areas with a surgical probe. Ninety-eight percent of these women could feel the probe when it touched the clitoris, but only 12 percent could feel its caresses inside the vagina, leading Dr. Kinsey to conclude—perhaps erroneously—that the vagina was not very sexually sensitive.

The Modern View

A decade after the G-spot made the rounds of the TV talk shows, physiologists and sex researchers have had time to take another penetrating look at the physiology of women's sexuality and to hunt for hard evidence of the elusive spot. But it's fair to say that the whole business still remains controversial. Some noted sex specialists, such as Loyola University psychiatry professor Domeena C. Renshaw, M.D., have concluded that, at least until better evidence is presented, "the G-spot must remain unacceptable as a scientific fact." Other researchers conclude that if it exists at all, the G-spot is not nearly as widespread as its proponents claim. One study of over 100 women found that only 10 percent had anything resembling such a secret erogenous zone. Then again, in another survey of 1,245 professional women, 65 percent reported that they had a sensitive area in their vaginas resembling the G-spot, and almost three-quarters of these women also said they'd experienced orgasms when it was stimulated.

Zwi Hoch, M.D., director of the Center for Sexual Therapy, Education and Research at Rambam Medical Center in Israel, lays out what seems to be a sensible bottom line in all this. "Evidence in support of the 'G-spot'—defined as a discrete anatomical structure located on the anterior vaginal wall, which swells upon being tactilely stimulated—is inconclusive," he notes. "However, it seems reasonable to accept that women possess a zone of tactile erotic sensitivity on the anterior vaginal wall, which in many of them may extend to the entire anterior wall and to the posterior vaginal wall."

And this is supposed to be news?

How to Find Whatever It Is

Anyway, whatever you call it, and whatever it is, it certainly wouldn't hurt to try to find it. Since it's difficult to locate while lying on your back, some investigators suggest that women try to locate the area while seated on the toilet. For one thing, the first sensation many women experience when the spot is stimulated is an urgent need to urinate. Try exploring the upper front wall of the vagina by applying firm upward pressure with a finger. With sufficient stimulation, the area may begin to swell, feeling like a small lump or bean to the touch. Some women also find that it helps if they apply firm downward pressure with the other hand on the abdomen, just above the public bone, at the same time.

During intercourse, many women report that it's easier to "hit the spot" if she's on top, so that she can control the targeting of the man's erect penis. Other women find that the rear-entry position also works well. Some women say using a diaphragm, on the other hand, can interfere with G-spot stimulation.

If you discover that you're sexually sensitive in this area, consider it a new addition to your repertoire of erotic pleasure. But please don't conclude that you're neurotic, undersexed or inadequate if you can't find any such thing. As the good Dr. Kinsey said long ago, "There is nothing more characteristic of sexual response than the fact that it is not the same in any two individuals."

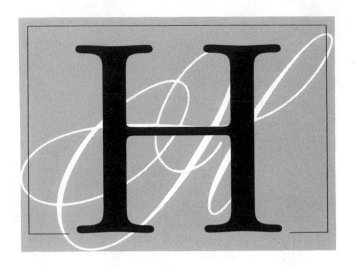

HANDICAPS

In the touching 1978 movie *Coming Home,* about a soldier who returns from Vietnam in a wheelchair, viewers were confronted with the sexual needs and problems of someone struggling with a physical disability. It was, perhaps, a breakthrough moment in cinema history, because we so often forget that people in wheelchairs, or those who have spinal cord injuries or are suffering from multiple sclerosis, cerebral palsy or any other handicap, are also real people whose sexuality is as important to them as yours is to you.

"People struggling with disabilities tend to be perceived as asexual, but they probably have an even greater need for physical intimacy than those who are not disabled," says Sandra S. Cole, Ph.D., professor of physical medicine and rehabilitation at the University of Michigan Medical Center in Ann Arbor and president of the American Association of Sex Educators, Counselors and Therapists. "Disease or injury can have a profound impact on one's self-esteem, body image, gender identity and sense of masculinity or femininity."

There are also a thousand daily slings and arrows that make finding sexual satisfaction far more difficult when you're struggling with a handicap.

"For instance, one thing that's as much a sexual handicap as not getting an erection is transportation," Dr. Cole says. "If you can't get around, you have a much tougher time finding a partner, and you often wind up living a more reclusive life. And since sexuality is an avenue toward intimacy, the imposition of a life devoid of intimacy may have a devastating effect."

Having a disability does not make you a nonperson. You still have needs, including sexual needs, and you need to acknowledge them unashamedly, she says.

"I'm a very sex-positive, pro-active kind of person, and I think people with disabilities have to say 'Yeah, it's a bitch, but life goes on,'" Dr. Cole says. "People *do* succeed in finding partners. They *do* find sexual satisfaction in their lives."

Ways to Cope

Generally, Dr. Cole says, when it comes to communicating their sexual needs, "the burden is really on the person with the disability. It may seem a little harsh to say this, but it's really *their* responsibility to educate their partners, to 'desensationalize' the disability so their partners can see through it to the person who's behind it. Actually, people who have disabilities do this well, because that's how they survive."

Fairly often (for instance, for many men with spinal cord injuries), erection is just not possible. In such cases, men need to learn to expand their sexual repertoire to include nonintercourse sex. (Which is actually good advice for *everybody.*)

In some ways, people with disabilities have a small advantage here, because when there's sensory loss in one part of the body, some other part of the body often becomes doubly sensitive. This means there may be a highly erogenous hot spot hidden in some nook or cranny of the flesh, just waiting to be kissed or caressed.

"Also, we sometimes forget about hugging and holding and warm, tender feelings, which are a far more important part of intimacy than intercourse," says Dr. Cole.

On the other hand, she adds, it's a little too easy for rehabilitation specialists to say "Well, if your penis doesn't work, just nibble on her ears." Men who have been strongly socialized to think that erections equal manhood are sometimes devastated when they can no longer get one on cue. If getting an erection is of central importance, there's an increasingly wide array of medical methods for creating an erect penis, whether it be through surgery, injections or an implant. (See "Erection Problems.") And many young men with spinal cord injuries, who can't sustain an erection or have an orgasm, can even impregnate their wives through a technique called electroejaculation (which triggers ejaculation by means of a low-voltage jolt of electricity).

Four Kinds of Disabilities

It's beyond the scope of this book to go into all the various disabilities in any detail. But basically, specialists divide them into four general categories, each with its special sexual challenges.

Type 1: childhood nonprogressive. Type 1 disabilities are those that begin before puberty and don't get progressively worse, like deafness. People with this type of disability grow up being "different" and often internalize the shame of society or the overprotectiveness of parents, either of which can have a negative effect on their sexuality. For such children, healthy, warm and loving support is critical. "But most important is to consider the child as a sexual person from the very beginning," says Dr. Cole.

It's also important to be sensitive to unexpected problems they may face in their sexual development. For instance, the most common chronic disability in the United States is deafness. But since the average deaf child achieves a reading level of between the fourth and fifth grade, their sexual education may be impaired because there's a shortage of sex education material for kids of that age.

Type 2: childhood progressive. This type of disability begins in childhood but gets worse. It includes things like muscular dystrophy, cystic fibrosis and childhood-onset diabetes. Often these kids wind up with a poor body image, a feeling of being constantly sick and an inability to think of their bodies as capable of sensual or sexual pleasure. As they age, their expectations of physical, emotional and sexual health tend to gradually decline. For them, a healthy sex life is as much a psychological challenge as it is a physical challenge.

Type 3: adult nonprogressive. These disabilities occur during adolescence or adulthood and don't get worse; they include things like spinal cord injuries or severe burns. People who have these disabilities usually have already experienced normal sexuality, so in many ways it's easier for them to return to normalcy than for those who don't know what that is. Still, such injuries can be devastating to one's sense of self-worth, and depression (which is known to smother sexual desire) is frequently a problem. In one study of spine-injured men, it took two to three years for them to reestablish a healthy sex life, although many still complained they had problems getting erections.

Type 4: adult progressive. These disabilities are caused by degenerative diseases, such as heart disease, cancer, arthritis and adult-onset diabetes. Generally, these conditions come on slowly, allowing a person to make a slow, easy adjustment to the changes in their sexual life. (For more, see "Aging," "Arthritis," "Cancer," "Diabetes" and "Heart Attack and Heart Disease.")

Headache

We have been taught that a headache surrounding sexual activity is a problem that is purely psychological, purely an excuse and purely female," says neurologist Jerome Goldstein, M.D., director of the San Francisco Headache Clinic.

But in reality, none of the above is true. Throbbing headaches that occur just before or during sex—known as benign sexual headaches, or *coital cephalagias* in high medicalese—are caused by real physical problems. They're not an excuse, because people who have them would usually *like* to have sex as much as anybody else. (Which is not to suggest that a "headache" isn't sometimes used dishonestly as a convenient means of avoiding a sexual encounter.) But most surprising of all, sexual headaches are actually four times more common among men than women. The typical sufferer, in fact, is not the frigid, fussy housewife of the cartoons but a middle-aged man who is slightly overweight, has mildly elevated blood pressure and may have a family history of migraines but is otherwise psychologically well adjusted.

Four Strains of Pain

Actually, researchers have found there are several different types of sexual headaches, each with its own cause and cure.

Muscle contraction headaches. This type is caused by tensing of the muscles during sex; these headaches are usually focused in the head and neck and gradually intensify as excitement rises. At orgasm, they may culminate in skull-splitting pain so severe it can cause nausea, vomiting or vision changes. For some people, learning muscle relaxation techniques has proved helpful. Ask your doctor to refer you to someone who teaches these techniques.

Vascular headaches. Caused by the increase in blood pressure during sex, these headaches can be scarier. They're usually characterized by a sudden, severe, almost explosive pain that occurs at the moment of orgasm. For people with this type of headache, says Dr. Goldstein, the prescription blood pressure drug propranolol (sold as Inderal) can be very helpful. So can other medications used to treat migraines. ·

Postural headaches. These are thought to be caused by low cerebrospinal fluid pressure, which occurs due to tiny tears in the membranes surrounding the spinal column. They usually occur while having sex in a sitting or standing position. The simple solution: Lie down during sex. That usually takes care of it. Still, if you experience this type of headache, you should discuss the problem with your doctor.

Drug-related headaches. As the name implies, these headaches are caused by having sex under the influence of alcohol or drugs. It's well known that alcohol, especially red wine, can trigger vascular or migraine headaches and that other "recreational" drugs (like cocaine or marijuana) can cause headaches by raising or lowering blood pressure. The solution: Make your bed a drug-free zone.

Dr. Goldstein hastens to add that most of the time, sexual headaches are unpleasant but relatively harmless. Only rarely are they caused by some really serious underlying problem. Still, sudden, severe headaches during sex, especially if they're accompanied by nausea, vomiting or wooziness, should be brought to the attention of your doctor.

Heart Attack and Heart Disease

First comes the heart attack. Then comes the fear of sex. Never mind that it's groundless, never mind that it's irrational. For all too many people who have suffered the trauma of a heart attack, the fear barrier is very real. A sense of terrible, lonely fragility holds them back from the healing warmth of sex. What could be more frightening than the thought that you might have another heart attack, or even die, during intercourse?

That's why so many people—between 50 and 75 percent, by some estimates—either curtail their sex lives or completely draw the curtains on sex after a heart attack. (Often it's the spouse, not the patient, who's most reluctant to resume sex, studies have shown.)

It doesn't help that there's often a major communication gap between cardiologist and patient on the subject of the patient's sexuality, says Chris Papadopoulos, M.D., chief of cardiology at South Baltimore General Hospital. Cardiologists just haven't been very good at giving patients specific, practical advice about sex during recovery, and patients haven't been very good at asking for it. Part of the problem, says Dr. Papadopoulos, is that cardiologists tend to be as uncomfortable talking about sex as anybody else. And even though many patients view them as experts on sex, often they're really not terribly well informed. The result: One survey showed that of 135 postcoronary patients, almost half got no information at all about how soon it was safe to resume sex after surgery.

Still, because of recent research into the matter, a good deal is now known about the sexual aftermath of heart attacks and heart surgery—and much of it is reassuring.

Overcoming the Biggest Fear

For one thing, the biggest fear—that you'll die during intercourse—is "highly unlikely," Dr. Papadopoulos says. "It's understandable that lots of people may think this, based on what they've read or seen on TV, but in most cases this is not a significant risk." In fact, according to a panel of six prominent cardiac rehabilitation specialists, about 80 percent of recovering heart attack patients can safely resume having sex; 20 percent should limit sex to some extent.

The reason: Despite its physical ecstasies, sexual intercourse actually requires much less energy than most people think. In one classic study, a group of middle-aged men, all of them married for more than 20 years and all convalescing from heart attacks, wore 24-hour Holter (electrocardiogram) monitors at home, which recorded the secrets of their hearts during ordinary activities, including sex. This study showed that the men's heart rates at orgasm averaged only about 117 beats per minute, with an average heart rate for the period 2 minutes before and 2 minutes after orgasm averaging 98 beats per minute.

Other studies have also confirmed that—at least among middle-aged people making love with their usual partner, in a familiar setting—the top heart rate rarely exceeds 120 beats per minute, and then only briefly (usually for about 10 or 20 seconds during peak excitement). It's not unlikely that you'd get your heart that excited while playing doubles tennis or even mowing the lawn. Not terribly romantic, perhaps, but comforting all the same.

Another oft-cited study on the subject, conducted by Japanese researchers, looked into the causes of 5,500 sudden deaths. (These were sudden deaths in the general population, not specifically in heart attack survivors.) Thirty-four of these people died during sex, including 18 from heart attacks. But here's the kicker: Thirty of them were having sex with someone other than their spouse (and that person averaged 18 years younger than their spouse). And all of those who died during intercourse had blood alcohol at or near intoxication levels. You can fill in all the other exotic details, but the general drift of this study seems clear: Monogamous sex is fairly safe, but torrid affairs, especially with younger partners, can be murder.

Back to Basics

How long should you wait after a heart attack or heart surgery to resume having sex? "It's really not safe to make blanket recommendations about how soon it's safe to resume sex after heart surgery, since every case is different," says Dr. Papadopoulos. Studies have shown that cardiologists advise patients to wait anywhere from two or three weeks to two or three months, depending on their condition.

In one study of 134 bypass patients, Dr. Papadopoulos found that the average time after surgery before they resumed sex was 7.8 weeks. Ninety-one percent of those who were sexually active before the operation resumed having sex afterward. Half the patients reported having sex as frequently after the operation as they had before it, 40 percent said they made love less often, and 10 percent said their frequency actually increased afterward.

Other specialists feel that your physical condition, rather than the mere passage of time, is a better measure of your readiness to resume life as a sexual being. "A patient who is able to climb two flights of stairs at a brisk pace can be considered sufficiently fit to have sexual intercourse," according to Armand J. Wohl, M.D., chief of cardiology at Grossmont Hospital in La Mesa, California. Other doctors say you should be able to walk a city block at a brisk pace without discomfort before attempting sex.

For people who are particularly apprehensive about sex after heart surgery, a treadmill exercise test or even wearing a Holter heart monitor for 24 hours (including during sex) can give more precise information to the cardiologist and a sense of reassurance to the patient, Dr. Papadopoulos says.

It makes sense to be prudent, but sometimes we forget: There's a deep magic, and lots of healing medicine, in the sense of emotional closeness and tenderness we get from sexual contact with our mates. It doesn't necessarily have to involve intercourse—cuddling, touching, even just talking can be the best remedy for the depression, anxiety and loneliness that often come on the heels of a heart attack. Avoiding sex because you're concerned about your health is not always a good idea. Sometimes, in fact, it's a terrible idea.

Don't Let Medications Sideline You

It's possible that your return to sexual normalcy could be delayed by the medications you're taking. Many drugs given to people recovering from a coronary condition—drugs to treat high blood pressure, in particular—can interfere with sexual functioning. Sedative hypnotics (like Valium or lithium), the high blood pressure drug reserpine (Sandril, Serpasil), as well as barbiturates and alcohol, can smother your interest in having sex at all. Depression, which is common in the first three months after surgery, can also sap all interest in sex. But ironically, antidepressant drugs can also take their toll on libido.

If you suspect that drugs may be causing sexual side effects, try to discuss this frankly with your doctor. Sometimes switching drugs or lowering the dosage of your present medication can take care of the problem.

Coping with Angina

What about people who *haven't* had a heart attack but who suffer from angina (chest pain due to heart disease) during sex? Such a situation requires the advice of a physician and should be evaluated with cardiac tests, including an exercise stress test, a Holter monitor recording and perhaps coronary angiography, Dr. Papadopoulos says.

However, in one study of 35 patients with stable angina pectoris, a cardiologist's simple advice was able to take the pain and apprehension out of sex for nearly all of them. At the beginning of the study, 29 of these folks reported that they were sexually active, although 19 of them complained that they usually developed chest pain or palpitations during sex. All of them, and their spouses, worried about this and reported it interfered with the frequency and enjoyment of intercourse. Their cardiologist advised them to warm the bedroom and the sheets and to avoid intercourse soon after a meal or a bath (since heat and overeating stress the heart). They were also advised to take a common angina drug (isosorbide dinitrate, or Isordil) 10 minutes before sex. Afterward, all but 2 reported they were able to have sex without pain.

Cardiologists often advise taking an angina drug shortly before sex to reduce both the pain and the apprehension. It's well known that *time to angina*—the amount of time it takes, given a certain amount of exertion, to produce pain—is lengthened by nitroglycerin and other vessel-dilating angina medications. Unfortunately, at higher doses, some of these drugs—beta-blockers, for example—can also cause erection problems.

Heart-Safe Sex

In general, Dr. Papadopoulos says, people recovering from heart attacks or surgery should follow these guidelines.

Take it easy. The first time you have sex after your surgery, go gently, and don't attempt intercourse. Warm, unpressured, nongenital touching is best. Indulge in these gentle pleasures over the course of a week or so, and if there's no chest pain, shortness of breath or palpitations, it's safe to move on to intercourse.

Rest first. Avoid sex when you're tired. Many men find that the best time for lovemaking is first thing in the morning or just after a nap, when they're well rested (and may already have the woman abed).

Slip into something comfortable. It's best to have sex in familiar surroundings—preferably at home in your own bed. Don't have sex when the room temperature is too hot, too humid or too cold. Warm up the bed sheets before sex, because a cold bed stresses the heart.

Don't treat it like dessert. Don't have sex right after a heavy meal, which also puts an added burden on the heart. It's best to wait 2 or 3 hours after eating before having your sweetie. It's also unwise to have sex after indulging in alcohol—wait at least 3 hours.

Forget gymnastics. Choose a sexual position that's comfortable and familiar. Cardiologists used to advise patients to avoid the top position, but recent research has shown that (in terms of energy cost) sexual position makes no particular difference. (Still, people with still-tender surgical incisions from a bypass find it less painful to try the bottom position, or side by side.) If you have shortness of breath while lying down, trying sitting in a chair with your partner in your lap, Dr. Papadopoulos suggests.

Listen to your body. Be alert for these warning signals of cardiac distress, and always report them to your doctor.

- Rapid heartbeat and rapid breathing that persist for 10 or 15 minutes after intercourse
- A feeling of extreme fatigue that lasts to the next day
- Dizziness, light-headedness, irregular heartbeats, blackouts or chest pain during or after sex

Herpes, Genital

The bad news about genital herpes is that it's caused by a particularly tricky virus, and—at least for now—it can't be cured. (Gonorrhea and syphilis, which are caused by bacteria, *can* be cured.) The first outbreak is usually the worst, but the virus often causes recurrent outbreaks for many years after the initial infection.

The good news is that although it's a genuine hassle, genital herpes is usually not serious, and the discomfort it causes can be fairly well controlled with the drug acyclovir (Zovirax). In fact, "for most people, herpes is not much more than a minor inconvenience," says Robert T. Ross, M.D., a medical epidemiologist at the Centers for Disease Control's Division of Sexually Transmitted Diseases.

The Unspeakable Itch

Genital herpes infections usually start out as a suspicious, mildly itchy rash around the genitals. Then they blossom into small, fluid-filled blisters on the penis, scrotum or inner thighs (in men) or on the inner or outer lips of the vagina, inside the vagina or around the rectum (in women). The blisters eventually burst open, evolve into burning, itching, ulcerated sores and finally scab over and heal without leaving scars. Infections usually show up about a week after contact with an infected person (although sometimes they don't show up for months) and generally last for one to three weeks.

For some people, these outbreaks can be extremely unpleasant. A particularly hellish episode can make it painful to urinate or even to walk and leave you feeling tired, feverish and without appetite. For others, though, the symptoms are so mild they're never even reported to a doctor. There may not even be any symptoms at all—which is why nobody really knows how widespread the disease is.

"Herpes has a wide range of manifestations—many people don't even know they have it, although they may still be able to transmit it," explains Dr. Ross. "The natural history of the disease is that a person becomes infected, the lesions go away, but the virus persists. But everybody who's infected will have an antibody to it—that's how we tell if a person has ever been infected."

And when doctors measure the prevalence of herpes antibodies in the population—the "footprints" of the disease—the numbers are truly astounding. By some estimates, over 40 percent of the population has been exposed to herpes.

Dangers to Women

Women exposed to the herpes virus have special reason for concern. Although it's never been conclusively proven that genital herpes actually *causes* cervical cancer, there is a statistical link: Women with these infections are much more likely to develop cancer of the cervix than women who are herpes-free. Doctors often recommend that infected women have a Pap test every six months. Cervical cancer is easy to detect and is easy to cure if it's caught early.

Pregnant women with herpes have a more serious matter to consider: Infants who contract genital herpes from their mothers are at risk of developing permanent damage to their nerves and eyes, and many of these babies—by some estimates, 50 percent—will die.

Although frequent checkups and delivery by cesarean section can reduce the risk of infecting the baby, if you're pregnant and have herpes it's critical that you let your doctor know this from the start. Many doctors also recommend that if either you or your partner has a history of herpes, you should avoid intercourse during the last trimester to avoid the possibility of an active vaginal infection at the time of birth.

Meet the Culprit

The cause of all this unpleasantness is usually a highly contagious virus called herpes simplex type 2. (Every once in a while, genital herpes can be caused by the type 1 strain of herpes simplex, a cousin virus that usually infects the mouth, causing blisters and cold sores. Herpes zoster, which causes shingles and chickenpox, is a different animal.) Although it infects the genitals, type 2 herpes is not necessarily passed through sexual contact. It can be passed from a cold sore on the lip down to the genitals, or from a sore lip to an eye by means of a fingertip. It can ride a wet towel or even a wet fork.

Because the virus is so very contagious, you should avoid all sexual contact during an outbreak. Don't even cuddle. Don't share towels, and if you've got sores in your mouth, don't share utensils. If you've *ever* had a genital herpes infection, you should always use a condom during sexual intercourse, even if you can't see any sores. That's because this crafty virus will begin shedding (making you contagious) for a few days before the sores appear and for a few days after they heal. This means that you may still give your sex partner a valentine of herpes, no matter how hard you try not to.

What exactly makes this virus so persistent? It has, it seems, developed a truly ingenious way of protecting itself.

After the first outbreak, the herpes virus retreats to a favorite hiding place in an obscure cranny of the spine called the dorsal nerve root ganglia. There it lies dormant for months or years—even, in some people, forever. For most people who have been infected, periodic herpes outbreaks (usually around the site of the original infection) become an unpleasant part of life. One small consolation prize: Over time, these recurrences usually decrease in frequency and ferocity.

It's still not clearly understood what touches off recurrent episodes. Some herpes sufferers say exposure to sunlight, fever, emotional stress, illness or (in women) menstruation increases the likelihood of an outbreak. But one study suggests the widespread belief that stress touches off herpes outbreaks may be unfounded. In a three-month study of 64 people infected with genital herpes, University of Florida researchers failed to find any connection between emotional stress and later outbreaks. Most of the subjects were students, and the researchers noticed dramatic increases in psychological stress on the day before tests and on *the day* the subjects' herpes broke out. But they found no evidence at all that emotional stress *preceded,* or touched off, the outbreaks. "These data do not support the popular idea that emotional stress triggers recurrences of genital herpes," the researchers concluded.

Acyclovir to the Rescue

No matter what the cause, the herpes virus tends to become a regular visitor. And at least for now, the best drug available to send it packing the first time it shows up is acyclovir, an antiviral agent developed by Burroughs Wellcome and approved by the Food and Drug Administration in 1982. The bottom line on acyclovir, says Dr. Ross, is this: "Usually the drug reduces the duration and severity of the initial episode. However, except for people who have very frequent recurrences, it has only a minimal effect on recurrent episodes, and most doctors don't prescribe it for that purpose."

If you get started on the drug within five or six days after noticing symptoms for the first time, acyclovir can reduce the pain and discomfort and speed up the healing of the sores by anywhere from four to nine days, according to a review of acyclovir studies published in the *Journal of the American Medical Association.* The drug also can significantly reduce the viral shedding time of infections, meaning (at least in theory) that you're not contagious quite as long.

Unfortunately, the drug doesn't seem to reduce the risk of recurrent outbreaks. And if you use it during one of these recurrent episodes, it only shortens the healing time by a day or so. If your symptoms are only mild, it's probably not worth the trouble.

Symptomatic Relief

During those periodic outbreaks there are a few ways to get some relief without taking prescription drugs, according to Joseph J. Apuzzio, M.D., associate professor and director of maternal-fetal medicine in the Department of Obstetrics and Gynecology at the University of Medicine and Dentistry of New Jersey/New Jersey Medical School.

- Take a sitz bath (sitting in shallow tepid water for about 5 minutes) two or three times a day.
- Apply cool compresses of Burow's solution—an astringent (drying agent)—to the infected area four to six times a day. Or try using an ice bag.
- To reduce pain and fever, take aspirin or acetaminophen (Tylenol).
- If the pain is really severe, you can ask your doctor to prescribe an anesthetic cream.
- Wear loose-fitting cotton underwear to allow air to soothe the sores and to avoid chafing.
- In general, keep your genital area clean and dry. After a shower, pat (don't rub) yourself dry, and use a separate towel to avoid spreading the virus to uninfected areas. Or use a hand-held hair dryer set on cool.

HIGH BLOOD PRESSURE.

See Medications

HOMOSEXUALITY

Everyone has an opinion about homosexuality, often a strongly held one. But whatever yours may be, at least one thing is certain: Homosexuality exists. To one degree or another, it can be found in nearly every society around the world and has been documented in many ancient societies throughout history. It also exists "in virtually every animal species that has been exhaustively studied," according to Richard C. Pillard, M.D., a psychiatrist at Boston University School of Medicine and a noted expert on homosexuality.

Based on the findings of the late Dr. Alfred Kinsey and others, most experts now estimate that around 4 percent of American males are exclusively homosexual throughout their lives. Around 10 percent are thought to be more or less exclusively homosexual for at least three years of their adult lives. And many more have had homosexual experiences: In his sample of over 5,000 American men, Dr. Kinsey found that 37 percent had had at least one sexual encounter to orgasm with another male.

Among women, the numbers are a little lower: Around 2 or 3 percent of adult women are thought to be exclusively homosexual (lesbian) throughout their lives. Interestingly enough, in studies of other modern cultures ranging from Central America to the Philippines, quite similar percentages of the population have been shown to be homosexual.

The Trouble with Labels

But that's where the simple part of the story ends. What *causes* homosexuality, whether or not it's "natural," even what homosexuality *is*—those are more difficult questions to answer.

The simplest way to define homosexuality is as "a sexual preference for partners of one's own gender." But like everything else about human sexuality, this preference is usually not an either/or situation. Lifelong heterosexuals sometimes fantasize about same-sex encounters, but that doesn't necessarily make them "latent homosexuals," as people used to say. (In one survey of 171 heterosexual men, a third reported having same-sex fantasies at least occasionally.) And most lifelong homosexuals have had sex at least occasionally with partners of the opposite sex. (One review of the literature found that 60 or 70 percent of homosexual males had had sex with a woman at least once, and up to 80 percent of lesbians had occasionally had sex with a man.)

As Dr. Kinsey summed up the situation long ago: "Males do not represent two discrete populations, heterosexual and homosexual. The world is not to be divided into sheep and goats. . . . The living world is a continuum in each and every one of its aspects. The sooner we learn this concerning human sexual behavior, the sooner we shall reach a sound understanding of the realities of sex."

To more accurately depict the "realities of sex," Dr. Kinsey devised a seven-point scale (now known as the Kinsey scale) that showed the full range of human sexual preference. At one end of the scale (zero) were people who were exclusively heterosexual throughout their lives; at the opposite end (six), those who were exclusively homosexual. In between those two extremes lay the vast and varied gray area of everybody who did not precisely fit into either category. One of Dr. Kinsey's great findings was that this in-between group was amazingly large, ranging from people who'd had one brief, out-of-character sexual encounter to those who were equally content with male or female partners (bisexuals).

Causes Unknown

Nobody really knows what "causes" homosexuality. Then again, nobody really knows what "causes" heterosexuality, which goes to show how little we really know about sex at all.

There has been, of course, a long-running debate about the origins of homosexuality. Are gay people "just born that way," as many gays claim? Does their homosexuality spring from something in their upbringing? Or are nature and nurture both involved? There's no firm answer yet, but over the past decade, researchers from a variety of fields have begun turning up compelling new evidence that there may be some innate, biological difference between gays and straights.

Some of these findings are really intriguing.

In late 1991, for example, a researcher at the Salk Institute for Biological Studies in San Diego reported what appears to be the first real evidence of an innate difference between the brains of homosexuals and heterosexuals. Neuroscientist Simon LeVay, Ph.D., reported that in a group of heterosexual men that he autopsied, one tiny cluster of neurons in the hypothalamus (a deep structure of the brain known to be involved in regulating sexual behavior) was more than twice as large as the same structure in the brains of a group of women and homosexual men. Since the homosexual men had died of AIDS, some critics charged that these brain differences might have been caused by the disease. But when Dr. LeVay autopsied a gay man who'd died of lung cancer, he found the same thing.

A variety of studies have also shown that being gay tends to run in families— suggesting, perhaps, that there may be some genetic component to sexual preference. In one recent study of homosexuality in twins, researchers from Boston University School of Medicine and Northwestern University reported that if one identical twin is gay, the other is almost three times more likely to be gay than if the twins are fraternal. Because identical twins share the same set of chromosomes, the study raises the intriguing possibility that there may be a "gay gene" that is as yet undiscovered.

Other studies have shown that male homosexuals are much more likely to have bisexual or homosexual brothers than heterosexual males. Some studies have shown that about 22 percent of male homosexuals report that their brothers are also gay; only about 4 percent of heterosexual males say their brothers are gay. (The familial nature of female homosexuality is much less clear; some studies have shown no such correlation at all.)

On the other hand, critics raise the obvious point that twins and siblings also share a similar upbringing, so their sexual preference could be explained as easily by the parenting they got as by their genes. And although most identical twins share the same sexual preference, not *all* of them do. What about the twins who are different? So far, the explanation for these anomalies is just not clear.

One intriguing line of study currently under investigation by a number of researchers is that homosexuality may be related to exposure to sex hormones during pregnancy. Animal studies have shown that female babies exposed to testosterone either in the womb or as tiny babies tend to exhibit more aggressive, "masculine" behavior. Homosexual men and women are also considerably more likely to be left-handed than their heterosexual peers—and handedness has been linked to sex hormone levels during brain development.

One theory holds that male homosexuality may be related to maternal stress during pregnancy. The reasoning: It's known that stress inhibits the production of sex hormones, and it's sex hormones that sculpt fetal tissue into a male or a female body. Studies with laboratory animals have shown that maternal stress during pregnancy sometimes "feminizes" male sexual behavior, apparently by affecting testosterone production.

This theory—like all the others—remains intriguing but unproven.

What about Upbringing?

One school of thought holds that homosexuality has nothing to do with biology at all. For much of this century, it was widely believed among psychoanalysts that male homosexuality has to do with the male child's inability to break free of his mother and identify with his father. The combination of a smothering, dominant mother and a weak or distant father resulted in the child developing an inner identification with femaleness, the theory suggests.

The trouble is that although there are plenty of gay men who grew up in this kind of family, plenty of heterosexual men did, too.

"My clinical experience suggests that while the early environment has considerable influence on the manner in which sexuality is expressed, it has indiscernible influence on the sex of the love object," observes psychiatrist

Richard Isay, M.D., chairperson of the American Psychiatric Association's Committee on Gay, Lesbian and Bisexual Issues and the author of *Being Homosexual.*

"There is no evidence," Dr. Isay maintains, "to suggest that gay men can revert to heterosexual behavior without great difficulty and without becoming anxious or depressed."

Even so, many parents of homosexual children agonize over what they might have "done wrong." Although the evidence strongly suggests they should not blame themselves, they may need help and support. A good place to contact is Parents and Friends of Lesbian and Gays, a national support group. Write to Box 24565, Los Angeles, CA 90024.

In the end, all these fascinating theories may prove to be partly true and partly false. It could very well be that there are many different developmental paths that lead a person to become a homosexual, and no one theory will explain it all. What really matters is that homosexuals are people and should be treated that way.

Perhaps Freud, for once, should be given the last word in all this. In response to a letter from the mother of a homosexual son in 1935, Freud wrote back: "Homosexuality is assuredly no advantage, but it is nothing to be ashamed of, no vice, no degradation, it cannot be classified as an illness; we consider it to be a variation of the sexual development."

Hormone Replacement Therapy

Estrogen is such wonderful stuff it almost deserves to be called a wonder drug. During puberty, it orchestrates the radiant unfolding of a girl's womanhood; during adulthood, estrogens are involved in everything from promoting the suppleness of skin to touch perception, from cardiovascular health to increasing the body's readiness for sex.

That's why, when it ebbs away slowly (after menopause) or drops suddenly (after a hysterectomy in which the estrogen-producing ovaries are removed), it's often sorely missed. Declining estrogen levels often cause vaginal tissues to grow thinner, drier and itchier (a condition called atrophic vaginitis), so many older women complain that intercourse is painful. Sexual desire often begins to fade. Some older women develop stress incontinence (dribbling urine when they laugh or sneeze) because of estrogen-related changes in their genitourinary system. And of course, hot flashes, night sweats and insomnia, also related to hormonal changes, may make life even more miserable. (For more, see "Menopause.")

Hormones Can Help

Not all women have these problems after menopause, of course. But for those who do, hormone replacement therapy (HRT) may be worth considering. (It's also sometimes called estrogen replacement therapy, or ERT, but since a variety of hormones are used today, HRT is the more accurate term.) The missing hormones are replaced by means of pills, shots, vaginal creams, skin patches or a BB-sized pellet inserted under the skin.

"Ninety percent of the women who get started on a replacement therapy program and stick with it for four to six months show a pretty remarkable reversal of their symptoms," says Judith H. Seifer, Ph.D., R.N., clinical professor of psychiatry and obstetrics/gynecology at Wright State University School of Medicine in Dayton, Ohio. "In general, I'd say to women who are considering it: Give it a six-month commitment. Don't be afraid. Give it a try, and stick with it."

Some women can't take replacement hormones, even if they want to, because of preexisting health problems. These include a previous blood clot, active thrombophlebitis, which often shows up as varicose veins, and preexisting cancers or disorders of the liver or gallbladder.

But for women whose doctors consider them candidates for HRT, the potential benefits of replacement hormones are many.

- HRT "reliably relieves" hot flashes and night sweats and restores dry, itchy vaginal tissue to a much more youthful state, according to Barbara B. Sherwin, Ph.D., codirector of the McGill University Menopause Clinic at Jewish General Hospital in Montreal. Many women who complain that intercourse is painful are able to enjoy it again after they start taking hormones.
- A number of studies have shown that HRT can revive a woman's sexual desire, particularly if androgens (male hormones) like testosterone are added to the mix.
- Many women just feel better when they're taking replacement hormones. They report an improved sense of overall well-being and more energy, almost as if HRT were a kind of "mental tonic."

- One of the biggest benefits of HRT is not sexual at all: Many studies have shown that it greatly reduces a woman's risk of developing coronary artery disease. One study tracked 48,000 nurses who had gone through menopause for ten years. The women who were taking estrogen were 44 percent less likely to die of a heart attack than the women who were not taking hormones. Even women who took estrogen for only part of the decade had a 17 percent lower risk.

   Although it's not entirely clear what causes this truly amazing reduction in cardiovascular risk, it is known that estrogen raises blood levels of HDL cholesterol (the "good" kind) by 30 percent or so, while at the same time lowering LDL cholesterol (the "bad" kind) by about 20 percent.

- HRT also cuts the risk of hip fractures due to osteoporosis (brittle, porous bones) by an estimated 60 percent. This is significant because the second most common cause of death in women over 72 is complications from a fractured hip.

Considering the Risks

With all that good news, though, there has to be a downside, and there is.

- There continue to be worries about HRT's role in increasing the risk of cancer of the endometrium (lining of the uterus). Estrogen stimulates the growth of the breasts and the uterus during puberty—but exposing these tissues to a lifetime of growth-stimulating hormones may be unhealthy, some doctors believe. Today, however, estrogen is almost always prescribed in combination with progesterone, another female hormone, which appears to eliminate the additional risk. (Women who've had a hysterectomy, of course, don't have to worry about uterine cancer because they don't have a uterus.)

   Also, adds Dr. Seifer, it's important to remember that endometrial cancer is very treatable once it's discovered.

- Some studies have shown that unopposed estrogen (that is, estrogen taken without progesterone) increases breast cancer risk. But again, there's no evidence that women taking both estrogen and progesterone have an increased risk—in fact, there's some suggestion that it may even protect against breast cancer.

   "Estrogen does not cause breast cancer," explains Dr. Seifer, "but if a tumor is estrogen-responsive (and the majority of them are), taking estrogen will cause the mass to grow."

- As a practical matter, one of the biggest drawbacks of HRT is that a woman who still has her uterus will begin to menstruate again. The bleeding isn't very heavy, or crampy, but it's an inconvenience all the same—the very thing most older women were so relieved to be finally done with!

    However, in the newest form of HRT (taking only two pills, once a day, every day), the periods go away after nine months to a year.

- Among the other minor side effects of estrogen, nausea is the most common. Some women may also retain water, and the breasts may become tender. Estrogen also raises blood pressure in some women, and progesterone, despite its benefits, makes some women irritable.

What's the Verdict?

Which brings us to the tricky part. If HRT takes away hot flashes, improves genital health, makes you feel sexier, reduces your risk of heart disease and osteoporosis—while at the same time slightly increasing your risk of uterine cancer—should you use it? What it comes down to is a weighing of risks against benefits—a complex analysis that only you and your doctor can make.

If you do opt for HRT, you have a number of decisions to make.

There are probably as many forms of HRT as there are doctors to prescribe them, but one of the most common forms in use today is a combination of estrogen and progesterone. Typically, this cyclic HRT regimen involves taking estrogen in monthly cycles—25 days of estrogen, plus 7 to 10 days of progesterone during the final days of the estrogen, followed by 5 or 6 days of taking no hormones at all. That's a whole lot to remember, of course (and one of the main reasons women drop out of HRT programs). Newer forms of HRT currently under development— already being prescribed by some doctors, in fact—involve taking just two pills, once a day, every day, and that's that.

The Role of Androgens: Still a Puzzle

In recent years, an increasing number of doctors have been prescribing an HRT regimen that combines some form of estrogen with androgens, or male hormones (usually testosterone). Why would a woman want to take a man's hormones? Well, *male hormone* is a misnomer, actually, because small amounts of testosterone are produced in a woman's ovaries and adrenal glands. It's testosterone, researchers now believe, that inflames the libido in both women and men.

In one study, postmenopausal women who complained that they had little or no interest in sex, even when they were already taking estrogen, were given a testosterone/estrogen combination. Within three months, most reported a startling increase in their interest in sex, their enjoyment of sex play and the frequency with which they initiated sex with their husbands or lovers. Other studies have shown it also gives women a better sense of general well-being and gives them more energy than estrogen alone.

If you're interested in learning more about the libido-boosting potential of androgens, this is another option to discuss with your doctor.

Once you start on any HRT program, it's important to see a doctor regularly. Physicians recommend that women taking hormones see their doctor once a year, at a minimum, and get an annual Pap test, mammogram and blood work to check lipid levels. Many doctors give prescriptions for only 12 once-a-month refills, to gently encourage compliance, and it's a good idea to take the hint.

HYSTERECTOMY

Not so very long ago, most doctors believed that women who said sex just wasn't as enjoyable after their hysterectomy were simply imagining things. "Where there are changes in libido or sexual satisfaction following hysterectomy, the cause of these changes is undoubtedly psychogenic," concluded one study that was quoted for years after it first appeared in the *American Journal of Obstetrics and Gynecology.* In other words, "it's all in their heads."

But times have changed.

"We just don't know in any authoritative way what percentage of women experience some change in their sexual responsiveness after a hysterectomy — but some women certainly do," says sex therapist Shirley Zussman, Ed.D., a director of the Association for Male Sexual Dysfunction in New York City and former president of the American Association of Sex Educators, Counselors and Therapists. And many of those changes have to do with the physical or hormonal effects of the operation.

One study of about 1,400 women who had undergone hysterectomies, conducted by the Centers for Disease Control in Atlanta, found that more than half these women reported no change in sexual desire after the operation, 9 percent reported a decrease in desire, and 9 percent said their sex drive and enjoyment actually *increased* afterward. On the other hand, a series of studies in Great Britain found that between 33 and 46 percent of women reported they enjoyed sex less, just weren't as interested in it or had more trouble reaching orgasm after having a hysterectomy.

It's hard to know quite what to make of all this. And, doctors say, it's almost impossible to predict how any given woman will respond to the operation. But in general, it shouldn't be surprising that some women experience sexual aftereffects. After all, a hysterectomy is the surgical removal of the uterus and other attendant parts of a woman's reproductive system—and sex and reproduction are not entirely unrelated (although until fairly recently many doctors believed that the uterus and cervix had nothing at all to do with sexual pleasure).

Just to clarify: The most common version of the operation, a *total hysterectomy,* means the surgical removal of both uterus and cervix. Another common procedure, a hysterectomy with *bilateral salpingo-oophorectomy,* means the ovaries and fallopian tubes are also removed. A *radical hysterectomy,* the most extensive operation of all (usually performed for invasive cervical cancer), means the removal of, in addition to these organs, the upper third of the vagina and the lymph nodes. These organs are removed either through an incision in the abdominal wall, which leaves a scar and requires a longer recovery, or through the vagina, which leaves no scar, causes fewer complications and is likely to result in a faster recovery. (For a number of medical reasons, not all hysterectomies can be done through the vagina.)

Sexual Side Effects

Although the surgery is sometimes performed because of life-threatening problems like uterine or ovarian cancer, more often it's done as an elective procedure meant to improve the quality of a woman's life. It may help relieve pelvic pain or reduce heavy menstrual bleeding, for example.

Getting rid of pain and bleeding can be a real boon to a woman's sex life. But other times, the side effects are not quite so positive. If a woman is going to experience some postsurgical sexual problems, Dr. Zussman says, these are the likeliest ones.

Loss of the "deep orgasm." Most women reach orgasm through stimulation of the clitoris, that tiny, shallowly buried tongue of flesh over the entrance to the vagina. But it's been known for many years that some women experience orgasm through some other, deeper mechanism. For them, deep penetration of the penis, to the point where it makes direct contact with the cervix, touches off the flood of orgiastic ecstasy. This is not a vaginal orgasm, because the vaginal walls have little feeling; it appears to involve rhythmic contractions of the uterus and the muscles of the pelvic floor.

For women who experience orgasm this way, the loss of the cervix and the uterus may be acutely felt. One woman wrote to the surgeon who'd performed her hysterectomy: "The greatest change since surgery is this. Before, each time the penis was pushed hard against the cervix, I would feel intense excitement deep inside me, huge waves of pleasure. . . . This was by far the most exciting part of sex, the real climax. I've tried to be satisfied with the orgasms I get from stimulation of the clitoris. . . . Maybe I'll get used to it in time, but it isn't nearly as good, and I feel very sad."

For women who feel that they experience orgasm in this way, Dr. Zussman says, it's quite likely a hysterectomy *will* negatively affect their sexual pleasure. Few doctors quite know how to tell women this, she says. Instead, they simply say that the operation is unlikely to have any sexual aftereffects at all.

Some women agree to the operation on the basis that it will not have an impact on their sex lives. "I think this is inaccurate informed consent," Dr. Zussman says. Possible loss of sexual pleasure is no reason to avoid hysterectomy for cervical cancer or some other serious disorder, she says, "but in borderline cases, it might be one reason a woman would turn to alternative treatments, and certainly a reason to seek a second opinion."

If your main complaint is heavy menstrual bleeding, you may be a candidate for a relatively new alternative to hysterectomy called *endometrial ablation.* In this procedure, instead of removing the uterus, the uterine lining (endometrium) is burned away by lasers or cauterization. Ablation is quicker, cheaper and less likely to produce unpleasant aftereffects than a hysterectomy — although its sexual side effects have so far not been carefully studied, according to Stephen Corson, M.D., clinical professor of obstetrics and gynecology at the University of Pennsylvania School of Medicine. Eight or nine out of every ten women who have endometrial ablation don't need to have a hysterectomy later. One unexpected bonus: Ablation often greatly reduces the symptoms of premenstrual syndrome. "The reason for this befuddles me and everyone else," he says.

Hormonal changes. Women who have their ovaries removed may experience sexual changes caused by a decline in hormone levels. The ovaries produce not only estrogen and progesterone, the two main female hormones, but also androgens (male hormones), which fuel sex drive. Typically, these women complain about a loss of vaginal lubrication during arousal and a shrinking and drying-out of the vaginal tissues. Some women also complain that they don't feel aroused as often and may have trouble reaching orgasm. Advances in hormone replacement therapy have gone a long way toward soothing these problems, though. (See "Hormone Replacement Therapy.")

Psychological troubles. "For most women, there's a very definite psychological reaction to the loss of the uterus, because it represents being young and feminine and desirable—even though the reproductive years may be over," Dr. Zussman observes. "This may seem a little strange, since the uterus is something that exists only in perception; it's never actually *seen,* like the breasts. But somehow it's central to many women's sense of their own womanhood."

Grief over this loss may lead to depression, which can smother a woman's interest in sex, she says.

Speeding Your Sexual Recovery

Returning to sexual self-confidence after a hysterectomy really begins *before* the operation. First, seek a second opinion to make sure the operation is necessary. It's been convincingly argued that many hysterectomies are unnecessary—some doctors say the figure may be as high as 90 percent—so it's important to make sure that yours *is* necessary. Also, if a woman has lingering doubts over whether her surgery was necessary at all, her psychological recovery is likely to be more difficult, Dr. Zussman says. But if she's convinced the operation was needed, her recovery is much less likely to be complicated by rage, anger, self-doubt or depression.

Second, inform yourself. One study in New Zealand showed that when women were given an informative booklet before the operation, so that they understood exactly what was to be done and how it would affect their sex lives, it helped immensely. In this study, 52 percent of the women said there was no change in their sex lives after the surgery—and 42 percent said their love lives actually improved.

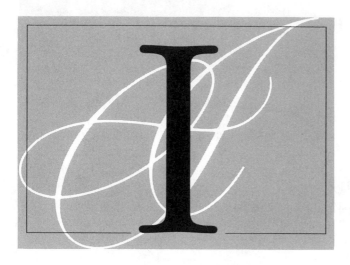

ILLEGAL DRUGS

Cocaine, marijuana and a handful of other illegal drugs have the reputation for being love potions. Sigmund Freud, an early cocaine user, considered the drug an aphrodisiac, and sexual stimulation is one of the side effects listed by pharmaceutical companies who manufacture cocaine products for use as topical anesthetics. Pot smokers have made all sorts of claims about marijuana's ability to enhance orgasm, delay ejaculation or heighten sexual sensation.

The trouble, of course, is that these drugs are expensive, often habit forming and illegal. And when it comes to sex, they have Jekyll-and-Hyde personalities. In the beginning, in small amounts (at least for some people), they often do live up to their reputation as love drugs. But with chronic use, the sexual side effects flip completely. Heavy users have trouble performing sexually and often lose all interest in sex. Eventually, "nearly all chronic high–dose cocaine users become sexually dysfunctional," notes Arnold M. Washton, Ph.D., executive director of the Washton Institute on Addictions in New York City. And marijuana, although not as castrating as cocaine, is not quite the benign party toy it's often thought to be, either.

Cocaine: Empty Glitter

"Cocaine affects the brain in many complicated ways, but one thing it does is to stimulate brain dopamine, a neurotransmitter that acts as a kind of natural aphrodisiac," explains James A. Cocores, M.D., medical director of Outpatient Recovery Centers at Fair Oaks Hospital in Summit, New Jersey. Excited by cocaine, the brain dumps massive quantities of dopamine into the system, evoking a sense of glittery euphoria and sexual desire. The first time they use it, most people (although not all) report that it enhances both their erotic desire and their sexual performance. Some users who inject cocaine have described multiple orgasms, prolonged endurance and even spontaneous orgasm, according to some reports. And smoking freebase cocaine, or crack, "greatly exaggerates all these effects," Dr. Washton says, because higher doses are delivered to the brain when they travel through the lungs rather than the nasal passages.

But the body quickly tires of all that frenetic, artificial stimulation. A condition called *dopamine deficiency* develops, in which dopamine is burned up so rapidly that the body doesn't have time to manufacture any more. And when the supply is depleted, all its sex-enhancing properties turn into their opposite. Usually the first thing to go, Dr. Cocores says, is performance—men start having trouble getting an erection, and women can't seem to lubricate properly or can't reach orgasm. Eventually, desire itself begins to fade away.

Cocaine affects the body in another way, too: By touching off a rush of adrenaline, it kicks the heart into overdrive (tachycardia, or rapid heartbeat) at the same time it boosts blood pressure. And when you add sexual excitement (or exercise) to the burden on an already excited heart, the result can be dangerous, perhaps even deadly.

Says Dr. Cocores: "Sex and cocaine are not a healthy combination."

The good news: Cocaine-induced sexual dysfunction usually goes away after two or three weeks of complete abstinence from the drug.

More bad news: Cocaine has been linked to neurological abnormalities in babies born to users. The mechanism by which this damage is done has never been quite clear, but one recent study by researchers at Washington University School of Medicine in St. Louis suggests a novel answer: Coke sticks to sperm cells like a sort of toxic glue, without affecting the sperm's speed of travel or its ability to penetrate an egg. When a sperm cell *does* fertilize an oocyte (immature egg), it carries with it a potentially dangerous dose of drug, like a terrorist carrying a suitcase bomb onto an airliner.

These studies were conducted *in vitro* (by mixing sperm and coke together in a lab dish); it's not even known for sure whether cocaine is present in the semen of users. However, a wealth of other evidence suggests that it is. Also, the researchers suggest, it's not only the father who needs to be concerned about his coke use around the time of conception. "It is also possible that the spermatozoa bind to cocaine if it is present in the reproductive tract of the female," they observe. Either way, the image of a human life tainted with poison from the very moment of conception is almost inexpressibly sad.

Pot as "Mood Amplifier"

While the sexual side effects of cocaine are fairly consistent, the reported effects of marijuana are all over the map. Some people claim it helps men last longer or enhances the enjoyment of orgasm; others say it has no effect at all or that it only works sometimes. In one survey of 251 college students, about half said it increased their sexual desire and enjoyment. But others disagree.

There are a couple of reasons for these seeming contradictions. For one thing, *marijuana* is a vague term—there are over 90 varieties of THC (tetrahydro-cannabinol, the active ingredient in pot), and they may all have slightly different sexual side effects. Some cannabinoids may inhibit sex, others may enhance it—nobody really knows (only one variety of THC, the delta-9 type, has been well studied). For another, pot's effect on sex may be hard to predict because it simply "amplifies" a person's preexisting state of mind. If you're already feeling sexy, it will probably make you feel sexier—but if you're feeling silly, it will just make you feel sillier.

The most consistently reported effect is an enhanced sense of touch, which may partly account for pot's alleged erotic powers. Marijuana also tends to give the illusion that time is passing more slowly, which could be why some people report more enjoyable orgasms.

Pot's Effect on Fertility

But it's wrong to conclude from all this that pot is a harmless sexual aid. Cannabis contains some of the same tars that are in tobacco smoke, including the potent carcinogen benzopyrene, so regular use may increase your risk of lung cancer. It can also disrupt hormonal balances and interfere with fertility in both men and women.

Although occasional marijuana use doesn't seem to affect a man's fertility, prolonged use can reduce testosterone levels, suppressing sperm production and sex drive. One study showed that young men who smoked pot at least four days a week for six months had lower testosterone levels, and 35 percent had lower sperm counts, and 10 percent were completely impotent, according New York

City pharmacist M. Laurence Lieberman, author of *The Sexual Pharmacy: The Complete Guide to Drugs with Side Effects.* Other studies have shown that young men who are chronic pot smokers are more likely to have malformed sperm cells than nonsmokers. In women, pot seems to interfere with fertility by inhibiting ovulation.

"The safest advice for the couple contemplating pregnancy is for the husband to refrain from marijuana use," says Ernest L. Abel, Ph.D., professor of obstetrics at Wayne State University in Detroit. (Don't forget that it takes a man's body about 70 days to produce a mature sperm cell, so if the two of you are trying to get pregnant, you'd better knock it off a couple of months before you start trying.)

INTERCOURSE

In her massive study of female sexuality, *The Hite Report,* author Shere Hite discovered something that should probably come as no great surprise to most women: Sexual intercourse is actually a fairly clumsy and ineffective way for a woman to reach orgasm. By some enigma of nature, the clitoris is tucked away in such an odd, aloof location that it's often not stimulated directly enough (or long enough) during intercourse to take a woman "over the top." And man-on-top, missionary-position intercourse is probably the least effective method of all.

In fact, many sex therapists contend that couples tend to greatly overemphasize intercourse—as if every sweet ritual of love were just an insignificant prelude to The Main Event. As if intercourse were the only thing that qualifies as "real sex." There are many more effective ways to send a woman (briefly) to heaven than intercourse—at least intercourse as it's ordinarily practiced.

But surely none of us is about to give up on intercourse, no matter what sex therapists have to say about it. Perhaps the most satisfying solution is simply to take another look at it and learn how to do it more sweetly (and effectively).

Three Rules of Lovemaking

A multitude of problems could be avoided if we all followed three simple rules for intercourse, says Jude Cotter, Ph.D., a psychologist and sex therapist in private practice in Farmington Hills, Michigan.

1. Women first. The woman should be allowed to reach orgasm *before* the man. She may get there through whatever arousal patterns she needs—by stimulating her clitoris with a finger (his, hers or both), through oral sex, with a vibrator or whatever. But she should always be allowed to get there first. This is not mere chivalry; it's physiology.

"When the guy is done, he's done—it's all over," Dr. Cotter explains simply.

After orgasm and ejaculation, men's bodies need a period of recovery before they can repeat the performance, and the older the man is, the longer it takes. A teenager may need a minute; a 50-year-old requires hours. Women, on the other hand, require no such recovery time; many can reach orgasm repeatedly without ever needing a rest.

"Also, if a guy is having erectile problems, he obsesses; he worries; he gets performance anxiety," Dr. Cotter says. "But very few things can give a man confidence like seeing her come. If she comes first, that takes away 90 percent of his fears."

2. She decides when it's time for penetration, not him. The woman should determine when penetration will take place—whether she assumes the on-top position or he does.

"You ask a guy how he knows that a woman is ready for penetration, and he says, 'She's wet, or her nipples are erect,' " Dr. Cotter says. "But a woman can lubricate before she even undresses, and sometimes her nipples are erect because she's freezing. Other women *never* get erect nipples. The fact is, the only one who knows for sure that she's ready is *her.*"

That's why the woman, not the man, should be the one to direct the proceedings, he explains. Male sexual response, Dr. Cotter is fond of saying, is like a light bulb: You turn it on, and it's hot almost instantaneously; turn it off, and it's cold in a matter of seconds. A woman's response cycle is more like an iron: You turn it on, and then you wait and wait and wait until it heats up; and after you turn it off, you wait and wait and wait until it cools.

"If you superimpose these two sexual curves on each other, about 80 percent of the female response cycle is left out," he explains. But by allowing the woman to take the lead, she's more likely to be able to satisfy herself—and also to satisfy him.

3. It should always be the woman who guides her partner's penis in. The woman should control how rapidly things proceed to climax. Allowing her to guide him in is just another way to make sure this happens. Also, even if he is not fully erect by the time she is ready, she can use his penis as a dildo, rubbing and stroking it against herself so that he is almost bound to have an erection before too long and then is able to penetrate her.

In general, Dr. Cotter explains, these rules acknowledge something most people don't realize: It's the man, not the woman, who is more sexually fragile. As William Masters, M.D., codirector of the Masters and Johnson Institute in St. Louis, once remarked, "The female has an infinitely greater capacity for sexual response than a man ever dreamed of." It is he, not she, who is more likely to have trouble fulfilling his side of the sexual bargain. And as a man ages, getting an erection becomes increasingly difficult (almost all men, no matter what their age, have trouble getting an erection at least sometimes). And as a couple ages together, it's much more likely that their sex life will decline—not because of her, but because of him.

"When a couple practices these simple rules for intercourse, though, it wipes out almost all those sexual problems," Dr. Cotter contends.

INTRAUTERINE DEVICE (IUD)

The Dalkon Shield gave all other IUDs a bad rap. True, there's no way to go back into history and erase the horrors of that particular device, which looked as cute and fanciful as a little plastic fish but turned out to be deadly. Although it was at one time the biggest-selling IUD in the world, the Dalkon Shield resulted in 33 deaths and thousands of miscarriages in the United States alone. Its manufacturer was ultimately driven into bankruptcy under the weight of more than 14,000 lawsuits.

But that celebrated tragedy overshadows something much less sensational, but much more comforting, about IUDs: Except for the Dalkon Shield, they're considered quite safe and very effective. In fact, both the World Health Organization and the American Medical Association consider IUDs to be one of the safest and most effective birth control methods currently available.

How Do They Work?

The IUD is a little contraption made of plastic (and sometimes copper as well), usually shaped like a T, that's inserted by a doctor all the way up inside the uterus. A string attached to the device trails through the cervix and about 2 inches into the vagina, where it can be used to check the IUD's placement and withdraw it when the time comes. And that, pretty much, is that. When a woman wants to make love, she doesn't have to remember to do anything—which is one reason IUDs are so effective.

"Although modern IUDs have been used and studied for two decades, the precise combination of mechanisms by which they prevent pregnancy remains unclear," one research team recently concluded. Suffice it to say that in a variety of complicated ways, they make it more difficult for the egg to be fertilized, or interfere with the movement of egg or sperm, or alter the lining of the uterus in a way that makes pregnancy less likely. In any event, they work.

"Of all the nonpermanent birth control methods available to women, including the Pill, the IUD has the highest efficacy at preventing unwanted pregnancies," says Ronald T. Burkman, M.D., chairman of the Department of Obstetrics and Gynecology at Henry Ford Hospital in Detroit. Out of 100 women using copper-containing IUDs (the most effective kind), about 2 will get pregnant during the first year, compared with 3 or 4 women using the Pill, Dr. Burkman says. (Other estimates put failure rates for the IUD and the Pill at just about the same level—roughly 3 pregnancies per 100 women during the first year, given typical patterns of use.)

Only Two Types Left

One of the unpleasant legacies of the IUD scares of the 1970s and 1980s is that, as of 1991, there are only two types of IUDs available in the United States. Many others, even those widely believed to be safe, were withdrawn by manufacturers who feared a feeding frenzy of lawyers.

The Progestasert. Made by Alza Corporation, this IUD is a plastic device shaped like a T, which slowly releases the female hormone progesterone. Among other things, progesterone increases the thickness of cervical mucus, making it more difficult for sperm to penetrate the cervix. This device must be removed every year and replaced with a new one. But, according to some doctors, this is a hidden benefit—women who use them are forced to have a yearly checkup and Pap test.

The ParaGard, or Copper T 380A. Made by GynoPharma, this type is sometimes called "the 380" and is also a T-shaped device made of plastic, with copper sleeves attached. (It's not fully understood why copper increases an IUD's effectiveness, but it does—IUDs with copper are roughly twice as effective as those without.) Researchers report that the ParaGard has the lowest failure rate of any

IUD so far developed and can be left in place for four years. This is a special advantage in a different way, because most infections occur during the first month or so after the IUD is inserted. Doctors maintain that leaving it in place for four years means that overall, the risk of infection is decreased.

Boosting Effectiveness

Planned Parenthood suggests that you can increase the effectiveness of your IUD if you remember to do two things.

Regularly check the IUD string. If it feels longer or shorter than it was after it was first inserted, it may be that the IUD has shifted position and needs to be moved back into place. Check with your doctor—and use some other kind of birth control in the meantime.

During times when you are most fertile, double your protection by also using condoms or spermicidal foam. For women whose cycle averages 28 to 32 days in length, the most fertile period can be approximated as cycle days 11 to 20.

Also, don't hesitate to contact your doctor if you have severe cramps or abdominal pain, pain or bleeding during sex, fever, chills or an odorous vaginal discharge. These are all signs that something's gone wrong. And if you miss a period and think you're pregnant, see a doctor immediately—because if you are, the IUD needs to be removed. Allowing a pregnancy to continue with an IUD in place can result in serious, perhaps fatal, infection. (About half these pregnancies will result in spontaneous abortion.)

The Best Candidates—and the Worst

The best candidate for an IUD, says Dr. Burkman, is a woman who has already had a child, is in a "mutually monogamous relationship," needs a highly effective form of birth control and has no history of pelvic inflammatory disease, or PID (a general term meaning infections that invade the reproductive system).

Anna is typical of such women. She is now 35, is happily married, has a sparkling 2-year-old and thinks she may want another someday (but not yet!). Her gynecologist suggested an IUD after she had problems (migraines, weight gain) while taking the Pill and could no longer use a diaphragm after her first pregnancy. Says Anna: "Speaking as a woman with no other birth control options, I think the IUD is terrific! It's completely spontaneous—you don't have to take a pill or put anything on every time—and there's no discomfort. Also, there's just one major expense, when it's inserted, and that's it for the next four years."

On the other hand, IUDs are most likely *not* a good choice for women who have multiple sex partners or who have not had children. That's because women with multiple partners who use IUDs are more likely to develop PID, which can result in infertility. (More on this later.)

Other Drawbacks

Like every other form of birth control, IUDs come equipped with drawbacks and risks. Just remember this, though: Overall, IUD use poses less of a risk to a woman's health than getting pregnant, according to Planned Parenthood.

Possible drawbacks include:

Bleeding. It's common for women to have heavier periods that last longer while using an IUD. Also, many women spot a little between periods, especially during the first few months. Disturbances in bleeding are the most common reason women quit using their IUD.

Pain. This is the second most common reason women quit using their IUD. It's not uncommon for the IUD to cause pain during insertion and for a few days afterward, but if it persists, don't hesitate to have it checked by your doctor. Pain could mean the uterine wall has been perforated, that you've gotten an infection or that the IUD has slipped out of place.

Explusion. Quite a few women—up to one in four, according to some estimates—can't retain the IUD in their uterus, and it pops out or slips out of position. This is more common among women who've never been pregnant. It usually happens in the first few months after insertion or during menstruation. It's estimated that up to 20 percent of the time the expulsion goes undetected and the woman runs the risk of pregnancy without knowing it. Many doctors recommend that women who use an IUD have checkups at least once a year, just to make sure everything's in place. Also, during her period, a woman should check her tampons to see if the IUD has fallen out.

More Serious Risks

All those problems are fairly minor. There are a few others, though, that are much rarer but more serious.

Perforation of the uterine wall. Sometimes the IUD breaks through the wall of the uterus—usually when the doctor is inserting it. Every year, about 40 out of every 100,000 IUD users are hospitalized because of this or because the device migrated into the peritoneal cavity (an abdominal space outside the uterus). If this happens, surgery may be required to remove it.

Pelvic inflammatory disease. One of the biggest worries about IUD use is the increased risk of developing pelvic infections that ascend through the uterus into the rest of the reproductive system, where they may result in infertility. The key thing, a variety of studies have shown, is not so much that IUDs increase the risk of these infections *by themselves*. It's that when a woman using an IUD picks up a sexually transmitted disease, it's more likely to invade her deeper reproductive system than if she weren't using an IUD. Some researchers believe that the mechanism of increased risk is the string that's attached to the IUD and protrudes from the cervix, which may provide microorganisms with a royal road into the uterus. Whatever the reason, though, women with more than one current sex partner shouldn't use an IUD, because they are at higher risk of picking up sexually transmitted diseases.

On the other hand, if you're a monogamous homebody, and so is your partner, IUDs don't seem to raise the risk of infection or infertility. Says Dr. Burkman: "It's sometimes said that the risk of infertility is increased with IUD use, but if you look at the monogamous married couples who use IUDs, this risk disappears."

It's important to remember something else, too: Unlike barrier contraceptives such as condoms or a diaphragm, IUDs don't offer any protection against sexually transmitted diseases. Which is one more reason why women with more than one partner should probably find some other form of birth control.

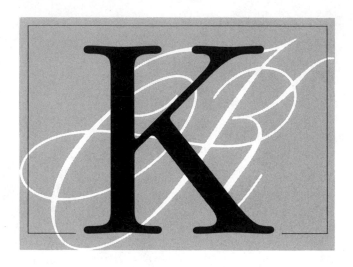

KEGEL EXERCISES

Sexual intercourse is not an athletic event. Still, making love *does* involve muscles, and muscles that are trim and taut are usually more responsive than ones that are flabby. That's the basic theory behind the Kegel exercise, a way of strengthening certain key muscles called the pubococcygeus (PEW–bo–kak–se–GEE–us) muscles, or PC for short. Many therapists believe that pumping up the PC muscles can help enhance sexual pleasure by strengthening orgasm and increasing your awareness of sexual sensations—whether you're a man or a woman. For women, Kegels have the additional benefits of helping to restore muscle tone after childbirth and preventing or correcting weak pelvic muscle support.

The exercises were developed by gynecologist Arnold Kegel, M.D., who, during the 1950s, began recommending them to women who had problems with stress incontinence (involuntary spillage of urine during orgasm or when coughing, sneezing or laughing). Many of these women later reported that not only were they better able to retain urine, they also got more enjoyment out of sex. This shouldn't be too surprising: The PC muscles, which are slung between your legs to provide a sort of floor for the pelvis, are the muscles you use to shut off the flow of urine, and they also produce deep, pleasurable contractions during orgasm.

Find It, Then Flex It

Women can find their PC muscles by sitting on a toilet, spreading their legs a little and then trying to start and stop the flow of urine without moving their legs. The muscles you squeeze to shut off the flow are the ones you're after. Men can find their PC muscles the same way (they just don't have to sit down) or by squeezing their buttocks as if trying to withhold an imaginary bowel movement. Try not to contract your stomach or thighs at the same time; keep the contractions focused on those key deep muscles.

There are quite a few variations on the basic Kegel exercise, but the beauty of all of them is that they can be done almost anywhere—while waiting in line, stopped at a red light or waiting for the aperitif to be served. Just don't tell anybody what you're doing.

One program recommended by the Arlington Center for Marital and Sexual Concerns in Columbus, Ohio, includes both fast and slow Kegels. To do a slow Kegel, just squeeze your PC muscles, hold for a slow count of five, then release. Relax for 5 seconds, then repeat. A quick Kegel simply means tightening and relaxing the PC muscles as rapidly as you can, five times.

At first, during slow Kegels, you may notice that it's hard to keep the PC muscles squeezed tight for the full 5 seconds. And your fast Kegels may not be very fast or very regular. But stick with it, and your muscular control should improve within a week or so. Pay attention during love play, too, and see if you notice a difference.

Pull In, Push Out

Women can try another variation called the "pull in, push out" Kegel. First, imagine that you are trying to suck in water through your vagina, pulling up your entire pelvic floor in the process. Then reverse the process, bearing down as if you are expelling all that imaginary water. That's it.

The Arlington Center recommends that you try repeating each of these exercises three times, three times a day, and from there work your way up to 50 to 100 repetitions a day. If that's not realistic, try doing them as often as you think of it for a month or so, and see if you notice any change in your sexual responsiveness. Women can actually check for improvement by inserting two lubricated fingers into the vagina and squeezing. If you notice more pressure on your fingers than you did before you started the exercises, you can start calling your PC muscles Arnold.

KINSEY

Alfred C. Kinsey, D.Sc., was a bony-faced zoology professor at Indiana University who in 1938 was asked to teach a course on marriage to students. To his astonishment, he discovered that many of their questions about sex simply couldn't be answered. At that time, there were only 19 studies of human sexual behavior in the entire scientific literature, most of them small and poorly designed. There were plenty of moral injunctions about sex, and lots of theories, but very little actual data. As Dr. Kinsey was later fond of remarking, in 1938 more was known about the sexual behavior of farm animals than of humans.

To rectify the situation, he set out on what was to become one of the greatest scientific adventures of modern times: an attempt to gather, in carefully structured, face-to-face interviews, the complete sexual histories of 100,000 people, men and women, young and old, heterosexual and homosexual, educated and uneducated, of all social classes, from towns, cities and farms across the United States. It was the first time anyone had attempted to exhaustively catalog, and then statistically analyze, the great and mysterious variety of human sexual experience, and to do so (as far as possible) without making moral judgments. Dr. Kinsey set out not to describe what people ought to do, or think they ought to do, but what people actually *do*.

The findings of Dr. Kinsey and his colleagues formed the basis of two books, *Sexual Behavior in the Human Male,* published in 1948, and *Sexual Behavior in the Human Female,* which appeared in 1953.

"A Violent Storm"

The publication of these books, Dr. Kinsey's longtime collaborator Wardell B. Pomeroy later recalled in a memoir, "raised one of the most violent and widespread storms since Darwin." The findings of the Kinsey Reports, as they came to be known, showed that men and women were far more sexually active than almost anyone had previously believed, that sexual behavior (even what might be called perverse or "abnormal" sexual behavior) was far more varied and widespread than anybody thought and that even children had sexual lives. He reported, for instance, that 85 percent of men had had intercourse before marriage, that 30 to 45 percent of husbands had been unfaithful to their wives, that 62 percent of women had tried masturbation and that 37 percent of men had had at least one homosexual experience to orgasm as an adult.

Many of his findings seemed to fly in the face of every accepted sexual convention. *Life* magazine called Dr. Kinsey's findings "an assault on the family as a basic unit of society, a negation of moral law and a celebration of licentiousness." Newspapers denounced the books in editorial pages and refused to cover them on the news pages. Church leaders railed that the books were amoral, immoral, even communist. Dr. Kinsey's supporters, by contrast, claimed he had "done for sex what Columbus did for geography."

Today, the shortcomings of Dr. Kinsey's work are widely acknowledged. They do not present a picture of the whole range of human sexuality but are disproportionately skewed to the behavior of white, middle-class midwesterners and college students. Some critics have charged that too many of his interview subjects were prisoners or sex offenders, hardly stellar examples of "normal" sexuality. And because the people he interviewed were all volunteers (who may well have been more interested than most people in discussing their sex lives), his samples weren't really representative of the population as a whole.

Perhaps the most serious charge leveled against Dr. Kinsey, one that is still occasionally heard today, is that he was actually promoting some "hidden agenda" of sexual libertinism and secretly meant to drop a bomb (cleverly disguised as 1,646 pages of graphs, charts and scientific data) that would touch off a sexual revolution.

There's no doubt that the publication of his findings *was* followed by a sexual revolution—many of whose leaders acknowledged their indebtedness to Dr. Kinsey. *Esquire* magazine dubbed him the Patron Saint of Sex, and sexologist Morton Hunt referred to him as "the giant on whose shoulders all sex researchers since his time have stood." He *did* forever alter our ideas about human sexuality, at least partly by redefining our notions of what is sexually "normal." He *did*, in effect, change the world.

Sickly, Shy, Scholarly

But the picture of Dr. Kinsey as a wild sexual libertine, a screaming propagandist for the "if it feels good, do it" generation, bears little resemblance to the man himself. As a young man, he was intense, scholarly, sickly and shy—the quintessential nerd. Raised in a strict, religious household, he never had a single date with a girl throughout high school or during his undergraduate years at college. He was about as far from being "sexually liberated" as you can get—in fact, he married the first girl he ever dated.

Actually, for much of his early life he was far more interested in his greatest love—the gall wasp—than he was in girls. As a graduate student at Harvard, and later as a young assistant professor at Indiana, Dr. Kinsey became so obsessed with collecting specimens of this obscure insect that eventually his collection numbered more than four *million* specimens, many of them painstakingly measured and cataloged. When he later gave it to the American Museum of Natural History in New York, it was the largest collection of its kind ever given to the museum. As Pomeroy later observed, Dr. Kinsey was by nature "a *collector,* and perhaps the most unusual one this nation of collectors has ever seen." He collected wasps, irises, classical recordings, recipes for rum drinks—and, of course, stories about the most intimate experiences of human life.

Dr. Kinsey's Legacy

As a collector, he did his job well. Even today, more than 40 years after the first Kinsey Report was published, his work remains probably the most frequently cited body of data in the literature of sex research. He failed to reach his grandiose goal of interviewing 100,000 people (only about 18,000 interviews were completed at the time of his death), but he succeeded in compiling more sexual information—by far—than anybody before or since. In retrospect, some of his numbers have proven too high, others too low. But by providing a foundation of knowledge on which others could build, he paved the way for later researchers and the new science of sex therapy, pioneered by William Masters, M.D., and Virginia Johnson, of the Masters and Johnson Institute in St. Louis, and others.

For the rest of us, his work remains valuable simply because it helped unveil the sexual truth about ourselves—whether we liked it or not.

KISSING

Kissing is a kind of touch that has as much range as a big-city orchestra. It can be a perfunctory peck on the cheek, so asexual that balding Communist party apparatchiks aren't ashamed to do it on TV, or it can be so explosively erotic it's about as close to intercourse as you can get. French kissing (what's sometimes called "soul kissing"), in which one's tongue deeply penetrates a lover's mouth, is an almost perfect mimic of intercourse itself. In fact, the late Dr. Alfred Kinsey reported, a few women become so aroused by French kissing that they're able to climax without any genital stimulation at all.

The lips, the tongue and all the wet caverns of the mouth are richly supplied with nerve endings, making them exquisitely sensitive to the touch. (Because they're nearly as sensitive as the genitals, in fact, it's no wonder that mouths and genitals, the two most inflammatory hot spots of the body, often wind up in direct contact during sex.)

The erotic potential of the lips and tongue has not been lost on the animals. Most mammals, even some fish, birds and lizards, will dally in oral sex play for long periods of time—hours, sometimes—before actual intercourse takes place. They make sensuous contact with their lips and tongues ("kissing," you might say), they lick each other all over, they nuzzle, they nibble, they bite. In fact, humans who (for whatever reason) *don't* kiss or lick each other during sex are the exception among all the mammals.

Lots of people prefer to make love face-to-face, so they can kiss. Some people like to kiss intermittently, others almost continuously, on the lips, on the face or all over.

According to the sixteenth-century Tunisian love manual *The Perfumed Garden,* the only sort of kiss that's really appropriate during intercourse is the French kiss. But the sixteenth century was a long time ago, so feel free to write an amorous new chapter of your own.

Scandalous Smooches

Kissing is not quite the "universal language of love," as is sometimes (rather sappily) said. There are a few societies where kissing is completely unknown, and others where it's considered disgusting and unsanitary (such as among South Africa's Thonga people).

In many other parts of the world, kissing in public is not considered quite so innocuous as it is here. In the United States, the sight of a young couple smooching in public evokes a dreamy smile from most passersby, but in parts of Asia, India and some Arab countries, it is considered scandalous or is expressly forbidden by law. (That's known as "oral chastity" in China.) In fact, as recently as 1978, a Hindi motion picture called (in English) *Love Sublime,* which depicted several rather chaste kisses between a man and his wife, touched off a national scandal in India, followed by a national debate over censorship.

What does it all mean? Perhaps only that the sexual nature of kissing is not lost on anybody. Kissing, the ancient Chinese felt, belongs in the intimate, erotic world of the Jade Chamber (sexual relations), so that kissing in public was felt to be almost like having sex in public.

The Kiss of Death

Unfortunately, these days something else must also be mentioned about kissing. Although the AIDS virus exists in highest concentration in blood and semen, it's also been found (in much lower concentrations) in saliva. Dry kissing, or kissing on the cheek, is not considered dangerous. But most public health officials, including the U.S. Surgeon General, now warn that wet kissing, when the lips, gums or other mouth tissues are raw or broken, could potentially transmit the AIDS virus. For people who test HIV positive (that is, positive for the human immunodeficiency virus, which causes AIDS), and for everybody else who has reason to be unsure about a partner, deep French kissing is not a good idea. Kissing on the genitals can also be risky for both men and women, due to the virus's presence in semen and vaginal fluids. (See "Safer Sex.")

Again: The chances of getting AIDS from deep kissing are quite remote—studies have shown that people who live in the same house with HIV carriers, sharing the same kitchen utensils, don't get AIDS unless they also do risky sexual acts with them. But even if the risk if slight, it's unwise to take any chances.

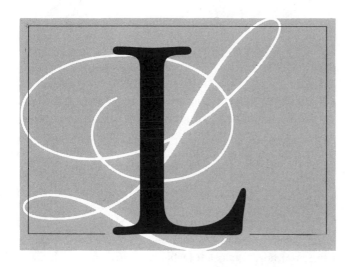

LESBIANISM.

See Homosexuality

LUBRICANTS

Here's the most important thing to remember about sexual lubricants: Never use an oil-based cream or jelly (like baby oil or petroleum jelly) when you're also using a latex condom or a diaphragm. According to the Kinsey Institute, studies have shown that these products destroy latex with incredible speed, boring it full of microscopic holes—holes large enough to allow free passage for the AIDS virus—within 60 seconds. Within minutes, oil-based lubricants eat holes in latex large enough to allow sperm to pass through, rendering your barrier contraceptive about as impregnable as a colander.

Instead, use a water-based lubricant such as K-Y Jelly or Lubrin inserts, both of which are safe to use with latex contraceptives and are available without a prescription in drugstores or grocery stores. Another water-based lubricant favored by Robert Birch, Ph.D., director of the Arlington Center for Marital and Sexual Concerns in Columbus, Ohio, is a commercial concoction called Astroglide, which Dr. Birch says is better than K-Y Jelly because it lasts longer. (It's available from Astro-Lube, P.O. Box 9788, North Hollywood, CA 91609.) And don't forget the oldest and sexiest of water-based lubricants, also available without a prescription: saliva.

Superstars of Slippery

Normally, an aroused woman will produce enough natural lubrication to make intercourse silky and sweet. Many men, in fact, think that when a woman is wet, she's ready. But it's important to remember that lubrication is only one of the first signs of a woman's arousal; usually she requires a good bit of foreplay before she's actually ready for intercourse.

Also, men sometimes interpret a woman's lack of wetness as a sign that he doesn't turn her on. But sometimes she may have trouble producing enough natural lubrication for painless penetration for reasons that have nothing to do with him. Older women, especially, often have trouble getting wet enough for intercourse because, after menopause, reduced levels of circulating estrogen inhibit the vagina's ability to produce natural lubrication during arousal.

That's important, because among humans, women provide most of the natural lubrication for sex. In other animals, it's different: The male contributes a slippery preejaculatory fluid—a sort of natural K-Y Jelly—manufactured by an obscure part of the sexual anatomy called the Cowper's glands. Stallions, rams, boars, male goats and other animals "may dribble or run continuous streams of such secretions as soon as they approach a female in which they are sexually interested," according to the late Dr. Alfred Kinsey. Although the Cowper's glands are much more poorly developed in humans, many men produce a drop or two of this dewy lubricant (sometimes called "gland-come") shortly before they actually ejaculate. (It may contain a few overeager sperm cells, which is one reason it's wise to put on a condom well before you ejaculate.)

For women who have trouble getting wet enough for intercourse, or lovers who simply want to add a little spice to their lovemaking, there are lots of lubricants to explore. Sex therapists say clients especially like Albolene cream, massage lotion or coconut oil, in addition to the ones already mentioned. For clients in therapy, Dr. Birch recommends coconut oil. (Remember, though, this is a no-no if you're using barrier contraceptives.) You can buy it in a health food store, put it in a bottle and put the bottle in a pan of hot water to keep it warm while in use.

It may take a little experimenting to find the lubricant you like best—but it's hard to imagine a more interesting science project.

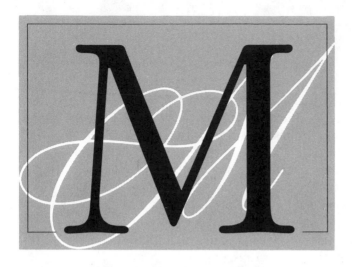

MASSAGE

With a warm, quiet place and a bottle of scented oil, you can spread pleasure over every inch of your partner's body," says Gordon Inkeles, best-selling author of *The Art of Sensual Massage, The New Massage* and other books.

What a pity that we so seldom do it!

Even people who love each other and have been happily married for years tend to forget 95 percent of the vast and varied vocabulary of touch. After a few years of marriage, the way we touch each other tends to be reduced to one of two things: We touch each other either in a completely sexless, perfunctory way (a peck on the cheek, a pat on the back) or in a way that is as sexual as you can get. Often, when a man touches his wife at all, it's basically a way of asking a question: Do you want to have sex? First comes the touch, then the kiss, then a fast-forward to orgasm.

Even when we get sexual, the places that we touch each other tend to be limited to a couple of square inches of skin the dimensions of an airmail envelope. Whole kingdoms of the body, and of sensuous pleasure, go unnoticed. Says Inkeles: "It's entirely possible that a woman who's been married for years has never been touched behind the knee, or between the toes, by another adult since childhood." Our whole culture, in fact, is so starved for touch that sometimes people will have sex when all they really want is to feel the delicious warmth of skin against skin.

Massage as Sex-Enhancer

But all is not lost—you and your lover can learn the exquisite pleasures of touch and rediscover each other in the process.

It's called massage.

Don't be intimidated by that word. There are forms of massage that require lots of training, and maybe even a few courses in human physiology, but that's not what we're talking about here. We're simply talking about using touch to give your partner pleasure and then unashamedly *receive* it (which is also the goal of satisfying sex). *That* kind of touch doesn't take any particular training at all, although it does require that you care for each other.

Massage is a potent "sex-enhancer," says Inkeles, because it induces deep relaxation by rapidly dissipating the negative effects of stress. People tend to have sex as a way of blowing off physical tension. But a far better approach is to slip into a state of deep relaxation *first,* through sensuous massage, and then make love.

For one thing, the ascent to orgasm (which, momentarily, involves extreme body tension) is much more dramatic if you first go *down* into a state of deep relaxation, rather than starting from a state of semiaroused agitation, says Martha Brown, a registered massage therapist in Charlottesville, Virginia. It's almost like adding another 50 feet to the top of the roller-coaster ride.

For another, Inkeles explains, part of the complex physiology of stress involves a gradual buildup of acidic wastes in the muscles. When you're under sustained stress, without any accompanying physical release, your muscles stead-ily fill with lactic and carbonic acid, in readiness for "fight or flight." But instead of doing either one, you just sit there at your desk as those wastes accumulate in your body. Allowing all that acidic gunk to pass out of your system naturally might take days or weeks—but deep massage can force it out of the muscles in a matter of minutes and in this way induce a sense of deep, languorous relaxation. Studies of Olympic athletes have shown that 15 minutes of deep massage can have a profound effect on the acid content of muscles, says Inkeles. Massage also pumps oxygen into the muscles, which is tremendously invigorating.

"The biggest obstacle to great sex," Inkeles says, "is stress." And sensual massage is one of the oldest and most reliable stress-reducers in the world.

Sensual massage, whether or not it's overtly sexual, is also just a delightful way to express affection. It's a way of exploring the forgotten frontiers of your partner's body and in the process vastly expanding your repertoire of touch. And it's a way of finding out what makes your lover feel good and what doesn't.

The How-To Part

Preparing for a sensuous massage is like setting the mood for love. It doesn't have to be terribly involved. Just find a space in your life where you're sure you won't be interrupted—the bedroom is fine. Take the phone off the hook. Lock the door. Put the clock in the drawer and forget about time. Don't focus on giving your lover a massage for any particular amount of time—just do it for as long as it feels good. (It's worse to persist if you feel bored or resentful.)

It's nice to use massage oils, because they feel great and tend to make the skin more sensitive to touch. In biblical times, to anoint meant to massage with oil, and in Mediterranean cultures 5,000 years ago, people probably used ordinary vegetable oil scented with a few drops of lemon, Inkeles says. Safflower oil still works fine, and it's cheap. Others prefer coconut oil, which is light, nongreasy and odorless. It's best to warm it a little before use. Try putting it in a plastic squeeze bottle for convenience. Instead of oil, some people like to use cornstarch, which is so silky to the touch it almost feels wet.

Other things to remember:

- Generally, says Brown, people tend to touch each other during massage in the same way *they* like to be touched. The result: Women tend to massage men too gently, and men tend to massage women too firmly. The solution: Just keep asking for feedback. "How does this pressure feel?" "Should I bear down harder?" "Is that too soft?" The only unforgivable sin of massage is to make your partner feel uncomfortable. Says Inkeles: "One moment of pain destroys an hour of good massage."
- People tend to hold lots of tension in their faces, especially people in public life. Try massaging the forehead, jaw muscles, temples. Use strokes that "smooth out" or go across the lines on the face. Another great spot to focus on: the feet.
- Women tend to hold tension in their neck and shoulders, men tend to hold it in the small of their backs, Inkeles says. Give those areas special attention.
- Any place where the skin is thin is especially sensitive, such as around the ankles and the insides of the arms and neck.
- You really don't need any fancy equipment to give a great massage, but sometimes a vibrator can be used for spice. Try strapping the device to the back of your hand, so that your fingertips transmit the good vibrations.

Sensate Focus in Sex Therapy

The marvelously sensuous magic of massage has not been lost on sex therapists. In fact, a form of massage has been a key part of many sex therapy programs for the past 20 years. First developed by William Masters, M.D., and Virginia Johnson, of the Masters and Johnson Institute in St. Louis, *sensate focus* exercises (sometimes also called *nondemand pleasuring*) are a way for couples in sexual distress to break free of mutually reinforcing avoidance. But even people who are not having sex troubles can use these exercises to great effect.

Basically, nondemand pleasuring works like this: A couple gets naked together in a quiet, romantic place and takes turns caressing each other's body. (Usually, at least to begin, the couple is seated, with the receiver sitting between the giver's legs.) There's just one rule: The breasts and genitals are off-limits, and so is intercourse. There is no pressure to push forward to orgasm, no pressure to achieve anything or get anywhere, no pressure to "return the favor." There's no place to go except into the sensuality and stillness of the present moment.

MASTECTOMY

"Who would be attracted to a disfigured woman?" asked one mastectomy patient sadly, shortly after her breast was removed due to a malignant tumor.

She's not alone. The enormous literature on the aftereffects of breast surgery has shown that about a third of women go through a difficult period of sexual and psychological readjustment after the operation. Even though surgeons have learned to conserve as much of the breast as possible and sometimes reconstruct the breast during or after the cancer surgery, some women slip into a depression that lingers for months. Others can't shake a feeling that they are somehow less a woman, less feminine, less sexually desirable, than they were before. They may feel mutilated or damaged or plagued by an odd feeling that their bodies are deformed or lopsided.

The process of coming to terms with the loss of a breast has even been likened to mourning for a lost loved one: First there's denial, then anger, depression, despair and finally (if all goes well) acceptance. Many women dread the possibility of such an experience—an American woman now has roughly a one in nine chance of developing breast cancer (the most common cancer in women) some-time in her life. Still, according to at least one expert, all this may have gotten just a bit too much press.

"The fact is that the majority of women cope well with the stress of cancer surgery and the loss of a breast," says Leslie R. Schover, Ph.D., staff psychologist at the Center for Sexual Function at the Cleveland Clinic Foundation in Ohio. "Losing a breast does not mean you're no longer a woman; I think that's kind of an antique notion, a big exaggeration."

What's emerging from the most recent studies, Dr. Schover says, is the realization that the best predictor of postsurgery sexual satisfaction is overall psychological health and a happy relationship. It's the women who are in trou-bled relationships or who already had sexual or psychological problems before the surgery who are most likely to have trouble afterward.

The Culprit: Chemo

Actually, says Dr. Schover, the most common culprit in sexual problems after breast surgery is probably not loss of a breast at all—it's side effects caused by the hormonal therapy or chemotherapy that often follows the surgery.

About 40 percent of breast cancers are *hormone-responsive*—meaning that their rate of growth is altered by the female hormones estrogen and progesterone. So some breast cancer patients have their ovaries removed or begin taking drugs to alter their hormone status after the surgery to prevent the potential spread of the cancer. But in a younger woman who hasn't yet reached menopause, hormone therapy can bring about sudden, premature menopause. And this artificial menopause can have unpleasant sexual side effects—like pain during intercourse and loss of vaginal lubrication, not to mention hot flashes. When the ovaries are removed, sexual desire may also begin to fade because "male" hormones like testosterone, produced by the ovaries, are what inflame the libido.

Older women who've passed menopause but never had cancer can overcome many of these obstacles to satisfying sex through hormone replacement therapy, which restores the softness and wetness of vaginal tissues, among other things. (See "Hormone Replacement Therapy.") But because female hormones may stimulate the cancer if it's still lurking somewhere in the body, breast cancer survivors *can't* take replacement hormones. So they're often stuck with hot flashes and dry, painful intercourse. There are, however, some nonhormonal drugs for hot flashes, and vaginal lubricants can help combat dryness.

Chemotherapy can also be devastating. "If a woman has to have chemo-therapy, she loses her hair and feels nauseous, and it's terrible for her body image and self-esteem. By comparison, the issue of losing a breast might not be quite so overwhelming," Dr. Schover says. Chemotherapy can also cause ovarian failure, resulting in premature menopause and the very same kinds of sexual difficulties.

(Of course, let's not lose our way in all of this. These treatments, unpleasant as they may be, have saved countless women's lives. And for most people, life is better than death, whether or not we're lucky enough to be blessed with sweet, uncomplicated sex.)

Rebuilding the Breast

In recent years, great strides have been made in developing ways to reconstruct the breast after surgery. What was once considered nothing but a towering female vanity is now often covered (partly or fully) by medical insurance. Sometimes the breast is rebuilt by transferring a flap of skin from the abdomen or the back. (Until recently, silicone implants were sometimes used to give the breast fullness that was lost during surgery, but the Food and Drug Administration has banned these implants pending further study.) Even the nipple and areola (the dark circle surrounding the nipple) can be reconstructed from skin taken from elsewhere on the body, with tattooing used to complete the color match.

For all its impressive results, plastic surgery is not perfect. No matter what its original shape, a silicone implant tends to take on the shape of a baseball, may harden after scar tissue forms around it and is sometimes painful. The rebuilt breast also tends to be abnormally firm and has little erotic sensitivity. (That wonderful little nerve that provides the nipple with such exquisite responsiveness is severed during the surgery.)

Still, studies have consistently shown that women who have their breast (or breasts) restored after mastectomy feel better about their appearance, especially in the nude, than women who do not. The reconstruction is sometimes done months or even a year or more after the mastectomy. But some studies have shown that women who have the breast reconstructed at the same time the cancer surgery is performed are less likely to go through a period of depression, grief and sexual distress.

Ways to Help Yourself

If you're facing a mastectomy, it's good to know there are a number of things you can do to help you through the experience.

See a therapist. "When a woman has a mastectomy, she should definitely have at least one session with a sex therapist," says Jude Cotter, Ph.D., a psychologist and sex therapist in private practice in Farmington Hills, Michigan.

Dr. Schover agrees that if a woman has the means (such luxuries aren't usually covered by insurance), brief sexual counseling after a diagnosis of breast cancer can be helpful.

It's especially useful if the woman's sex partner can also attend the session, Dr. Schover adds. This helps to open up the channels of sexual communication between the two, and if any change in sexual technique is going to be required, the man needs to be informed about it.

In fact, a number of studies have shown that a woman's psychological and sexual recovery from breast surgery is greatly helped if her husband takes part in the whole process: participating in treatment decisions, visiting the hospital with her and being exposed early to the mastectomy or lumpectomy scar. Men, too, suffer through this; they're part of it. Men tend to favor one of their partner's breasts during sex play, Dr. Cotter points out—and may even gloomily blame themselves if that's the breast that developed a tumor.

Try sensate focus. Women who depend on nipple stimulation to get aroused may need to learn new ways to get turned on after surgery. Sex therapists often recommend sensate focus exercises, which increase the body's overall erotic sensitivity and may help you find a new highway to heaven. (See "Sex Therapy.")

Inform yourself. It's a good idea to inform yourself as fully as possible about the operation. If you intend to have the breast reconstructed after the surgery, it's a good idea to decide this beforehand and let your medical team know about it. In many cases, knowing beforehand can help the plastic surgeon save your nipple.

Reach for recovery. Many hospitals participate in the American Cancer Society's Reach to Recovery program, which matches up volunteers who had a mastectomy more than a year earlier with women who've just had one. Talking to somebody else who's had the same experience is one of the oldest, most reliable (and cheapest) kinds of therapy there is.

MASTERS AND JOHNSON

In 1953, at a hospital in St. Louis, a young obstetrician named William Howell Masters had the startling experience of seeing a newborn baby boy emerge from his mother's womb waving a tiny, full-blown erection. At the time, the late sex researcher Dr. Alfred Kinsey was under attack for suggesting (among other things) that human sexuality awakens very early in life, perhaps as early as preadolescence. But here was a baby who had an erection even before he drew his first breath!

An older physician gently explained that the erection was a reflex caused by pressure on the infant's head as it descended the birth canal. But three weeks later, Dr. Masters delivered another baby boy, this time by cesarean section. And that baby also had an erection.

"That's when I got interested in sex and decided to devote the rest of my life to studying it," Dr. Masters recently told a gathering of sex therapists and educators.

Drawn forward by a boundless curiosity about human sexuality, the most intimate of mysteries, he began a series of ground-breaking studies into what was then still largely an unknown field. During the 1940s and 1950s, Dr. Kinsey had laid the foundation for our understanding of sexuality, but his data were based almost entirely on sex histories (interviews). He only rarely studied or observed sexual behavior itself.

But Dr. Masters, along with his collaborator (and later his wife), psychologist Virginia Johnson, set out to take sex out of the realm of the interview and into the realm of empirical science. Between 1954 and 1965, under laboratory conditions, they stared unashamedly at over 700 people actually having intercourse, masturbating and otherwise expressing themselves sexually. They wired them up with electrodes to measure heart rate and breathing, used sensors to gauge the strength of muscle contractions and even designed wee cameras fitted inside plastic penises, which they then used to film the mysterious interior of the vagina. It was a place as alien, and as wonderful, as the dark side of the moon.

("Did you know that it's the woman who actually inseminates *herself,* and not the man?" Dr. Masters asked the gathering of sex experts. By means of those tiny penis-cameras, he and his colleagues were able to film semen pooling at the deep end of the vagina and then witness the woman's cervix actually dunking itself down into the pool in a series of muscular thrusts, almost as if it were a pair of thirsty lips lapping up a drink. "It's incredible—unbelievable!" he crowed.)

The Sexual Response Cycle

In 1964, Masters and Johnson established the Reproductive Biology Research Foundation in St. Louis, and in 1966 they published the classic *Human Sexual Response,* based largely on their laboratory research. The book was written in a particularly indigestible sort of medicalese—the *Saturday Review* called it "the worst-written best-seller of the century." But it was a best-seller nonetheless.

Little, Brown, the publisher, printed 30,000 copies, and they sold out in 6 hours, Dr. Masters recalls. "Did we get everything in the book right? Of course not," he admits today. Even so, it is still considered the first comprehensive study of the physiology of human sexual activity ever published.

Among other things, Masters and Johnson discovered that human sexuality awakens even before birth—baby boys have erections in the womb, six weeks before birth, and girl babies produce vaginal lubrication hours after they are born. They also described what has come to be known as the four-part sexual response cycle.

In the *excitement* phase, physiological arousal gradually builds: Muscle tension increases, the vagina begins to lubricate, blood vessels in the penis, clitoris and nipples become engorged with blood. The *plateau* phase is one of sustained excitement. Heart rate and respiration increase, the skin (also engorged with blood) begins to flush. All that arousal peaks and then explodes during *orgasm,* when muscles contract all over the body (especially in the genitals), engorged blood is released, and the male ejaculates. *Resolution,* the "afterglow" phase, is the body's gradual return to ordinary reality.

Sex Therapy Is Born

But Masters and Johnson didn't stop at merely describing human sexual behavior. In their next major book, *Human Sexual Inadequacy,* and many other books, they described what can go wrong in a sexual relationship and laid out their plan to cure it. In effect, they broke ground for the still-new science of sex therapy, and many of their methods (such as sensate focus exercises and the squeeze technique for premature ejaculation) are still widely used. In their highly successful model of comarital therapy, a troubled husband and wife are treated by a team of therapists, one male, one female. Generally, their program involves a two-week stay at the institute in St. Louis and a year of follow-up. Over the years, Masters and Johnson have trained many other therapists in their methods. (See also "Sex Therapy.")

MASTURBATION

Over the centuries, all manner of unspeakable inventions have been patented to put a stop to it: metal mittens; little cages with inward-pointing spikes, which a boy was supposed to wear over his private parts at night; even a device that jangled a bell in the parents' bedroom the moment a child's mattress began to shake.

Virtually every illness, mental or physical, has been blamed on it, including acne, various other skin diseases, epilepsy, bed-wetting, round shoulders, blindness, insanity, tuberculosis, asthma, rheumatism, stomach cramps, infantile paralysis, melancholy, impotence, hairy palms, rickets, "loss of vitality," hysteria and suicide. In insane asylums, there were once special wards for patients whose psychosis was supposed to have been caused by self-abuse.

Ingenious and complicated punishments have been devised to frighten people away from it. In the early Middle Ages, when churches distributed penitential books that described every sexual misdeed and prescribed punishments for each, the greatest stress of all was laid upon masturbation. St. Thomas Aquinas considered it a greater sin than fornication.

The Degeneracy Theory

Why, of all sexual transgressions, has masturbation been singled out for such specially scathing damnation? Maybe because it's so pleasurable and so common. Among the more than 5,000 men the late Dr. Alfred Kinsey interviewed, 92 percent said they masturbated. (Dr. Kinsey is sometimes accused of exaggerating the numbers, but in Shere Hite's study of male sexuality in 1981, she found the number to be closer to 99 percent.) Among women, Dr. Kinsey found, 62 percent said they masturbated at least occasionally.

Then on what *grounds* has most of humanity been made to suffer from sexual guilt and remorse? There have been many theories used to justify the claim that masturbation is bad—for instance, because it's "unnatural" (any sexual practice that didn't or couldn't produce babies was once considered immoral), or because it's infantile (it was reasoned that healthy adults should learn to practice intercourse instead). But during much of the eighteenth century, the most widely promoted explanation was "the degeneracy theory," laid out in a scholarly treatise by the Swiss physician S. A. Tissot in 1758. The basic idea was this: Semen is the most vital of all vital fluids—every drop of semen being derived from seven drops of blood—and by wasting it, you drained your body of vitality and laid yourself open to all manner of diseases and infirmities.

Unfortunately, much of the theory was based on bad science, explains John Money, Ph.D., professor of medical psychology and pediatrics at Johns Hopkins University and Hospital in Baltimore, in his book *Lovemaps*. Dr. Tissot observed that when men were castrated, they seemed to grow weak and "devirilized." He concluded it was loss of semen that was taking all the sap out of them. At the time, though, nobody yet understood that it was not semen but hormones produced by the testes that fueled the engines of male sex drive and virility. Dr. Tissot had also observed that prostitutes and their clients were often sickly—again blaming it all on wasted semen, not on widespread venereal diseases (which would not be discovered until a century later).

Anyway, the theory caught on like wildfire and soon spread to America, where one of its first public proponents was John Harvey Kellogg, a respected surgeon and health food faddist who introduced cereals and nuts as substitutes for meat (since meat was thought to inflame carnal desire).

"Few of today's eaters of Kellogg's Corn Flakes know that he invented them, almost literally, as antimasturbation food," Dr. Money observes. Kellogg, in fact, was the "degeneracy theory's most ardent antimasturbation advocate. For intractable cases of masturbation in boys he recommended sewing up the foreskin with silver wire or, if that failed, circumcision without anesthesia. For girls, he recommended burning out the clitoris with carbolic acid."

But such appalling attitudes are not lost in the sands of ancient history. As recently as 1940, a candidate could be rejected at the U.S. Naval Academy if he was found masturbating. And in 1959, a study showed that half the graduates of a Philadelphia medical school believed that mental illness is frequently caused by masturbation. More amazing still, one of every five *faculty* members at the same school believed the same thing!

The Up Side

To take an honest glance back through the history of human attitudes about masturbation is to be filled with sadness at all the guilt and pain we've needlessly inflicted upon ourselves. Because the bottom line on masturbation is this: Nobody has ever been able to show that it's harmful at all, whether physically or psychologically. The physical effects of self-stimulation aren't fundamentally different from those of any other kind of sexual activity, so how *could* it be harmful? In fact, today's sex therapists point to its many practical benefits.

- It can teach a woman how to reach orgasm—and in fact, many women first become orgasmic in this way. In Dr. Kinsey's sample, only 4 to 6 percent of the women who masturbated were *unable* to reach orgasm through self-stimulation (a much higher percentage than reach orgasm through intercourse).
- Rather than hindering a woman's ability to reach orgasm during intercourse, it can often help, by teaching her about her own sexual rhythms and preferences. ("Premarital experience in masturbation may actually contribute to the female's capacity to respond in her coital relations in marriage," Dr. Kinsey observed.)

- Older women who've passed menopause and don't have a sex partner often experience a gradual thinning and drying-out of vaginal tissues, which can make intercourse terribly painful once they do find a partner. One good way to keep the vaginal tissues soft, moist and pliable is to masturbate, preferably by using something like a vibrator in the vagina, therapists say.
- Because it's often fevered, guilt-ridden and quick, masturbation may teach a young man to ejaculate all too fast. Yet, carefully practiced, it can also provide terrific training in ejaculatory control. In fact, the squeeze technique, a kind of stop-and-start masturbation, is a widely used and highly effective form of therapy for men who ejaculate too rapidly to satisfy their lovers. (See "Premature Ejaculation.")
- Masturbation can also be used for mutual, rather than solitary, pleasure. It can be very instructive to watch your partner masturbate himself or herself to climax. It's one of the best ways for a woman to show her man precisely where her clitoris is and how she likes it to be stroked. Also, depressing as it is, mutual masturbation has gained a new kind of glamour in the age of AIDS. (See "Safer Sex.")

What Is "Excessive"?

Despite all this enlightened sexual happy talk, though, the truth is that most people still feel awfully guilty and embarrassed about masturbation and would probably be mortified if anyone found out they did it. Various studies have shown that despite the huge numbers of people who do it, many are filled with remorse and shame about it, have repeatedly tried to quit and worry that it might have some woeful long-term effect on their sex lives. A few have even attempted suicide because of it.

Even in the 1940s and 1950s, long after doctors admitted that the dire Victorian-age warnings about masturbation had been wildly exaggerated, they still maintained that "excessive" masturbation might be pathological. But what does "excessive" really *mean?* Nobody ever made it quite clear, so people reached the sort of conclusion they usually reach in such a situation: "I'm okay, it's you who's sick!"

William Masters, M.D., and Virginia Johnson, of the Masters and Johnson Institute in St. Louis, found that in a study group of several hundred men, everyone expressed concern about the insidious effects of excessive masturbation. But when asked to define "excessive," they invariably said it was more frequently than however often they themselves did it. One man who masturbated once a month said once or twice a week would be excessive. And another man, who admitted he indulged himself two or three times a day, said he thought that five or six times a day might lead to a "case of nerves."

The bottom line is that it's really quite impossible to say what "excessive" masturbation actually means, because the range of normal human sexual behavior is so dizzyingly vast. In fact, the frequency of masturbation is one of the most variable of all human sexual activities, Dr. Kinsey found. Some boys don't masturbate at all, others do it two or three times in their lifetime, others do it as frequently as two or three times a day for years at a time. It's not uncommon for men to continue to masturbate even after they're married, although the frequency generally drops off dramatically (averaging about once every three weeks).

And not one of them, it's safe to say, has hair growing on his palms.

MEDICATIONS

There are at least 200 medications that can interfere with your sexuality in one way or another. Drugs used to treat high blood pressure can interfere with a man's ability to get an erection or ejaculate or both. Antidepressants can stifle a woman's capacity to reach orgasm. And a whole slew of other drugs, even cold and allergy medications, can smother a person's interest in sex altogether.

"While doctors once attributed many sexual problems to psychological causes, today there is a growing awareness that more than half these conditions are connected to physical ailments or drug side effects," says M. Laurence Lieberman, a New York City pharmacist and author of *The Sexual Pharmacy: The Complete Guide to Drugs with Sexual Side Effects.*

According to a survey of urologists conducted by the Impotence Foundation, blood pressure medications were the most common offenders, with Inderal topping the list. Fully 60 percent of men taking these drugs reported some degree of sexual dysfunction, according to another nationwide survey. Other notorious troublemakers include diuretics, antidepressants, antihistamines, antipsychotics, tranquilizers, antispasmodics and ulcer medications.

What You Should Do

"If you suspect that a medication you're taking is causing sexual problems — and patients very often correctly make this connection — it's important to bring it to your doctor's attention," says E. Douglas Whitehead, M.D., associate clinical professor of urology at Mount Sinai School of Medicine and a director of the Association for Male Sexual Dysfunction in New York City. "Often the problem can be alleviated, or at least greatly reduced, by changing the patient to a different drug or by reducing the dosage." It may also be possible in some cases to use a combination of drugs at a lower dosage.

Which brings us to the good news: Today, there's an increasingly broad array of alternative drugs that have the same therapeutic effect as the drug that may be giving you trouble but are less likely to cause sexual problems. For instance, one study looked at the sexual side effects of three commonly prescribed blood pressure drugs: captopril (often sold as Capoten), propranolol (Inderal) and methyldopa (Aldomet). Among the men taking methyldopa or propranolol, there were numerous sexual complaints, including the inability to maintain an erection or a loss of interest in sex entirely. The most pronounced sexual side effects were found in men 51 years or older who were taking methyldopa or propranolol plus a diuretic (a common combination). But captopril emerged as the clear winner: Although it was equally effective in controlling blood pressure, it had few if any sexual side effects in most of the men surveyed.

There's no *guarantee* that having your doctor switch you to this alternative drug will make your troubles vanish. Sexual side effects just haven't been studied to any great degree. "The sexual side effects of pharmaceuticals are still among the most subtle, least discussed and most poorly understood consequences of the chemical arsenal used in modern medical care," says Lieberman.

Still, if your current medication seems to be giving you trouble, it might be useful to discuss an alternative with your doctor. What you should definitely *not* do is stop taking the drug without consulting your physician.

"Sometimes patients who suspect that a drug is causing sex problems will say 'I'd rather die happy than live and be unable to function sexually.' They'll simply stop taking the medication, or they'll stop taking it just before they go on vacation, to restore their sexual function for a few weeks," says Debbie Steele, R.N., nursing unit director of urology services at Sunnybrook Medical Centre in Toronto. "But that's playing Russian roulette with your life. If you're taking a heart medication or a blood pressure medication, you could have a stroke or a heart attack, and that would be tragic. You wouldn't die, you wouldn't be happy, and you wouldn't be able to have sex, either!"

When it comes to drug-related sex troubles, there's hope—but don't reach for it without your doctor's help.

MENOPAUSE

Hot flashes, night sweats, dizziness, stress incontinence: Not every woman experiences the full range of symptoms associated with menopause, but many come to know them only too well. Menopause is the time of life when a woman's ovaries stop producing eggs, and the hormones that orchestrate menstruation ebb away.

No matter what other symptoms they may have, most women must adjust to a variety of physical changes that may have an impact on their sex lives. In their massive tome *Human Sexual Response,* William Masters, M.D., and Virginia Johnson, of the Masters and Johnson Institute in St. Louis, detail those potentially challenging changes. They include a decline in vaginal wetness during sexual arousal, decreased vaginal elasticity, loss of interest in sex, lack of increase in breast size during sexual stimulation and fewer and sometimes painful contractions of the uterus during orgasm. Nearly all these changes can be explained by the decline in estrogen levels after menopause, according to Philip M. Sarrel, M.D., an associate professor of obstetrics and gynecology at Yale University School of Medicine.

When Dr. Sarrel and his colleagues interviewed 93 women who were going through menopause, they found that 68 percent of the women reported having some problems in their sexual lives. Of these, 77 percent reported a decrease in their sexual desire, 58 percent complained of vaginal dryness, 39 percent said intercourse was painful, 36 percent said their clitoris was no longer quite as sensitive as it once was, 35 percent said their orgasms weren't as intense as they used to be, and 29 percent said they no longer reached orgasm as frequently as they once did. Half the women said they were now having intercourse once a month or less.

The Bright Side

Still, menopause is not just one long, uninterrupted string of bad news. In one survey of nearly 2,500 middle-aged American women, only a tiny minority (3 percent) expressed regret about the physical changes wrought by menopause.

"Rather than a regrettable loss of reproductive function, these women expressed relief at the loss of concern over pregnancy, contraception and menstruation," notes investigator Sonja McKinlay, Ph.D., president of the New England Research Institute in Watertown, Massachusetts.

So there's an up side to the story.

A Long, Slow Process

Still, there's no denying that a majority of women experience some sexual sea change around the time of menopause. What many women don't realize, though, is that these changes don't *begin* at menopause. Although the average American woman usually reaches menopause at around age 51 (strictly speaking, menopause means not having a period for a full year), the ovaries' production of the female hormone estrogen begins shutting down roughly seven to ten years earlier (typically, in a woman's early forties).

The long, slow decline of estrogen production (known as *perimenopause*), which begins long before a woman stops menstruating, often isn't steady and gradual. More likely, estrogen levels will fluctuate wildly during this period of a woman's life. As a result, many women in their forties experience brief, mystifying episodes of vaginal dryness (caused by estrogen dips) that go away by themselves. If she doesn't realize that this is an early sign of impending menopause, a woman may mistakenly come to believe it's caused by a relationship problem and not merely a medical one. Her partner, in turn, may come to believe that her lack of wetness is caused by his inability to stimulate her or, worse, the end of her love for him.

"When communication is poor, vaginal dryness can lead to severe relationship problems in these couples," observes Gloria A. Bachmann, M.D., associate professor of obstetrics and gynecology at Robert Wood Johnson Medical School in New Providence, New Jersey.

A woman's periods may also grow more irregular during this time of life. They don't just stop on a dime at the age of 51; instead, the interval between periods becomes irregular, and usually the length of the entire cycle gradually grows longer. Women are often reminded to be on the lookout for abnormal bleeding during this time. Once periods haven't occurred for a year, it means that the ovaries' estrogen production has dropped too low to stimulate the lining of the uterus in preparation for pregnancy. (See "Menstruation.")

But there's one thing you don't dare forget during the last few years before menopause, while the menstrual cycles are beginning to disappear: *You can still get pregnant.* Don't stop using birth control until your periods have ceased for an entire year. Only then can you feel certain that you've gotten off the reproductive merry-go-round for good.

Tired Ovaries: The Early Warning Signs

If you're surprised to know that menopausal symptoms often begin showing up in a woman's early forties, consider this: Sometimes they show up as early as 36 or 37. In a certain type of ferociously driven, goal-oriented career woman, a collection of "classic" signs of perimenopause turn up at an amazingly early age, says Judith H. Seifer, Ph.D., R.N., clinical professor of psychiatry and obstetrics/gynecology at Wright State University School of Medicine in Dayton, Ohio.

"It's as if, in the hard-driving, Type A male, his heart wears out, but in these hard-driving women, their ovaries wear out," she says. The main thing they need to be told, she adds, is "No, it's not all in your head." Here are some of the symptoms that often show up.

A "very unique" form of insomnia. She falls dead asleep as soon as she hits the pillow and wakes up already on the run. Such women say, "I've got to sleep fast—I don't have time to waste," and manage to survive on 5 hours or less a night.

Short-term memory loss. A woman who never forgets anything, whose whole sense of self-esteem is based on her own competence, suddenly forgets the kids at the ballgame.

Difficulty receiving touch. Even though she may love him dearly, she begins to feel revulsion at her husband's touch. (Estrogen is known to affect touch perception, because it alters the levels of neurotransmitters.)

Stress incontinence. Since the genitourinary system is also affected by estrogen loss, many menopausal women have trouble retaining urine when they laugh or sneeze. When somebody starts telling a joke, they cross their legs.

When a woman in her late thirties describes such symptoms, many doctors don't think to check her estrogen levels, Dr. Seifer says. But if you suspect you might be experiencing early symptoms of perimenopause, have your doctor do a *maturation index* the next time you have a Pap test, she says. Basically, this is a very reliable test to see if the cervix is getting enough stimulation by estrogen. It doesn't cost a penny extra; it's simply a matter of putting an extra drop on the slide that's examined when the Pap test is put under a microscope.

His Side of the Story

Menopause doesn't affect only women. It takes two to tango, and the sexual and emotional side effects of a woman's change of life may also have an effect on her partner. In one survey conducted at Yale, Dr. Sarrel and his colleagues interviewed 50 couples in which all the women had passed menopause. Thirty-nine of the male partners (almost 80 percent) reported having sexual troubles of one kind or another.

Because their wives did not want to be touched, complained of vaginal dryness or suffered from vaginismus (a spasm of the vaginal muscles, making entry impossible), many of these men felt angry and rejected, Dr. Sarrel reported. Some said they were afraid they would hurt their wives, especially because the women had endured painful intercourse in the past but had not said anything about it. Five of the men had trouble getting erections at all after their wives began bleeding after intercourse.

Ten of the men complained that although sex was satisfying when their wives were younger, now they could no longer sustain an erection for as long as it took their wives to become aroused and lubricated. And a few could not even penetrate their wives' vaginas at all. Either she had severe vaginismus or the vaginal opening was so atrophied it had narrowed to the point he could not manage to get in. While he struggled to enter this apparently unwelcoming doorway, his erection would wilt.

What You Can Do

Some of these dispiriting problems can be overcome by learning to communicate, the experts say. Your partner may never know what hurts, or what feels good, unless you speak up.

There are also medical treatments that may help improve the symptoms that interfere with satisfying sex.

Talk to your doctor about hormone replacement therapy, which can restore vaginal wetness, revive a wilted libido, help with urinary problems and protect against coronary artery disease and osteoporosis. (See "Hormone Replacement Therapy.")

And here's a prescription that you may enjoy filling: One of the best methods for keeping the vagina soft, wet and youthful is regular sex. One study of 59 healthy women between 60 and 70 showed that those who had intercourse regularly had significantly less vaginal atrophy and wetter and more elastic vaginal tissues than women who were abstinent.

"Women who continue to be sexually active," says Dr. Bachmann, "either with a partner or through self stimulation, maintain a more nearly normal state of genital health than abstinent women."

If you have no sex partner, sex researchers suggest that you forget what your mother told you and masturbate. Preferably, says Dr. Seifer, this means "containing something in the vagina," such as a penis-shaped vibrator, which is much more helpful in preserving genital health than using a finger.

Do's and Don'ts

It also helps to avoid antihistamines and decongestants, which dry out mucous membranes, including the vagina. (Ask your doctor to suggest other drugs.) A few other medications, like antidepressants, antihypertensives and cardiac agents, can also worsen vaginal dryness.

It might be helpful to use a water-soluble vaginal lubricant like K-Y Jelly. One new alternative: A gel-filled tampon called Replens that's inserted into the vagina three times a week for continuous lubrication. It creates a moist layer of polymer cream that adheres to vaginal walls and actually redhydrates cells. It also helps protect against infections by normalizing vaginal acidity. (Replens is available over the counter in drugstores.)

Some women who are loath to get started on oral estrogen may wish to try estrogen creams such as Premarin, which can relieve vaginal dryness with fewer side effects. However, it's important to remember that estrogen creams should never be used as sexual lubricants, because they can be absorbed by a woman's partner through his penis. This has led, in a few cases, to a condition called gynecomastia, or abnormal growth of the breasts in men. Estrogen creams should be applied only at times when a woman knows she isn't going to have sex and should be used for only a few weeks.

Menopausal hormone changes disrupt the delicate pH of the vagina, increasing a woman's susceptibility to bacterial and yeast infections. Doctors recommend switching to mild (nondeodorant and fragrance-free) soaps and avoiding personal hygiene sprays, which can irritate dry, sensitive vaginal tissue.

And after a shower or a bath, be sure to dry yourself well, especially between your legs, because warmth and wetness are what bacteria and yeasts love most. You might even use a blow-dryer on the warm (not hot) setting. Wear cotton-crotch panty hose and underwear, which breathes better than nylon and keeps you drier.

Because menopause may cause the muscles supporting the vagina, uterus and bladder to sag, some doctors recommend Kegel exercises to increase the muscle tone of the pelvic floor. These easy-to-learn exercises can help you overcome stress incontinence, a common side effect of menopause, and also increase sexual responsiveness. (See "Kegel Exercises.")

You might also ask your partner to spend more time in foreplay. After menopause, it simply takes longer for a woman to become aroused and to lubricate sufficiently for painless entry. Slow down, and ask your partner to slow down. What's the rush?

Menstruation

If you see no reason to abstain from sex during menstruation, well, you've got plenty of company. Lots of couples think that's as ripe a time as any (especially if she's one of those women who are especially randy then). But if you just don't feel comfortable making love during that time of month, relax. Millions of other people feel the same way.

One of the most common objections is that it's messy, but if you both feel the urge, that's not an insoluble problem. Consider "that time of month" as a time for experimenting with making love in the shower, for example, or having an erotic encounter that doesn't involve intercourse. Or the woman can try wearing a diaphragm to dam the flow and then taking it out after intercourse. (If the diaphragm is your only birth control method, though, you'll have to use another kind of contraceptive as backup. Normally, a diaphragm should be left in place for 6 to 8 hours after intercourse; removing it right away increases your risk of pregnancy.)

Weird Magic and Ancient Taboos

Fortunately, medical science has found that there's no "right" or "wrong" when it comes to having sexual intercourse during menstruation—even though many ancient traditions had strict taboos against it. The Old Testament, the Koran and the Torah all frown upon it. (Lev. 15:19: "And if a woman have issue, and her issue in her flesh be blood, she shall be put apart seven days: and whosoever toucheth her shall be unclean until the even.") Among some Orthodox Jews, this taboo is still observed—in fact, if a bride is menstruating on her wedding night, one old custom requires that a young girl accompany the couple to the wedding chamber, just to keep the lovers chaste.

Many primitive cultures also have taboos against sex during menstruation, perhaps arising from dark fears about the "uncleanness" or magical powers of a menstruating woman. One South African clan believes that having sex with a menstruating woman will make a man's bones soft; others believe it will "kill" his blood, darken his skin and dull his wits.

A Higher Risk of Infection?

Surely menstrual blood is no more magic than any other kind of blood. But there may actually be a little bit of wisdom behind these ancient taboos. Normally, as a protective mechanism against bacterial invasion, the vagina stays fairly acidic (pH of 3.5 to 4.0). But during menstruation, blood's higher alkalinity slightly reduces the vagina's acidity (to a pH of 5.0 or so), making it more susceptible to vaginal infections. Menstrual blood flow also flushes away some of the mucus that normally plugs the cervix, making it easier for microbes to invade the uterus and the deeper reproductive regions.

If neither partner is infected with anything, there's no reason to worry that making love during her period will increase the risk of infection, say Philip M. Sarrel, M.D., and Lorna Sarrel, codirectors of the Sex Counseling Program at Yale University. But if he already has an infection, the couple should abstain from sex during her period. (Serious vaginal infections generally make themselves known by itching, burning, an unpleasant odor or vaginal discharge; they should be seen by a doctor right away.)

If the woman is carrying around some minor-league vaginal infection, her mate also runs a small risk of picking up urethritis—a painful, although usually not serious, infection of the urethra, or urinary drainpipe. The most serious worry of all, though, is AIDS. Since having sex during menstruation directly exposes the male to potentially infected blood, if she is a carrier of the human immunodeficiency virus (HIV) she must *not* have sex during her period. (See "Safer Sex.")

You *Can* Get Pregnant

Another unsettling health risk of intercourse during menstruation is a surprise pregnancy. Although most people think a woman can't get pregnant while she's having her period, that's not precisely true. Women who have very regular periods, and ovulate precisely at the middle of the cycle, probably won't get pregnant if they make love at any time during their period, say the Sarrels. But women who have irregular periods may run some risk. For instance, if you have a shorter cycle one month, make love on the last day of your period and ovulate five days later, there's an outside chance you might get pregnant. That's because sperm can survive in the fallopian tubes for up to five days.

Does Menstruation Make You Merry?

There's been a long-running medical debate as to whether women are more interested in sex when they're having their periods. But although numerous studies have looked into the question, nobody has produced any convincing evidence that all or even most women feel this way. Some women *do* feel randiest during their periods, some women feel sexier shortly before or shortly after menstruation, and others say their erotic moods have more to do with wine and roses than waxing or waning fertility. William Masters, M.D., and Virginia Johnson, of the Masters and Johnson Institute in St. Louis, point out that from an evolutionary point of view, it would make sense that a woman feels sexiest when she's ovulating, because that's when she's most likely to get pregnant. (Among many animals, that's the *only* time females demonstrate any sexual interest.) But despite its compelling logic, the evidence just doesn't show that the majority of women are most interested in lovemaking at midcycle. Like almost everything else about human sexuality, the truth seems to be much quirkier, and more individualized, than that.

Isn't it wonderful?

Mystery

William Masters, M.D., surely one of the reigning masters of sex research, told an interviewer a few years ago: "No one really knows anything about sexual functioning. Really. This little thing we put out is embarrassing in that it doesn't even scratch the surface." (The "little thing" he was referring to was the massive tome *Human Sexual Response.*)

No one really knows anything about sex, Dr. Masters maintained. How the nervous system contributes to sexual arousal, he said, "is a totally blank field . . . no one has ever written anything about it." Little is known about what happens to the heart and lungs during sex, either. What, precisely, is a woman's orgasm? How do hormones orchestrate arousal? *Why* do we become aroused, sometimes even against our own wishes? Why do some people become homosexual? Is it true that some women ejaculate? Why? What makes men different from women? What makes them the same?

It's wonderful to know that despite an explosion of research on human sexuality—despite all the impudent electrical probes, the graphs and charts, reports and studies and symposia by the ton—our sexuality, in many ways, remains as mysterious as the moonlit sea.

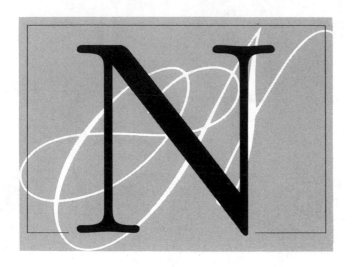

NOCTURNAL EMISSIONS

Nocturnal emissions, or wet dreams, are evidence of how deeply our sexuality is wired into us: Even while fast asleep, young boys often become so aroused that they ejaculate in their sheets. (About 40 percent of women, at least once in their lives, also have sex dreams so torrid they climax, but these are called nocturnal orgasms because, of course, women don't ejaculate.)

The late Dr. Alfred Kinsey found that 83 percent of men have nocturnal emissions at some time in their lives, with the highest incidence occurring during the late teens. About a quarter of 14-year-old boys and almost two-thirds of 17-year-olds wake up with sticky sheets about once every month or two (rarely more often than that) during this period of turbulent sexual awakening. Nocturnal emissions are, in fact, mainly a phenomenon of male adolescence—but they're not the *first* sign of sexual maturation. Usually, a boy will start having wet dreams a year or more after other adolescent changes have already begun taking place (like deepening voice, pubic hair and a sudden growth spurt).

Wet dreams gradually decrease in frequency during a man's twenties, with a few occurring after 30 and almost none after 40, Dr. Kinsey found. Still, he was able to document a couple of cases of men between 65 and 80 who still had an occasional wet dream—more evidence of the astounding range of human sexual "normalcy."

The modern explanation, advanced by William Masters, M.D., and Virginia Johnson, of the Masters and Johnson Institute in St. Louis, and others, is that nocturnal emissions simply provide a kind of physiologic safety valve for sexual tension. This view is apparently supported by the finding that it's mostly unmarried men who have wet dreams; after a man gets married (and presumably finds a steady, satisfying outlet for his carnal cravings), the wet dreams usually stop. The modern view also sounds a little more plausible (if less poetic) than the ancient Chinese explanation: Wet dreams, they believed, were caused by evil fox spirits, which change into beautiful women in order to rob men of their precious fluids in the night.

Braininess and Sex

One of Dr. Kinsey's most intriguing findings was that the brainier a man is (or at least, the better educated he is), the more prone he is to having nocturnal emissions. American men who went to college or were in the professions started having nocturnal emissions earlier in life than blue-collar workers, he found. They also continued to have wet dreams later in life and had them 10 to 12 times more frequently than their less-educated peers.

Why? It seems logical to conclude that more intelligent men are more imaginative and that they may be more accustomed to using their minds in an abstract way, including the practice of sexual visualization. Less-educated men, perhaps, are more inclined to need physical stimulation in order to become aroused to the point of ejaculation.

In general, nocturnal emissions are a form of human sexual behavior that religions have tended to treat rather more liberally than other, conscious sexual acts. In a sixth-century penitential, *Book of David,* nocturnal emissions were regarded as a kind of bush-league sin—as penance, boys were instructed to sing seven psalms in the morning and live on bread and water for one day. Some stuffy writers of the 1920s and 1930s, convinced that a child's religious duty included avoidance of wet dreams, suggested that children should attempt to control their thoughts before going to bed in order to prevent wet dreams or suggested that wet dreams could be controlled by the sort of pajamas children wore or the position they slept in.

But none of it seems to have done much good. Dr. Kinsey found that devout, church-going men had nocturnal emissions just as often as men who never went to church at all.

Norplant

Norplant, the newest birth control method approved for use in the United States, is in many ways a twenty-first-century contraceptive: It's safe, simple, long-lasting and virtually hassle-free. After one simple 15-minute procedure in a doctor's office, it takes care of your birth control worries for the next five years. It's amazingly effective—more effective, in fact, than any other birth control method except sterilization. But sterilization is permanent; Norplant is highly reversible. If you change your mind and decide you want to get pregnant, one 30-minute office procedure restores your fertility again almost immediately.

So what's not to love about it?

Well, like every other form of birth control, Norplant is not for everybody.

Some women may not be able to use it because of preexisting health problems, may be daunted by the idea of staying infertile for five whole years or (the biggest objection among teens) may shrink from the idea of bleeding between periods, one of the most common side effects.

On the other hand, "the typical satisfied user is an older woman who is sure she doesn't want kids for the next five years, who needs dependable, long-term contraception but isn't quite ready for sterilization yet," says nurse-midwife Linda Allen, of Planned Parenthood in Charlottesville, Virginia.

How It Works

Actually, although Norplant itself was approved for use in the United States only in late 1990, the technology behind it is not really new at all. It's only the delivery system that's new. The active ingredient is a synthetic female hormone called *levonorgestrel*—one of the active ingredients in many oral contraceptives in common use today. Instead of having to take a pill every day, though, a woman has six small capsules about the size of paper matches implanted just beneath the skin on the inner side of her upper arm—and that's that. The capsules, made of a type of silicone rubber called Silastic, diffuse the hormone into the bloodstream very slowly, maintaining levels that are high enough to prevent pregnancy for five years. (One other advantage: With Norplant, blood levels of hormone are kept at considerably lower levels than with most oral contraceptives.)

Implanting the capsules is quite simple. (Doctors prefer to do it toward the end of a woman's period, to make sure she isn't already pregnant.) A small incision (about ⅛ inch long) is made in the skin, and then the capsules are inserted in a fan-shaped array, so that they can all be removed through the same opening. You can't actually see the capsules once they're implanted, but you can feel them and sometimes see their outline on the surface of the skin. They shouldn't move around much at all, no matter how active you are. Taking them out is a little more involved and may take 30 minutes or more. If you want to keep using Norplant after your first five-year stint is up, a fresh set of implants can be inserted through the same incision.

Norplant seems to prevent pregnancy in much the same way oral contraceptives do, mainly by suppressing ovulation. It also thickens the mucous plug that keeps a lid on the cervix, making it more difficult for sperm to penetrate the uterus and tango with an egg. Norplant also suppresses development of the uterine lining—the endometrium—making it more difficult for the egg to become implanted in the uterine wall.

Excellent Track Record

According to various studies, the effectiveness rate of Norplant has ranged from 0.2 to 1.5 pregnancies per 100 woman-years. That means that, if a hundred women used Norplant for a year, 1.5 pregnancies, at most, would occur. (Actually, because the silicone capsule that is now used is thinner than the type used in the clinical trials, failure rates may be even lower. Oddly enough, though, some studies—although not all—have shown that Norplant's effectiveness rate decreases in women who weigh more than 150 pounds.)

By comparison, the effectiveness of the Pill is usually estimated at around 3 pregnancies per 100 woman-years, and condoms at around 12. Why does Norplant work so much better? One big reason: It's not "user dependent." In other words, you don't have to remember to do anything every time you want to make love, so human forgetfulness (and foolishness) is factored out of the equation.

Norplant and Norplant-2 (a newer version that requires two instead of six capsules but is effective for only three years) were developed and patented by the Population Council, an international nonprofit group. It's manufactured in Finland and is now licensed for use in 17 countries.

Costs vary, of course, but in Virginia, Planned Parenthood was recently charging $460 to insert the implants and $200 to remove them, and they recommend an annual exam costing up to $50 a year. Although Medicaid generally covers the cost, some women will undoubtedly find that a bit stiff.

The Up Side

Overall, about 80 percent of American women who get started on Norplant are still using it after a year, and after five years, 40 percent are still using it. By comparison, only half the women who get started on the Pill are still using it after a year.

Why? Because Norplant's advantages are many.

• You only have to make a single decision to get contraceptive protection that lasts five years.

• It's easily reversible. According to one study, half the women who had the capsules removed because they wanted to get pregnant had conceived within three months after the device was removed; 86 percent had conceived within a year.

• Many oral contraceptives contain estrogen, which can have unpleasant side effects in some women. Norplant doesn't contain any estrogen, so it's an alternative for the estrogen-sensitive.

• There seems to be no danger to babies conceived while their mothers are using Norplant. Follow-up studies on 15 such infants showed that all were normal.

• There are even a few unexpected door prizes to boot. Studies have shown that after a year of Norplant use, blood lipid and triglyceride levels decrease by 5 to 15 percent. Norplant increases the amount of hemoglobin in the blood and thus may offer some protection against anemia. Many Norplant users experience less menstrual cramping and pain. There's also some suggestion that Norplant may reduce the risk of endometrial cancer, just as the Pill does. (See "The Pill.")

The Downside

Of course, as with every other kind of birth control, Norplant does have some drawbacks.

• The thing Norplant users most often complain about is irregular menstrual bleeding. About 10 percent quit using Norplant during the first year for that reason.

Some women experience prolonged bleeding (that is, they bleed for more days than they normally would have, even though the total amount of blood lost is often smaller). Others may have bleeding or spotting between periods or may miss their period completely for a couple of months.

• About 5 to 20 percent of users get headaches, acne and a bit of discharge from the breasts. (The acne generally goes away once menstrual bleeding normalizes, which usually takes about a year).

• Unlike barrier contraceptives like condoms, a cervical cap or a diaphragm, Norplant doesn't provide any protection against sexually transmitted diseases.

• Because of preexisting health problems, some women shouldn't use Norplant. These include women with breast cancer, liver disease, unexplained vaginal bleeding or blood clots in the legs, lungs or eyes.

• Norplant's very newness could be a problem. It's been studied only since 1975, so—who knows?—it's possible there are long-term side effects that have not yet come to light.

This is a contraceptive option that's relatively new. If you're interested, discuss the pros and cons with your doctor.

NUDITY

Lots of parents worry that exposing their kids to casual nudity around the house, or allowing them to sleep in the parental bed, may have a disturbing impact on the child's sexual development. And over the years, a parade of psychoanalysts, child psychologists, therapists and other self-styled experts have stepped forward to offer advice to parents on the subject.

Freudians have suggested that kids exposed to parental nudity—even kids as young as six months to a year—might be terribly worried by the sexual fantasies and frustrations this evokes and perhaps even develop Oedipal problems as a result. (King Oedipus, of course, murdered his father and married his mother, and this conflict—where one parent is considered a potential lover, the other a rival—is thought to be a key phase of development among very young children, at least in Freudian theory.)

Other therapists have pointed out that if parents go to great lengths to cover themselves, children get the implicit message that there's something shameful about the body. And by repeatedly covering up some "forbidden" part of themselves, a parent may actually be calling greater attention to it—making the child obsessively curious about what's being hidden. If the parents were a bit more casual about nudity, they say, the child wouldn't be so interested. These therapists worry that by being *too* modest, parents communicate nothing but discomfort and anxiety about their sexuality, and this could lead to problems with adult sexual development when the children are grown.

A few other observers have expressed the opinion that, whatever your decision about nudity in front of the kids, the most important thing is that you feel comfortable about it. If you go out of your way to let your kids see you naked but you don't feel comfortable about it, the *discomfort* will be communicated to the kids. It's better to find your own—and your kids'—level of comfort, and let that be your guide, they say.

Don't Worry, Be Happy

The trouble with all these theories is that they're really nothing more than personal opinions, no matter how well adorned with footnotes. Until recently, there's been little attempt to provide any actual hard data on the subject.

One study, recently conducted at Old Dominion University, in Norfolk, Virginia, provides one of the first attempts to fill in the gaps. Psychologists Louis Janda, Ph.D., and Robin Lewis, Ph.D., asked 210 college students enrolled in a psychology course about their own exposure to parental nudity as children (up to 11 years old), how frequently they slept in their parents' bed as kids, about their parents' attitudes toward sex generally and about their own sexual development as adults.

Their conclusion: "The results suggest that childhood exposure to nudity and sleeping in the parental bed is not related to poor sexual adjustment. . . . Indeed, it appears that parents who have a casual attitude toward family nudity and who permit their children to sleep in their bed may have children with better self-esteem and who feel more comfortable with their sexuality."

Dr. Lewis and Dr. Janda go on to say, though, that exposure to nudity between the ages of 6 and 11 is "modestly related" to increased sexual activity later in life, for both girls and boys. Is that good or bad? Depends on how you look at it. These investigators favor the view that sexual behavior that's unburdened by guilt, anxiety or sexual dysfunction, even if it's sometimes a little freer than society generally condones, is probably a good thing. (We're not talking about wild promiscuity here; none of the students, no matter what their childhoods were like, said they were particularly inclined to having casual sexual encounters.) Other parents no doubt would feel differently and so might be more inclined to cover themselves up in front of the kids.

Despite the dire warnings of other experts, the psychologists also found that (especially for boys) sleeping in the family bed was related to greater self-esteem and less guilt and anxiety. In fact, every single student who spoke of it had positive recollections about relatively casual nudity around the house and about family bed-sharing. Said one: "It always gave me a feeling of security to know that if I had a bad dream I could crawl into bed with my mom and dad."

The psychologists go on to point out that it's not really nudity or bed-sharing, by themselves, that seems to lead to calm and happy sexual adjustment during adulthood—it's the whole attitude toward sexuality that permeates the household. "It seems," they say, "that the attitudes toward sex that the parents convey to their children may be more important to their subsequent sexual adjustment than any particular family practice."

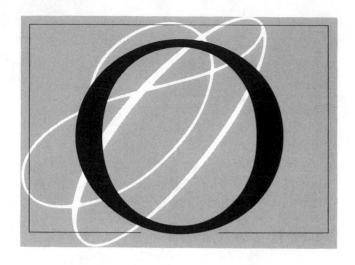

ORAL CONTRACEPTION.

See The Pill

ORAL SEX

People who have educated their tongues in the arts of love are overcoming a long-standing taboo in Western society. In Victorian times, oral/genital contact was considered so loathsome that in many states—even within the sanctity of marriage—it was illegal. Occasionally, somebody would actually be prosecuted for the crime of "copulation by mouth." (It's *still* illegal in some states, even today.)

In 1886, the unpleasant German psychiatrist Richard von Krafft-Ebing articulated the attitude of his times when he described a husband's "perverse impulse to commit cunnilingus" (mouth-to-vagina sex play). The good doctor seemed completely perplexed as to why anyone would even want to *do* such a thing: "These horrible sexual acts seem to be committed only by sensual men who have become satiated or impotent from excessive indulgence in a normal way."

Meanwhile, however, the average person (who had never even heard of Richard von Krafft-Ebing or his awful books) blithely blundered along, enjoying oral sex just because it seemed natural and felt good. Actually, the ordinary bloke was demonstrating a broader sense of culture than the eminent psychiatrist: There's evidence from ancient art and literature that oral sex has been practiced in almost every culture in history. The *Kama Sutra,* dating from the third or fourth century A.D., describes oral/genital contact in great and loving detail, devoting a whole chapter to fellatio (mouth-to-penis sex play). Tantric writings give elaborate, 12-part instructions for that particular rite of love, and ancient Peruvian pottery dwells on it with almost endless fascination.

It's Only Natural

Strictly speaking, of course, *oral sex* refers to any sexual contact involving the mouth, including kissing. Nor is it confined to humans. The late Dr. Alfred Kinsey observed that most mammals, when they're sexually aroused, will "make lip-to-lip contacts and tongue-to-tongue contacts and use their mouths to manipulate every part of the companion's body, including the genitalia." Among many animals, including horses and cows, this oral foreplay can go on for hours and hours before intercourse is even attempted.

Says Jude Cotter, Ph.D., a psychologist and sex therapist in private practice in Farmington Hills, Michigan: "We humans are mammals, and in all mammals, the male is very attendant to the vagina. He wants to see it, touch it, smell it, taste it—that's as true of humans as it is of horses, dogs or cats."

Back in the late 1940s, Dr. Kinsey made the interesting discovery that men from the higher social classes were more likely to indulge in oral sex—whether it was mouth kissing, breast kissing or cunnilingus—than those of the lower classes. Among married couples, he found that 60 percent of the men who'd been to college practiced oral/genital sex on their wives; among men who'd attended high school, only 20 percent did so, and only 11 percent of those who'd only attended grade school.

Thirty years later, surveys showed that these sweet enchantments of the mouth had escaped their confinement to the upper classes. In the mid-1970s, 100,000 women from a wide variety of social backgrounds responded to a sex survey in *Redbook* magazine. The overwhelming majority (almost 90 percent) said they gave or received oral/genital sex often or occasionally. And nearly all of them said they enjoyed it, either as an occasional spice or as a regular part of the menu of lovemaking.

The *Redbook* survey also revealed something else: "The women who had cunnilingus and fellatio the most often, and who enjoy it the most, are those who are most likely to say their sex lives and their marriages are excellent," observed social psychologists Carol Tavris, Ph.D., and Susan Sadd, Ph.D., who analyzed the survey results.

The Dissenting View

That's not to imply that in order to be sexually happy, you have to enjoy oral sex. (In fact, to self-righteously insist that your partner *must* favor you with oral sex is as boneheaded and dogmatic as anything Krafft-Ebing ever tried to cram down the throats of the masses.) It only means that the willingness to be sexually daring and imaginative seems to be strongly correlated with sexual happiness. The people who tend to like oral sex tend to be more deliciously uninhibited than those who don't. But not everybody likes it, including some people (male and female) who are sexually well adjusted in every other way.

"Although most studies show that 50 to 80 percent of women perform fellatio, only 35 to 65 percent find it pleasurable," reports June Reinisch, Ph.D., director of the Kinsey Institute, in her book *The Kinsey Institute New Report on Sex.* Sounds like a setup for trouble, and it is. Among the many complaints lovers have about each other, conflicts over oral sex (somebody wants it, somebody else doesn't want to give it) are among the most common. Dr. Kinsey even documented a few divorces that seemed to revolve around this question.

If your partner simply doesn't enjoy oral sex or is unwilling to give it cheerfully, you should respect that and not insist that he or she do so anyway. After all, coercive sex isn't even about sex; it's about power. And that's trouble.

On the other hand, sometimes people object to oral sex for reasons that are not entirely rational. Some people feel that it's unsanitary, for instance. But as long as you practice ordinary personal hygiene, "the truth is that there are more bacteria in the mouth than on the vagina or the penis," Dr. Cotter says. Women sometimes worry about the safety of swallowing semen. But a healthy man's semen is a harmless concoction of water, protein, fructose and minerals, and it isn't dangerous to your health. Although some people say spermicides have an unpleasant taste, it's not harmful to get them in your mouth, either.

Oral Sex and AIDS

A much more serious worry is the risk of contracting AIDS or some other sexually transmitted disease (STD) through oral sex. There's "plenty of clinical evidence" that many STDs can be transmitted via oral sex, including herpes, human papillomavirus (genital warts), gonorrhea, yeast infections and syphilis, according to Dr. Reinisch. Because the mucous membranes of the mouth are similar to the genitals, they make a safe haven for migrating microbes and pathogens, which is why STD specialists often routinely take a throat culture as well as a genital sample.

AIDS is the scariest risk, of course. If one of you is infected, the virus that causes AIDS (human immunodeficiency virus, or HIV) can be present in semen or vaginal secretions, and you must avoid any kind of direct contact with them. It's generally thought that the person *performing* oral sex is at higher risk, because he or she comes into contact with semen or vaginal fluids, and if there are cuts in the mouth, the virus can penetrate the body. The recipient, meanwhile, is only exposed to saliva (which is likely to have a far smaller concentration of the virus).

If you have reason to worry about your male partner, insist that he wear a condom during fellatio. And make sure that he puts it on well before he's fully aroused, because a few drops of preejaculate may escape from the penis well before full-blown ejaculation, and this clear, dewy fluid may also be infected. Women can lay a thin sheet of latex called a dental dam over their genitals and in this way protect their lover from direct contact with fluids. Dental dams (used to isolate infected parts of the mouth during dental work) are carried in many pharmacies now and sold on racks next to condoms. (See also "Safer Sex.")

Yes, it's true: All this talk of rubber paraphernalia is depressingly unsexy. Some people would just as soon skip the whole business rather than have to lick latex. But you might try using your imagination before giving up completely: You can simulate oral sex with an artful hand, lathered up with some silky lubricant. Or try silk. Try satin. Try feathers. . . . Just don't try anything foolish.

ORGASM

If you're quite convinced that you know what an orgasm is, consider this: Even researchers don't quite have a handle on it yet.

"Nobody has offered a universally acceptable explanation for what finally triggers orgasm," says Robert Birch, Ph.D., director of the Arlington Center for Marital and Sexual Concerns in Columbus, Ohio.

Studies that compared the well-known physiological part of orgasm (such as muscular contractions) with all those wonderful *feelings* people have during orgasm have found that the two don't necessarily correspond. A third of the women in one study confidently reported having had an orgasm, but monitors recording their physical responses showed they'd had no muscular contractions at all. The women were blissfully convinced they'd climaxed . . . but their bodies said they hadn't.

Even though it's now understood that orgasm is "a full body response," it still hasn't been clearly established where the sensations of female orgasm actually originate—in the clitoris, in the vagina, in the mind or all three. If it's centered in some deep, mysterious area of the genitals, then why can some women reach orgasm just by thinking sexy thoughts, without any physical stimulation at all? One sex researcher, after studying the matter for a decade, concluded wearily: "I think orgasm is a brain experience."

The whole process isn't really much clearer when it comes to men, either. Most men think orgasm and ejaculation are one and the same, but they're not; it's possible to have an orgasm and not ejaculate, although nobody understands quite how.

So which is it, the body or the mind? What *is* an orgasm, anyway?

The Sexual Response Cycle

The classic answer, drawn from the laboratory observations of William Masters, M.D., and Virginia Johnson, of the Masters and Johnson Institute in St. Louis, is that an orgasm represents the third stage of the sexual response cycle.

For a woman the first (excitation) phase is relatively slow—the muscles grow increasingly tense, the vagina begins to lubricate (normally, about 10 to 30 seconds after stimulation begins), its interior begins to dilate, and the clitoris and nipples begin to swell with dammed-up blood. Phase two (the plateau) is a continuation of this shivering buildup of tension—heart rate and respiration increase, the skin begins to flush, and the outer third of the vagina begins to swell dramatically.

All this comes to a dramatic climax at orgasm, when all that muscular tension and engorged blood are suddenly, ecstatically released.

A man goes through a similar, if much more visible, cycle. In the excitation phase, his muscles tense up, and his penis swells. In the plateau phase, his erection grows rigid. Then, just before ejaculation, there's a fleeting moment of *ejaculatory inevitability*—the feeling that he can't hold back any more. This is followed by a series of rapid muscular contractions (Masters and Johnson timed them at intervals of 0.8 seconds) that expels jets of semen out the urethra. After ejaculation, these muscles contract, less forcefully and more irregularly, a few more times. Women's orgasms are also accompanied by muscular contractions of the uterus (also at 0.8-second intervals) and of the outer third of the vagina—the so-called orgasmic platform. In men, and in some women, the sphincter muscles in the rectum also contract spasmodically during orgasm, right in sync with the genital contractions.

Vasocongestion—the damming-up of blood—produces the man's erection and causes the woman's labia to swell. Her uterus may also swell and, in some women, may actually double in size during arousal. The uterus returns to its normal size 10 to 20 minutes after orgasm triggers the release of all that trapped blood. If she *doesn't* climax, this return to normal takes far longer.

Focus on Feelings

The thing that's so wonderful about all this, of course, is the ephemeral *sensation* of orgasm. After all, you wouldn't be reading this book if sex amounted to nothing more than muscular tension and a temporary diversion of blood flow. Where do the feelings come from? Neurologists have discovered that during orgasm, there's a tremendous discharge of electrical energy in a deeply buried part of the brain called the limbic cortex—a crackling firestorm of activity similar to an epileptic seizure. The limbic cortex is the brain's pleasure center; rats will forgo food and sleep to press a bar that simulates sexual excitement by delivering a mild shock to this part of the brain.

It's also the part of the brain that controls awareness, according to Robert Heath, M.D., a neurologist at Tulane Medical School in New Orleans—which probably accounts for why people sometimes describe orgasm as if it were a journey into an alternate state of consciousness, complete with an almost psyche-delic warping of one's sense of time and space. The French call it *le petit mort* ("the little death")—a lovely allusion to that ineffable sense of having been transported to another, perhaps higher, realm.

Mysteries of the Female Orgasm

By comparison, a man's orgasm is a fairly straightforward affair. But after a century of debate and research, a woman's orgasm remains in many ways as mysterious as it ever was. It was Freud, of course, who insisted that only little girls and neurotic adult women reached orgasm by stimulation of the clitoris. Such immature, self-indulgent clitoral orgasms were to be put aside when a woman reached adulthood and she learned instead to respond only to vaginal orgasms produced by penile penetration.

This bit of Freudian blarney has been so thoroughly discounted that it's "far beyond the need for empirical disproof," according to Joseph LoPiccolo, Ph.D., a psychologist and sex therapist at the University of Missouri. Yet somehow it lingers on, attesting to the tenacious, sex-negative power of Freud on our culture—a wet blanket thrown over ten million beds.

The truth is that women experience orgasm in many different ways, and none of them is wrong. Many researchers believe that there's really only one kind of orgasm (triggered by stimulation of the clitoris, the centerpiece of sexual pleasure for most women). However, it can have many perceptual variations, depending on everything from wine and roses to the time of the month. For instance, the hormones estrogen and progesterone predominate at different times during the menstrual cycle, and since they cause the uterus to contract differently during arousal, they can also change a woman's experience of orgasm, according to Winnifred Cutler, Ph.D., cofounder of the Women's Wellness Center at the University of Pennsylvania Hospital in Philadelphia.

Other women insist that deep penetration of the vagina produces a "deep" orgasm that feels different from a clitoral orgasm. Still others say it's some indefinable blending of vaginal and clitoral stimulation that gets them to heaven. There are so many variations on the basic theme, in fact, that some sexologists have taken to using the term *orgasmic fingerprinting* to refer to each woman's unique and special experience during orgasm.

Faking It

Unfortunately, many women have trouble reaching orgasm consistently. Most recent studies have shown that about 10 percent of women are *preorgasmic,* meaning they've never experienced an orgasm at all. And at least 20 percent say they have orgasms only sometimes. Even love is no panacea: A University of Pittsburgh study found that 63 percent of women who said they were happily married had trouble reaching orgasm or becoming aroused.

Faking orgasm in order to make your partner feel good only makes the problem worse. For one thing, it incorrectly rewards him for doing the wrong thing, says sex therapist Lonnie Barbach, Ph.D., assistant clinical professor of medical psychology at the University of California, San Francisco, School of Medicine. Also, men are not as foolish as they may appear. If he knows you're faking it, he's inclined to grow more distrustful.

If you have trouble reaching orgasm, there are several things that may prove helpful.

One of the best ways for women to become orgasmic, sex experts say, is to practice conscious masturbation. Pay attention to your responses; try to learn precisely what it is that triggers orgasm for you, then carry this knowledge over to lovemaking with a partner. Masturbation is still a bit of a taboo in our culture, so you may have an inhibition to overcome. (One recent study showed that 40 percent of college-age women never do it). Nevertheless, a University of Iowa study, which reviewed 40 studies of treatments for inhibited orgasm, found that the most successful treatments involved the encouragement of masturbation.

Your partner may be able to help you achieve orgasm. Ask him to try the *coital alignment,* or riding high, technique, in which the man enters the woman from a higher angle, so that his pubic bone directly stimulates her clitoris by rocking up against it. At the same time, by avoiding deep thrusts, he can slow himself down long enough to satisfy her.

There are also a couple of good books for women who have trouble reaching orgasm: *For Each Other: Sharing Sexual Intimacy* and *For Yourself: The Fulfillment of Female Sexuality*, both by Dr. Barbach.

Multiple Orgasms: Can Men Learn How?

Once a woman does achieve orgasm, there's no stopping her. Masters and Johnson discovered lots of similarities between the sexual responses of men and women during arousal, but they also discovered one striking difference. Shortly after orgasm, men's erections wilt, and they quickly slip into a state of sexual unresponsiveness (the refractory period) that can last anywhere from a few minutes to a day or more. Women, on the other hand, are capable, at least in theory, of having a blissful succession of orgasms, one right after another. "The female has an infinitely greater capacity for sexual response than a man ever dreamed of," Dr. Masters once remarked.

Is it possible for men, like women, to become multiply orgasmic? Well, it appears that a few men already *are*. Both the late Dr. Alfred Kinsey and Masters and Johnson reported that a small percentage of men (most of them younger than 30) are able to climax repeatedly during a single sexual encounter. Out of the 5,000 men Dr. Kinsey interviewed, he found 380 who were endowed with this ability. "Very few adult males are able to reach more than 4 or 5 climaxes in any limited period of time," he wrote, "but an occasional teenage boy will reach 6 or more; and a quarter of the preadolescents for whom we have any record of orgasm were able to go beyond 5, and in some cases to as many as 10, 20 or more in a few hours' time." (On the other hand, teenage boys are notorious for exaggerating their sexual prowess, and Dr. Kinsey did draw his conclusions from interviews.)

More recently, a team of researchers took a closer look at 21 men whose partners confirmed they were multiply orgasmic. (Interestingly enough, most of these men were over 43, and 7 were 55 or older.) Their study disclosed that the men fell into two general groups. Thirteen of the men remembered having been multiply orgasmic ever since their first sexual encounter and long assumed *everybody* was like that. The other 8 men either had made the accidental discovery sometime later in life (including one skeet shooter who yelped "Doublee!"— the term for hitting two clay pigeons with a single blast—the first time he had a second orgasm) or had deliberately set out to teach themselves how to do so.

One of these self-taught lovers had learned the *squeeze technique* during sex therapy for premature ejaculation. Ten years later, he used the same technique to refine his control of ejaculation to the point where it was possible to repeatedly reach orgasm but not ejaculate. The squeeze technique involves masturbating to the very brink of ejaculation, then stopping, keeping the motionless hand firmly squeezed over the erect penis, then starting again and in this way learning ejaculatory control.

Some of the men used another technique, the researchers reported: Just before the moment of ejaculation, they stopped and deeply relaxed. At the same time, they clamped down with their pelvic muscles, as if they were shutting off the flow of urine (actually, a male Kegel exercise) in order to keep from ejaculating. It was during this moment of deep relaxation, while the ejaculation was being delayed, that the sensation of orgasm swept over them. Often the penis became so sensitive just after orgasm they had to either withdraw briefly or remain absolutely still before resuming thrusting. Then they'd build again to a peak of excitement and stop a second time, and so forth, sometimes achieving half a dozen or more orgasms at a time. (See also "Kegel Exercises.") Techniques for learning multiple orgasm are more fully described in a book called *Any Man Can,* by sex researchers William Hartman, M.D., and Marilyn Fithian.

Learning how to achieve multiple orgasms was not just some sort of sexual track-and-field event. The men all reported that they needed partners with whom they felt emotionally close, who were highly sensual, enjoyed prolonged lovemaking and kept signaling their continued interest. The goal, they all said, was not to have multiple orgasms but to have prolonged, enjoyable sex.

And one orgasm, sweetly achieved, is good enough for *that*.

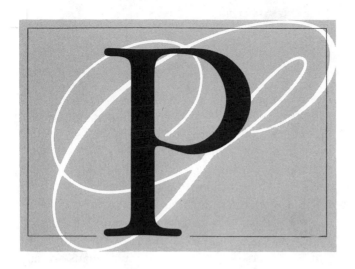

PAINFUL INTERCOURSE

It's not normal for a woman to have pain or discomfort during intercourse. Yet many women endure it, perhaps believing that painful sex is just the way things are supposed to be. Others blame themselves for some imagined sexual shortcoming. But self-blame, or stoic endurance, is not the answer.

"The first thing women need to be convinced of is that if intercourse hurts, there's something wrong," says Theresa Crenshaw, M.D., a specialist in sexual medicine and relationship therapy and past president of the American Association of Sex Educators, Counselors and Therapists.

Ten or 15 years ago, Dr. Crenshaw says, it was widely believed that when a woman experienced pain during intercourse, what was usually wrong was something in her mind—sex felt painful because she was filled with sexual guilt or anxiety, or repressed rage toward her partner, or something even more Freudian than that. But educated opinion has undergone a dramatic shift in recent years.

"We now know that there is almost always something *physically* wrong when a woman experiences painful intercourse—I would say, very conservatively, in at least 80 percent of cases," says Dr. Crenshaw. "There are often psychological problems surrounding the underlying physical problem, and there's no question that supportive psychotherapy can be helpful. But when a patient describes pain on penetration, you can almost always find a physical source if you look for it."

Consider that good news. Instead of having to wade into the deep realms of the psyche to find an answer and perhaps undergoing years of therapy, a woman may find that the whole problem is caused by something as simple (and treatable) as a herpes sore, a pelvic infection or even constipation. The important thing is to persist until you find an answer and get some satisfaction. Unfortunately, that may not always be easy.

"Women should be prepared for the fact that many physicians are not exactly at the crest of the scientific wave when it comes to dealing with dyspareunia [the scientific name for painful intercourse], and it may take considerable effort to find the correct diagnosis," says Dr. Crenshaw. "I would strongly recommend that women start by seeing a gynecologist, but if that doesn't help, they should continue to seek other professional opinion until they get a satisfactory answer. After all, your sex life is more important than your car, and if your car wasn't working you'd persist until you found somebody who could fix it."

One caution: If a physician recommends surgery (particularly if your pain is centered in the outer third of the vagina, rather than deeper inside), get a second or third opinion, Dr. Crenshaw says. Sometimes surgery is appropriate, but it also can simply make the problem worse.

Getting At the Cause

Part of the reason painful intercourse is so difficult to diagnose is that it's so often wrapped up in a disguise of psychosomatic (mind-caused) complaints. For instance, it's common for women with a history of painful intercourse to suffer from vaginismus, an involuntary spasm of the muscles surrounding the vagina that makes it difficult or impossible for a penis (or a tampon or anything else) to enter.

Vaginismus is "practically inevitable" if the pain persists for any length of time, even if the pain is actually caused by pelvic inflammatory disease (PID) or some other physical disorder, says Dr. Crenshaw. It's only natural: Vaginismus is the mind's way of protecting the body from pain, by slamming the vagina shut. Its message is: "That hurts, dummy, stop it!" (See "Vaginismus.")

But the main reason dyspareunia is so difficult to diagnose is that it can be caused by so many different conditions, ranging from minor infections to serious health problems like PID. In order to help your gynecologist get to the root of the problem as quickly as possible, Dr. Crenshaw says, it's important to pay close attention to the pain, noticing where and when it occurs, perhaps even keeping a little pain journal to help you remember.

Good questions to ask yourself: *When* does it happen—all during intercourse, or only intermittently? Does it change during intercourse? *Where* does it hurt—deep inside, or only around the vaginal entrance? Is it deep thrusting that hurts, or shallower strokes? If it's around the entrance, can you see anything (like a sore) around the painful spot? Does it occur during nonsexual activities like urination as well? If you have more than one partner, does it occur with all of them, or just one? Has this been going on for a long time, or did you first notice it recently?

It may be helpful, Dr. Crenshaw says, to try using some lubrication (like K-Y Jelly or the suppository Replens) and see if the pain remains. If not, it's likely that the problem has to do with lack of lubrication. In general, if there's some physical problem to blame, it's likely you'll feel pain under all different circumstances—with every partner, and during nonsexual activities as well.

Pain at the Vaginal Entrance

It's beyond the scope of this book to go into all the medical conditions that can cause painful intercourse, at least in any detail. What follows are brief descriptions of some of the most common causes, beginning with those generally associated with pain in the outer part of the vagina.

Yeast infections. These infections are one of the most common causes of burning and itching in the vagina. (See "Yeast Infections.")

Allergic reactions. It could be that your genital tissues are sore because of an allergic reaction to something you're using—a douche, a deodorant spray, a contraceptive foam, a bath soap or something else. If you suspect an allergic reaction, stop using the suspected product and see what happens.

Herpes sores. These typically produce sharp pain, and the sores are generally visible. The pain is likely to be intermittent, since it would only occur during flare-ups. (See "Herpes, Genital.")

Menopause. Whether naturally occurring or due to a hysterectomy, menopause may cause pain during intercourse because it leads to loss of naturally occurring vaginal lubrication. Try using Replens or another good commercial lubricant, or consider hormone replacement therapy. (See "Menopause" and "Hormone Replacement Therapy.")

Clitoral infections. Caused by an accumulation of smegma (a waxy secretion) under the fold of skin protecting the clitoris, these infections can cause painful irritation. The clitoris may also be painful because of rough handling by a partner.

Episiotomy scars. These scars can remain painful for months after childbirth and sometimes for even a year or more. (An episiotomy is a simple surgical procedure commonly done during labor to widen the vaginal opening and prevent tears in the surrounding tissue.)

Vulvar vestibulitis. This condition produces little wartlike lesions around the vaginal entrance. In about half of all cases, the warts go away by themselves within six months, according to Donald R. Ostergard, M.D., professor of obstetrics and gynecology at the University of California, Irvine. Some specialists feel that this syndrome may be associated with oral contraceptive use, so your doctor may recommend trying some other kind of birth control for a few months. Also, avoid irritating soaps, and try 1 percent hydrocortisone cream, available without prescription at your local pharmacy, Dr. Ostergard suggests. And be leery of surgery, which may only worsen the problem. If your doctor suggests surgery, get a second opinion.

Breastfeeding. Nursing mothers often complain that intercourse is painful. That's because breastfeeding releases a hormone called prolactin, which reduces estrogen levels in the body, thus thinning the walls of the vagina. Until the baby is weaned, trying using K-Y Jelly or some other commercial lubricant. (See "Pregnancy and Childbirth.")

Medication. Sometimes drug side effects may be involved. (See "Medications.")

Pain with Deep Penetration

If you feel the pain only with deep penetration of the vagina, other things may be to blame.

Constipation. One of the most common causes of pain during intercourse, and also one of the easiest to treat, is chronic or intermittent constipation, Dr. Crenshaw says. Typically, deep thrusting causes the most pain. Often the problem turns up in women with a retroverted, or "tipped," uterus, because such a condition tends to block the bowel. The solution: Using a stool softener, widely available in drugstores.

Arousal problems. Normally, during arousal, the inner two-thirds of the vagina opens up like a filling balloon, pulling the cervix up and out of harm's way. But when a woman is insufficiently aroused, the cervix stays in place and may get painfully battered by the penis during intercourse.

Pelvic inflammatory disease. An infection of the deeper reproductive system, PID is one of the most serious possibilities. Typically, dyspareunia caused by PID produces pain with deep thrusting. Lower abdominal pain is also a classic symptom of PID and is sometimes accompanied by spotting, cramping, painful urination or unusual vaginal bleeding. (See "Pelvic Inflammatory Disease.")

Mismatched Mates

Sex therapists sometimes forget that the word *dyspareunia* means "mismatched bedfellows," and it may be simply be that a woman's anatomy doesn't quite match her partner's, says Robert Birch, Ph.D., director of the Arlington Center for Marital and Sexual Concerns in Columbus, Ohio.

It's possible his penis is too large (either too long or too fat) to fit her vagina comfortably. If his penis is too long, Dr. Birch says, she can close her legs, creating an extra 2 inches for the penis.

More likely, though, it's his skill as a lover that needs some adjustment, not the size of his anatomy. The old saw "There are no frigid women, only clumsy men" applies. Quite often, Dr. Crenshaw says, the woman's partner simply needs to be more gentle and patient during foreplay, waiting until she's adequately lubricated before he attempts to enter her. In many cases, the woman finds intercourse painful because she can't get aroused (or hasn't gotten aroused by the time he enters her). Her lack of arousal may be caused by a variety of different things, but the result is the same: She's insufficiently lubricated, and it hurts.

He may not even know precisely where her clitoris is, or he may treat it too roughly. Sometimes if he keeps on thrusting after she's reached orgasm, she may lose her arousal, and her vagina may begin to dry. That can contribute to pain and irritation.

It may help to try intercourse positions that allow the woman a little more control (such as the woman-on-top or side-by-side positions). Let her be the one to control when she is ready for penetration and how deep or shallow the thrusting will be, Dr. Crenshaw suggests.

PELVIC INFLAMMATORY DISEASE

Pelvic inflammatory disease, or PID, is a general term for a genital infection that has spread into the deeper regions of a woman's reproductive anatomy—the uterus, fallopian tubes and/or ovaries. It's bad news—a serious, potentially life-threatening infection. It's also incredibly common. One in seven American women has been treated for PID, and about a million new cases occur annually, according to Guy Benrubi, M.D., associate professor in the Division of Gynecologic Oncology at the University of Florida at Jacksonville.

About 150 women a year die from PID, which is reason enough to take it seriously. But there's another worry, too: A bout with PID is known to greatly increase a woman's risk of becoming infertile. When invading bacteria penetrate the fallopian tubes, they often leave scars along the delicate inner lining, making it difficult (or impossible) for an egg to make its descent into the uterus, Dr. Benrubi explains. Occluded tubes also make it more difficult for voyaging sperm cells to make contact with a descending egg. The result is this terrible calculus: After one episode of PID, a woman's risk of becoming infertile is about 10 percent. After the second infection, it doubles, to 20 percent. If she gets it a third time, her risk soars to 55 percent. Overall, Dr. Benrubi estimates, PID causes somewhere between 125,000 and 500,000 new cases of infertility each year.

The other major worry about PID is that it increases a woman's risk of having an ectopic (tubal) pregnancy *sixfold*. The reason: Because the fallopian tube is often scarred by infection, the descending egg may get stuck and simply implant in the tubal wall. About 30,000 tubal pregnancies a year can be blamed on PID, Dr. Benrubi says. That's serious: Ectopic pregnancy, he says, "now accounts for approximately 15 percent of all maternal deaths and is rapidly becoming the most common cause of maternal mortality."

How to Avoid It

Suffice it to say that you want to avoid PID, if at all possible. The simplest way to reduce your risk: "Limit your number of sex partners, and know who you're sleeping with," Dr. Benrubi says.

That's because there's convincing evidence that having multiple sex partners increases a woman's risk of picking up one of the many microbes that can cause the disease. In one study, for instance, the number of hospitalizations for PID was three or four times higher among divorced and separated women (who are presumably more sexually adventurous) than among married women. And the peak incidence of PID is known to occur among women in their late teens and early twenties (a time of sexual experimentation and sometimes foolishness).

It also helps to use barrier contraceptives (such as condoms, a diaphragm or a cervical cap), which can offer some protection against the microbes that cause PID, Dr. Benrubi adds. You can increase your protection by also using a spermicidal cream or jelly.

Telltale Symptoms

PID can be caused by any one of a whole rogue's gallery of pathogens— *Neisseria gonorrhoeae* (the rascal that causes gonorrhea), *Chlamydia trachomatis* (the one that causes chlamydia), the ever-present *Escherichia coli* and a few other things. Back in the 1960s, the gonorrhea bug was the most common cause of PID, but today, the chlamydia bug is isolated in cervical cultures two to four times more often than the gonorrhea bug, according to Melvin G. Dodson, M.D., Ph.D., chairman of the Department of Obstetrics and Gynecology at Wright State University School of Medicine in Dayton, Ohio. Lots of times, more than one infectious agent is discovered, which is why treatment involves multiple, high-powered antibiotics (and often a hospital stay).

At least partly because it can be caused by so many different things, PID is notoriously difficult to diagnose. The symptoms may range from acute illness, with fever, lower abdominal pain and pelvic tenderness, to nothing but a little vaginal discharge. It's so difficult to identify that in one study, the diagnosis of PID made by trained gynecologists—who knew they were being studied—turned out to be incorrect 35 percent of the time. "All too often the diagnosis tends to be a dustbin for all sorts of nonspecific lower abdominal pain in young women," observes Dr. J. Malcolm Pearce, senior lecturer in obstetrics and gynecology at St. George's Hospital Medical School in London.

But here's the real kicker: In as many as a third of all cases, PID produces no symptoms at all. A woman may be walking around with an infection that's stealthily slipped into her uterus, without the slightest clue that it's there. As a precaution against such a sneak attack, Dr. Benrubi recommends that sexually active women be regularly checked for gonorrhea and chlamydia, the most common culprits. It's probably wise to add these additional tests to your annual checkup when you go in for a Pap test, he says.

Also, don't forget about your sex partner. If you're found to be infected, *he* needs to visit a clinic, too. In one study, partners of women with nonspecific PID had gonorrhea in 15 percent of cases and chlamydia in 12 percent of cases.

Additional Risks

A couple of other things can increase your risk of picking up PID.

IUD use. Among women who have more than one current sex partner, IUD use seems to increase risk. Although the mechanism is not fully understood, it's thought that the IUD's tail, which extends through the cervix into the vagina, may offer pathogens a route of entry into the uterus. The Food and Drug

Administration says IUD users have a three to five times greater risk of pelvic infection than nonusers, especially during the first few months after the IUD is inserted. Remember, though, that women who are in a mutually faithful, monogamous relationship are not thought to be at any additional risk. It's only women with more than one partner who seem to be at additional risk and should probably not use an IUD.

Douching. Too-frequent douching may increase the risk of PID, according to some recent studies. Nature keeps the vagina slightly acidic as a protective barrier against infection; but frequent douching alters its pH balance and makes it more prone to infectious invasion. In one multicenter study, a group of women with PID was compared with a group of women who were free of the disease. The researchers found that "those who douched three or more times per month were 3.6 times more likely than those who douched less than once per month to have confirmed pelvic inflammatory disease."

Miscarriage, an abortion, childbirth or cervical surgery. The cervix is the doorway to the uterus, and normally the door is closed. But certain things can partially open the door, making a woman especially vulnerable to PID. Be especially careful for a few months after these events.

The Pill: Possible Protection

On the other hand, it now appears that oral contraceptives offer *some* protection against PID. Women who use the Pill are less likely to develop the more severe forms of PID than those who don't—some studies have shown a 50 to 70 percent reduction in hospitalizations for women on the Pill, especially if she's been taking it more than a year. Several mechanisms have been suggested: The Pill decreases the amount of blood a woman loses each month, and menstrual blood encourages the growth of PID infections in some women. It also makes cervical mucus more difficult to penetrate, thus protecting the entrance to the uterus from invading pathogens.

PENIS

Even though the anatomy and function of the penis is as well understood as that of any other part of the body, "there is no organ about which more misinformation has been perpetrated," William Masters, M.D., and

Virginia Johnson, of the Masters and Johnson Institute in St. Louis, once observed. That amazing wad of flesh has been venerated in cults, reviled and misrepresented in folk legends and mutilated, decorated, hidden, exposed, adored and feared throughout the centuries.

Well, it's understandable. Unlike a woman's sexual anatomy, which is mostly hidden, the penis is about as blatant as you can get. It's kind of hard to ignore. Which is, perhaps, one reason people have come to believe so much nonsense about it.

Phallic Fallacies

In many cultures, it's believed that a man with a big nose, big hands or big feet also has an outsized penis. But it's not true. After comparing body size with penis size in 312 adult men, Masters and Johnson found almost no relationship at all between the two. In fact, they concluded, "the size of the penis has less constant relation to general physical development than that of any other organ of the body." In their study, the man with the most formidable penis (5.5 inches long when limp) stood 5 feet 7 inches and weighed 152 pounds. The man with the smallest one (2.3 inches when limp) was 5 feet 11 inches tall and weighed 178.

In cultures all over the world, people believe that the bigger a man's penis, the better able he'll be to satisfy a woman. (It's not only American men who tend to think this.) In fact, according to June Reinisch, Ph.D., director of the Kinsey Institute, the second most common reason men write the institute is about the size, shape or appearance of their penises. (Getting or keeping erections is number one.)

But for a couple of different reasons, sexual adequacy has almost nothing to do with penis size. For one thing, a variety of investigators have shown that while most limp (flaccid) penises may range from about 2.8 to about 5.6 inches long (measured from pubic bone to tip), erect penises don't differ nearly so much. A small penis swells proportionally more than a large one during erection. Masters and Johnson reported that one man whose flaccid penis measured a relatively modest 3.3 inches added 3.5 inches—more than doubling in size—when it was erect. Men with much larger penises did not increase nearly as much in size during erection. (In general, erections measure about 5 to 7 inches in length, they report.)

Why It Doesn't Matter

But more to the point, when it comes to pleasuring a woman, an enormously long penis is of no particular use. The most sensitive parts of a woman's sexual anatomy are the moist regions around the vaginal opening, including the clitoris, the labia and the outer third of the entrance; the deeper regions are poorly supplied with nerve endings and thus are fairly free of feeling. Being able to reach them with some epic organ is more or less useless. Besides, the vagina has been called an "organ of accommodation," which expands or contracts to suit virtually any size penis.

All of which comes down to this: Any number of studies have shown that while many men continue to be obsessed with the size of their penises, most women are wildly uninterested. When it comes to the physical attributes they value in a lover, women are much more interested in things like good muscle tone, white teeth or a nice rump than they are in penis size.

Large, Larger, Largest

At the risk of beating the subject into the ground, let's conclude the comparative math section by asking this age-old question: Is there any way to make a smallish penis bigger? The short answer: No. There are no muscles in the penis, so no amount of effort or exercise will change its size.

Just to clarify: There *are* muscles at the base of the penis that can be consciously flexed when a man has an erection, which briefly increases the erection's firmness. These same muscles also involuntarily contract during the expulsion of semen—making them somewhat odd, because they behave as both voluntary and involuntary muscles, according to Richard E. Berger, M.D., professor of urology at the University of Washington and coauthor of *BioPotency: A Guide to Sexual Success*. Still, the bottom line remains the same: Exercise does not a bigger penis make.

Dr. Reinisch sums it up neatly: "Not hypnosis, exercises, pills, creams, pumps, vitamins, injections or any other of the hundreds of products or services advertised in the backs of magazines or through direct mail will increase the size of the adult penis."

She adds this rather comforting observation, though: Some men may think their penises are smaller than their peers' simply because of the viewing angle. When you're peering down at it, your own equipment tends to look smaller than it would if viewed from the side (as one might glimpse a neighbor's in a public rest room).

Anatomy 101

Inside the penis are three long, narrow cylinders often described as being "spongy" because they're filled with sinuses, or cavities, that fill with blood during erection. Normally, they're limp and unassuming, like empty balloons, but during arousal, they fill with eight times the normal amount of blood and transform the penis utterly. Interestingly enough, humans are almost unique among primates in that they *don't* have a bone inside the penis. Penile bones (which apparently provide support for erections) are found among mammals in general, including shrews, hedgehogs, rodents, whales and bats. (For more, see "Ejaculation" and "Erection.")

Two of these cylinders, the corpora cavernosa, lie side by side along the top of the penis; the third, the corpus spongiosum, lies along the underside of the penis. All three of these expandable bodies are shrink-wrapped in an incredibly tough, fibrous coating called the tunica albuginea. In order for the penis to become rigid during erection, this wrapper must be unbroken; if there's a tear in it, the erection may veer off to one direction or the other. (Such tears, though rare, can usually be repaired by surgery.)

The urethra (the tiny pipe through which urine and semen pass) runs along the length of the penis. In order to keep you from urinating and ejaculating at the same time, the body has designed a clever valve system that closes off the neck of the bladder during ejaculation. The head of the penis, or glans, is the most exquisitely sensitive part of the penis because it's the most generously endowed with nerve endings. At birth, the glans is covered by a veil of skin (the foreskin, or prepuce). The inner surface of the foreskin contains glands that secret a lubricating fluid called smegma, which soothes the friction when the penis expands and retracts past its hood of skin. The foreskin is surgically removed during circumcision. (See "Circumcision.")

Perils of the Penis

Like every part of the body, the penis is heir to a few problems of its own.

Curvature. Lots of men have penises that list to the left or to the right— and there's nothing wrong with that, as long as it is not painful and doesn't interfere with lovemaking. But some men develop a condition called chordee (caused by the fact that the urethra is slightly shorter than the penis), which can result in severe, sometimes painful curvature. Chordee can usually be corrected surgically. A different type of curvature, which usually shows up after the age of 40, is caused by Peyronie's disease. (See "Peyronie's Disease.")

Hypospadias. About 1 in 300 boy babies is born with a condition called hypospadias, in which the urethra does not quite fuse together during fetal development. The result: Urine dribbles out somewhere down along the shaft of the penis, rather than from its tip. The physical deformity is usually relatively minor, but specialists say that if left unrepaired—or if it's repeatedly, badly repaired—the emotional damage can be great. Advances in microsurgery and pediatric anesthesia have made it possible to repair the deformity, with only overnight hospitalization, when the youngsters are less than one year old. If the operation is delayed until adulthood, the failure rate tends to be much higher.

Penis fracture. Believe it or not, it's actually possible (although difficult) to fracture a penis. This can happen only when the penis is erect and is rammed into an unyielding surface (like a woman's pubic bone during lovemaking, or even a bedpost or nightstand). Usually there's an unforgettable snapping sound, tremendous pain and swelling—sometimes the penis swells to three or four times its normal thickness.

Specialists say these terrifying symptoms are caused by damage to one or both of the corpora cavernosa and/or the tunica albuginea. You should swallow your pride and seek medical attention immediately; the damage can usually be surgically repaired.

Cancer. Cancer of the penis is quite rare—only about a thousand cases are reported nationwide every year. But it's very scary nonetheless: A quarter of these men die, and the rest may lose all or most of their penises. The good news: Penis cancer is almost invariably associated with poor hygiene, so all you have to do to protect yourself is keep your genitals clean. It occurs almost exclusively in men who haven't been circumcised, apparently because the intact foreskin tends to trap bacteria. But if you have no desire to be circumcised, simply take the trouble to wash yourself. In Sweden, where circumcision is rare but people tend to keep very clean, penile cancer rates are roughly the same as in the United States, where circumcision is common.

PERFORMANCE ANXIETY

Performance anxiety, one of the most common causes of sexual dysfunction, is an unpleasant demonstration of the negative power of the human mind. Men who begin to obsessively worry that they won't be able to get an erection, or whose minds are filled with memories of the last time they failed to get an erection, eventually *can't* get an erection. Likewise, women who worry excessively about being sexually responsive or who worry that they won't be passionate enough for their partner are apt to find that turning on turns into work. In either case, the person's fears, anxieties and self-doubts become so overwhelming they smother out everything else, even the powerful physiological impulses of sex.

Part of the problem is suggested by the very phrase *performance anxiety.* These people have come to see sex as a kind of performance, as if they were addressing the United Nations or playing in the World Series, rather than simply exchanging physical pleasure with another person. As if, instead of lying there in bed with their lover, they were surrounded by TV lights, crowds in the grandstands and the entire White House press corps. Once you start thinking of sex this way, it's only natural that you start worrying about "failure"—especially if you've "failed" in the past.

And it's only one more step to what William Masters, M.D., and Virginia Johnson, of the Masters and Johnson Institute in St. Louis, called "spectatoring"—mentally stepping outside yourself and watching your own performance. When you find a part of yourself sitting in the grandstands, watching yourself—almost as if there's a third person in the bed with you and your lover—you can't possibly be fully engaged in lovemaking. A part of you is looking down at the rest of you—judging, criticizing, even grading your every move. How could anybody really express themselves sexually, much less enjoy it, under such circumstances?

What Anxiety Does to Sex

The truth is that the anxiety produced by all this self-judging can be sexually devastating.

"When you're anxious, your hands get cold, and your palms get sweaty. That's caused by vasoconstriction—a narrowing of the blood vessels that supply circulation to the hands. Well, the same thing happens in the penis when you're anxious," explains Richard E. Berger, M.D., professor of urology at the University of Washington and coauthor of *BioPotency: A Guide to Sexual Success.* "But in order to get the blood flow required for an erection, what's required is *relaxation.*"

In performance anxiety, the mind has gotten in the way of the body. The trick is simply to get out of the way and let sex happen by itself. The body knows perfectly well what to do.

Instead, though, the typical man thinks of his penis as a tool, an object, that can be forced to work by sheer will, Dr. Berger says. After all, willpower and goal-orientedness are the way he accomplishes everything else in life, so why not sex? Unfortunately, the nerve pathways that trigger erections don't really work that way. You can't *will* an erection into being, no matter how hard you try.

All this may sound like a typically male conundrum, and it is. But not exclusively. "In today's world of equality, where everybody seems to be stressed-out and full of striving, women seem to suffer from performance anxiety as much as men," says Robert Birch, Ph.D., director of the Arlington Center for Marital and Sexual Concerns in Columbus, Ohio.

It may not be quite as obvious when a woman is overcome by sexual anxiety, but it can take all the joy out of sex just the same.

Forget Failure

Men or women who are truly troubled by performance anxiety may want to try short-term sex therapy. Basically, explains Dr. Berger, therapists do two things. First, they completely take the pressure off their clients by telling them to stop having sex for a while. And second, they teach them to relearn the gentle joys of physical sensation, without any pressure to reach the "goal" of orgasm or to score a perfect 10 on their performance. These sensate focus exercises are usually of gradually increasing intensity and spread out over a couple of months or so. Often they're highly effective. (See "Sex Therapy.")

At bottom, though, performance anxiety can perhaps be thought of as a paralyzing fear of failure. And overcoming *that* requires a whole change of heart. "In my view," says Dr. Birch, "one of the most important things is to learn the concept of 'fail-safe' sexuality—that there *is* no failure in a loving relationship."

PEYRONIE'S DISEASE

Peyronie's disease is a disorder in which the penis, when erect, is crooked. It looks normal when limp, but when it's rigid it may veer off to the left or the right, head for the sky or become erect only halfway up its length, making it painful, difficult or even impossible for a man to enter his lover's vagina. Over half the men with Peyronie's have enough trouble making love that it qualifies as a genuine sexual dysfunction. Nearly all find it terribly distressing— even "devastating," in the words of one urologist.

This odd, localized deformity is caused by patches of scarring, or fibrous plaque, on or around the spongy shafts (the corpora cavernosa) inside the penis that fill with blood during an erection. It's like "a long balloon trying to expand with a piece of tape on one side," explains Philip Hanno, M.D., chief of urology at the Philadelphia Veterans Administration Hospital. If the plaque is on top of these shafts, the erection bends back toward the belly; if it's on the left side, the erection veers to the left, and so forth. Peyronie's may also show up as a tight, constricting band around the shaft of the penis—as if the balloon had a tourniquet around its middle. There may also be spots along the penile shaft that seem to have lost their sensitivity.

It's not really known how common the disorder is (lots of men would probably rather suffer in silence than see a urologist about it, so nobody knows the numbers), but it's much more common than once thought. Urologists who specialize in male sexual problems probably see four to six men with Peyronie's a month, says Michael P. Small, M.D., clinical professor of urology at the University of Miami Medical School in Coral Gables, Florida.

Not All Curves Are Equal

Still, not *every* man with a curved penis has Peyronie's disease. Penises, like hands and faces, come in an astonishing variety of styles, and some simply have a bit of swoop in them. That's not a deformity; that's *you*. Curvature of the penis may also be caused by other conditions, such as a congenital disorder (usually not serious) called chordee.

But Peyronie's is different because it's not a lifelong condition, instead appearing fairly suddenly, usually when a man is in his fifties or sixties. Often it's painful (especially during the first six months or so). And usually, it produces scar tissue that can be felt. Generally, the plaque is on top of the penis and can be felt as a ridge or knot just beneath the skin there.

The only way to tell for sure if it's Peyronie's is to see a urologist or other specialist in sexual dysfunctions. Embarrassing as it may seem, it's often helpful if you bring along a snapshot of your erect penis to help the physician get a better fix on the problem. Then high-tech testing methods such as radiography or diagnostic ultrasound can be used to precisely pinpoint the location and extent of the scarring.

Enigmas of the Penis

Peyronie's disease, unfortunately, has pained and humiliated men for centuries (it was named after the physician to Louis XV of France), but it's still not very well understood. What causes the accursed plaques to form is simply unknown. And the course of the disease is also impossible to predict: About half the time, men mysteriously get better without any treatment at all. The pain gradually goes away, and then, over a period of several years, the bend straightens out all by itself—a spontaneous remission of the penis, so to speak. (This is why too-hasty reactions to a crooked erection, such as surgery, are usually unwise.) In other cases, it will simply stay the same or gradually get worse.

No Quick Fix

The good news about Peyronie's is that it's usually not terribly serious (except for the emotional distress it causes). The bad news is that it's not easily fixed. Any number of treatments have been tried over the past 200 years, but most of them are thought to be of questionable value. For one thing, it's almost impossible to tell what really works, since so many men get better if they do nothing at all. As one urologist points out, "Natural improvement is easily confused with therapeutic success."

Sometimes urologists have patients take vitamin E or aminobenzoate potassium (Potaba) to reduce the inflammation. Or they give patients radiation therapy, which softens the plaque and often helps the pain but doesn't improve the erection. Sometimes diathermy (heat treatments) is used. In another new treatment that's been used with some success, collagenase (an enzyme that breaks down collagen) is injected into the affected area to dissolve fibrous tissue.

Still, "none of these therapies has been notably successful," according to John Gregory, M.D., medical director of the Deaconess Institute for Sexual Medicine in St. Louis. "Their use is therefore difficult to justify except to demonstrate physician concern for the patient, while allowing time for the condition to stabilize."

The Nesbit Tuck

All of which seems like an awfully expensive and uncomfortable way to kill a little time. Still, if you and your urologist have waited long enough to become convinced that the problem is not going to go away by itself, you might consider surgery. Several new procedures have produced considerably more reliable results than vitamins or heat treatments.

In one such operation, called the Nesbit tuck, a diamond- or ellipsis-shaped patch of healthy tissue is removed from the normal side of the penis, and then the opening is sutured shut. This straightens out the erections, although it makes the penis a little shorter in the process. (For that reason, in cases of severe curvature, the procedure can't be used.) Still, says Dr. Gregory, the surgery is "highly successful in correcting curvature and rarely causes erectile impotence." A man's fear, anxiety and depression over all this *may* cause impotence, however—which is why most urologists like to team up with a sex therapist in such cases, to help ease the man through what is likely to be a rather unsettling experience.

THE PILL

In the first few years after the Pill was approved, it proved to be so effective, and so easy to use, that it was widely credited with touching off the sexual revolution. (Remember the sexual revolution of the 1960s?) The Pill was seen as the perfect no-muss, no-fuss solution to the messy problem of pregnancy: Just remember to take your teeny little pill, and you were worry-free.

Then, during the mid to late 1970s, a rash of reports suggested that oral contraceptives might increase a woman's risk of cardiovascular problems, high blood pressure, breast cancer, cervical cancer and a host of other frightening complications. The Pill's popularity plunged. Even today, although oral contraceptives provide virtually foolproof contraception to millions of women worldwide, plenty of women are still frightened of the Pill.

"But comparing the pill of today with those available in the 1970s is comparing apples to oranges," says Judith H. Seifer, Ph.D., R.N., clinical professor of psychiatry and obstetrics/gynecology at Wright State University School of Medicine in Dayton, Ohio. "The new pills are very, very safe. We see perhaps one-sixtieth of the health problems we used to see in women taking them. Oral contraceptives have been greatly refined over the years, and their potency has been vastly reduced. For young, sexually active women, they're the safest reversible form of birth control you can get."

It's true that there are some women who *shouldn't* take the Pill—mainly those who smoke and/or are over 35. Others who should not take the Pill include those with active liver disease and those with a history of breast cancer or migraine headaches. Still, experts say, the risks associated with the Pill are minimal. Risk factors that should be discussed with your doctor include smoking, obesity, diabetes, chronically high cholesterol levels and age. In fact, experts agree that for younger, nonsmoking women, using the Pill is safer than not using any birth control at all (since childbirth itself poses a significant risk to your health).

Most studies show that for every 100 women taking the Pill for a year, there will be two or three pregnancies—one of the highest effectiveness rates for any form of birth control except permanent sterilization (tubal ligation). But don't forget that these estimates are for *typical use* (meaning she makes lots of mistakes). One classic scenario: A woman decides to go off the Pill, doesn't have a backup contraceptive like condoms handy, makes love anyway and—bingo! Baby. This is a very real problem, because studies show that more than 50 percent of women who start using the Pill quit within the first year. So if you plan to quit, have a backup birth control method handy. On the other hand, if you're very, very careful and remember to take every single tablet, oral contraceptives can have an effectiveness rate of one pregnancy per 1,000 women. In other words, they're practically foolproof.

Power and Perils of the Pill

Oral contraceptives prevent pregnancy by sending chemical messages to the reproductive system. Those messages are varied and complex—suppress ovulation, make it difficult for sperm to get through, change the lining of the uterus so a fertilized egg can't implant. But they all translate into one clear message that comes through loud and clear: "Pregnancy prohibited." These chemical messages are sent in the form of synthetic versions of the sex hormones estrogen and progesterone.

But like every other form of birth control, the Pill is not perfect. One big advantage, though, is that so much is known about its shortcomings. In fact, since it was first introduced, no single pharmacologic agent has received as much scientific scrutiny. Researchers have studied the Pill from a wide variety of angles.

Cardiovascular problems. Early studies suggested that women on the Pill were at roughly four times greater risk of having a heart attack than women who were not taking it. But lower-dose versions and more careful studies have greatly changed this dire picture. The risk is somewhat greater in older women and those who smoke.

Breast cancer. There have been a fair number of studies that have suggested a link between the Pill and increased risk of breast cancer—and a fair number that have shown no increased risk at all.

"Everybody is confused," Dr. Seifer admits. "But what we do know is that you don't want to relentlessly stimulate breast tissue with estrogen. Estrogen stimulates breast tissue; that's why one of the first signs of pregnancy is breast tenderness. But progestin can oppose that—if anything, progestin-only pills offer *protection* against fibrocystic breast disease (which may or may not predispose a woman to breast cancer)."

Blood pressure. Oral contraceptives elevate blood pressure in many women, though the increase is usually mild and returns to normal a few weeks after the Pill is discontinued. In the Walnut Creek Contraceptive Drug Study, involving 11,672 women, oral contraceptives were linked to a pressure elevation of 6 points systolic and 1 to 2 points diastolic. In a British study involving 46,000 women, it was found that users were 2 to 2½ times more likely to develop high blood pressure than nonusers.

That's why it's important to have your blood pressure checked regularly when you're taking oral contraceptives. (This shouldn't be any problem, because most doctors won't give prescriptions for any longer than six months—partly so that you'll come in for a blood pressure check, Pap test, breast exam and pelvic exam.)

Cervical cancer. In one review of the medical literature, five studies demonstrated some link between Pill use and increased risk of cervical cancer, and seven studies found no increased risk.

"The evidence on cervical cancer is about as confusing as it is on breast cancer," Dr. Seifer says. "But I really think cervical cancer has more to do with lifestyle issues—like having many partners and unprotected sex—than it does with taking the Pill."

Danger Signs

One way to protect yourself, should problems ever develop while you're taking the Pill, is to memorize the following danger signs. If any of these ever occur, it's important that you see a doctor *immediately*.

- Severe abdominal pain
- Severe chest pain, shortness of breath
- Severe headache
- Dizziness, weakness or numbness
- Loss or blurring of vision, or speech problems
- Severe pain in the calf or thigh

Minor Worries

Along with the big worries, there are a handful of minor ones you're much more likely to encounter.

Mood changes, nausea, headaches, bleeding and breast tenderness. These are fairly common side effects. Some of this goes away with time, though. "One of the biggest problems we have is with impatience," says Dr. Seifer. "Women we've switched to the new low-dose pills will come in complaining that they've had a little bleeding and say, 'Can't you just give me the old pills back?' But the bleeding goes away in three to four months—you've just got to wait until your body gets used to it."

No protection. One of the biggest drawbacks of the Pill is that it doesn't offer any protection against sexually transmitted diseases (STDs). Barrier contraceptives, such as condoms or a diaphragm, create a physical barrier, or shield, that protects the cervix and uterus against AIDS, herpes and other STDs.

Many doctors recommend that young, sexually active women on the Pill *also* use condoms.

Reduced desire. Many women find that the Pill reduces their sex drive.

"One of the things we learned from the 1960s and 1970s was that the Pill has a cumulative effect on libido," says Dr. Seifer. "Often a woman would be on the Pill 12 to 18 months before she started losing her sex drive. We'd take her off, and it would be 10 to 12 months before she started feeling like herself again."

Today, though, with lower-dose oral contraceptives, explains Dr. Seifer, "in a young, sexually active woman who has no other libido problems, it's unlikely that the Pill will affect her sex drive at all."

New Choices

Back in the early 1970s, oral contraceptives contained up to ten times as much estrogen and progestin as those in use today. There's a lot of variation now, because more than 60 varieties are currently available. Some modern versions of the Pill now contain no estrogen at all. These progestin-only pills (sometimes called POPs, or *minipills*) were introduced about ten years after the original combination Pill, which contained both estrogen and progestin, and are slightly less effective than combination types. But they have special advantages, too.

"Women need to understand that it's the estrogen that causes the vasoconstriction and all the cardiovascular complications," explains Dr. Seifer. "Progestin-only pills don't affect the vascular system." Because they do not increase cardiovascular risk, minipills are especially suited for older women, who are at greatest risk of heart attacks and stroke.

One drawback: "Some women are progestin-sensitive; they cannot tolerate progestin," Dr. Seifer says. "They get cluster headaches, tend to feel bloated and irritable and have terrible PMS (premenstrual syndrome). But if you're one of those women who can't take a progestin-only pill, you'll generally know it within three to four months."

Added Benefits

Not all the side effects the Pill produces are negative, however.

In addition to their effectiveness as a birth control device, oral contraceptives have also been shown to have multiple, additional health benefits—a sort of unexpected bonus.

Oral contraceptives are known to decrease the risk of endometrial (uterine lining) and ovarian cancer and decrease the incidence of benign breast disease, endometriosis, pelvic inflammatory disease (PID) and PMS.

According to researchers, users of combined oral contraceptives have half the risk of ovarian or endometrial cancer, compared with women who've never used them. And in some studies, the Pill reduces a woman's risk of PID (a potentially serious infection of the deeper reproductive tract) by 50 to 70 percent, especially if she's been taking them for at least a year. Also, some women report milder, less crampy, more regular periods, lower incidence of ovarian cysts and fewer PMS symptoms.

The French Abortion Pill

Birth control pills are so effective at controlling female fertility that it was perhaps inevitable that someone would invent one that went beyond *preventing* pregnancy and could actually *terminate* a pregnancy that had already occurred. Such a pill, called RU486 by its promoters and the "abortion pill" by detractors, was developed a few years ago by French researcher Etienne-Emile Baulieu, Ph.D., a biochemist at the University of Paris–Sud School of Medicine.

The RU486 pill works by blocking the hormone progesterone, which prepares the uterus for implanting a fertilized egg. With the hormone blocked, the uterine lining does not thicken, so the tiny egg (smaller than the period at the end of this sentence) washes away during menstruation. The action of the RU486 is somewhat similar to that of the progestin-only minipill, except that it does all this within 10 hours—so that a woman who feared she might have gotten pregnant the night before could take it as a "morning after" pill. (It's also being tested in France as a once-a-month birth control pill.)

One Israeli study showed that when this pill is taken during the first f weeks of pregnancy, it induced complete abortion in 60 to 85 percent of ca When combined with drugs that stimulate uterine contractions, abortion are 95 to 99 percent. RU486 is controversial because it seems to muddy the line between contraception and abortion—and for that reason, it is still illegal in the United States.

Pregnancy AND CHILDBIRTH

The main point of sex (biologically speaking) is to make babies. But babies tend to have such a profound effect on a couple's love life—beginning months before they're even born—that some people think of pregnancy as the beginning of the end of sex.

Well, it's not really that bad. It's simply that once a baby is on its way, things are bound to change. You've just got to try a little harder to make a place in your life for sex, just as you've learned to make a place for the baby.

The changes often show up during pregnancy. Typically, it begins when the woman—fatigued, nauseous, her body reeling with hormonal riptides—starts to lose interest in sex. Her husband, meanwhile, is likely to be as randy as ever. In one 1991 study of 112 Swedish couples, 40 percent of the women said they experienced a lessening of sexual desire during the first and second trimesters of their pregnancies. By contrast, only 9 percent of the husbands reported a loss of desire during the first trimester, and only 17 percent during the second. It's a situation ripe for conflict.

"Communication is the key to defusing anger and resentment and establishing understanding, warmth and support" during this difficult time, says Susan Hetherington, Dr.P.H., a certified nurse-midwife and psychiatric nurse and professor in the Department of Psychiatric and Community Nursing at the University of Maryland School of Nursing at Baltimore. You've got to keep talking to each other—and touching, hugging and snuggling. "Couples shouldn't forget that intercourse isn't the only way of being sexual," she says. "Massaging, ching, oral sex and masturbation should all be considered an acceptable part ur sexual life."

Fortunately, nature seems to even the balance during the third trimester. In the Swedish study, *both* women and men (75 percent and 64 percent, respectively) reported losing interest in sex during the latter part of the pregnancy. Other studies have reported quite different patterns of change in the woman's (or the man's) sex drive during pregnancy. In fact, quite a few women say that sex during pregnancy was the best in their lives—at least partly because they didn't have to worry about getting pregnant, for once!

Go Ahead, Enjoy

Can having sex during pregnancy harm the baby in any way?

"If there are no problems in the pregnancy, there's absolutely no reason why couples should abstain from sex, even up to the very end of the third trimester," says Dr. Hetherington. "After all, pregnancy is not a disease, it's a normal event, and there's no evidence it's harmful to the fetus."

Studies have compared babies born to women who had sex throughout a pregnancy with those born to women who stopped having sex at some point during the pregnancy—and no significant difference was found in any measure of the baby's health, according to June Reinisch, Ph.D., director of the Kinsey Institute. Although one study in the late 1970s suggested that intercourse late in pregnancy might increase the risk of infections of the amniotic fluid and placenta, that study has been largely discredited, Dr. Hetherington says.

In fact, in some societies, female orgasm (which triggers the release of oxytocin, a hormone that stimulates uterine contractions) is used to help initiate childbirth. When a woman has reached full term and is ready to deliver, the midwife simply leaves her alone with her lover, and they have sex as a sweet little prelude to parenthood. (Women who have a history of premature deliveries are generally advised to abstain during the final phase of pregnancy, though, because sex could trigger birth prematurely.)

There are a few times when you *shouldn't* have sex during pregnancy, however. If there's vaginal bleeding or pain or leakage of amniotic fluid, you should abstain from sex and see your doctor immediately, says Dr. Hetherington. Leakage means that the woman's membranes may have ruptured and that delivery could be imminent. It also means that the barrier that protects the baby could be broken, leaving it vulnerable to infection.

What about Condoms?

Couples also sometimes worry that having sex might increase the risk of infecting the fetus with a sexually transmitted disease (STD). A pregnant woman should *never* have sex with anyone she knows or even suspects of being infected with an STD, such as syphilis, gonorrhea, herpes, genital warts or (of course) AIDS. If the mother became infected, it could have tragic effects on the baby— even if her own symptoms were relatively minor.

"But if a couple is mutually monogamous, and they're both disease-free, there's really no reason to worry," says Dr. Hetherington. Some doctors used to advise that couples wear condoms during pregnancy as a precaution against STDs, but that's really excessive, she says. All pregnant women who are getting competent prenatal care will be checked for syphilis, gonorrhea and other STDs (often twice).

After the Baby Arrives

After the baby arrives, couples are generally told to abstain from sex until the six-week checkup. But lots of people ignore this advice—studies have shown that 40 to 60 percent of couples don't wait that long to start making love again. How soon is it safe to start having sex after childbirth?

"If the woman didn't have an episiotomy [surgical expansion of the vagina] or a cesarean [abdominal delivery], it's okay to resume having sex almost immediately after childbirth, although there will be some vaginal discharge for a week or so. It's highly variable, and it's really up to the couple to decide," says Dr. Hetherington. "If there's been a cesarean, women can resume having sex within a week or two. Theoretically, an episiotomy is supposed to heal within three weeks, but I've found that some women still find sex painful after four months." Some studies, in fact, have shown that a year after childbirth, 16 percent of women who had vaginal deliveries with episiotomy still found intercourse painful.

Women who are breastfeeding also often complain that intercourse is painful. The reason: Breastfeeding reduces the body's levels of estrogen, which helps stimulate vaginal lubrication. This leaves the vagina dry and sensitive to the touch. The situation should improve once the baby is off the breast.

Back to Basics

For those first lovemaking sessions, it's important to go slowly and gently and to use plenty of lubrication. Lubricate the vagina and penis with a sterile, water-soluble gel, such as K-Y Jelly, to ease entry. It's also helpful if the man gently and slowly explores the vagina with his finger before entering, because this helps to relax the muscles, increases sexual stimulation and may ease her anxiety about pain.

One more thing: Remember to use some kind of birth control, unless you want kids spaced nine months apart. It's *not* true that a woman who's breastfeeding can't get pregnant. Breastfeeding does inhibit ovulation, thus making a woman less fertile. But shortly after she stops breastfeeding exclusively (sometimes giving the baby a bottle), ovulation begins again, Dr. Hetherington explains. The trouble is, you can never tell when the first ovulation occurs — waiting for a period doesn't work, because you may get pregnant and never have one at all.

It's also important to remember, if she's breastfeeding, that virtually everything she ingests can pass through her breast milk to the baby. That's why oral contraceptives are not recommended for breastfeeding women. (One exception: The minipill, which contains only progestin, is considered safe, Dr. Hetherington says.) Generally, barrier methods such as condoms with spermicidal foam or an IUD are recommended.

The First Year

Many couples don't really realize that the frequency of their sexual contact is likely to remain at a fairly low ebb for as much as a year or more after the baby arrives. In one University of Maryland study of 126 couples with newborns, at least 60 percent of them reported having intercourse "less" or "much less" often when they were interviewed a year after the baby's birth.

"The biggest problems are fatigue and discomfort," says Dr. Hetherington, "but if couples can find a place in their lives for sex — if they work hard to find time to be together when they're not tired, stressed-out and uncomfortable — these problems are solvable."

It helps to use your imagination and not focus so exclusively on intercourse, she says. Touching, kissing, snuggling, caressing — there are lots of delightful ways of communicating intimately without penis-in-vagina sex. You can also learn to incorporate masturbation into the whole sexual scenario. She can masturbate him, orally or by hand, if intercourse is too painful for her.

"Lots of couples have trouble accepting masturbation, but they need to give themselves permission for that," says Dr. Hetherington. "It's an important and useful method of finding sexual satisfaction, just another kind of sexual activity."

As to fatigue, there are solutions. Juggle your priorities, and see if you can afford some help around the house. The man needs to learn to help out with the housework as much as he's able, and the woman needs to learn not to criticize him when he doesn't do things the way she would.

And both of you should consider making love *after* a good night's sleep, not before.

Premature Ejaculation

Premature ejaculation (coming too quickly) is an amazingly common sexual problem for men. Fortunately, though, it's also one of the easiest ones to fix.

"For most sexual problems, I don't start seeing good results until after three months to a year of therapy," says sex therapist Shirley Zussman, Ed.D., a director of the Association for Male Sexual Dysfunction in New York City and former president of the American Association of Sex Educators, Counselors and Therapists. "But with a relatively uncomplicated problem like premature ejaculation, many therapists get good results — perhaps even taking care of the problem completely — within three months."

She's referring to weekly therapy sessions combined with at-home practice — but plenty of men have also overcome the problem by mastering the techniques described later in this chapter, without any help from a therapist at all.

What Does It Really Mean?

The term *premature ejaculation* sounds forbiddingly precise — as if you have it or you don't, like malaria. Actually, though, the term is so vague that therapists have argued for years over the correct definition. Some authorities say a man is a premature ejaculator if he's unable to keep his penis inside his lover's vagina during intercourse for a minute, or 1½ minutes, or 2 minutes (or whatever) before ejaculating. Or he's got it if he's unable to last a certain number of strokes (50 or 100, say) before ejaculating. Years ago, William Masters, M.D., and Virginia Johnson, of the Masters and Johnson Institute in St. Louis, suggested that a man has premature ejaculation if he reaches orgasm before his partner more than half the time.

Well, let's just throw all those definitions out the window. They're outdated anyway, and they cause more problems than they solve. (The late Dr. Alfred Kinsey reported that 75 percent of men ejaculate within 2 minutes of vaginal penetration — so by at least one of those definitions, only a quarter of men are "normal," which makes no real sense at all.) Premature ejaculation really just means you can't last as long as you'd like to; you don't have as much voluntary control over when you ejaculate as you wish you did. *Ejaculatory control* is a better way of talking and thinking about the problem, rather than setting up some arbitrary cutoff point that separates "normal" from "abnormal."

Rapid ejaculation is not *always* a problem, by the way. Some couples have simply learned to work around the man's hastiness. The woman may learn to reach orgasm a bit more quickly, to synchronize their love play. Or the man may become quite skillful at bringing her to orgasm without actually penetrating her, then go for it himself. People make all sorts of arrangements, and if both of you are sexually satisfied with your way of doing things, there's no real reason to change.

"Sometimes 'premature ejaculation' is a problem that's not a problem," says Robert Birch, Ph.D., director of the Arlington Center for Marital and Sexual Concerns in Columbus, Ohio. "If he pleasures her for a long time without penetration, until she reaches orgasm, and then he reaches orgasm himself, no matter how rapidly—so what? Where's the problem? There are many sexual concerns that don't have to be concerns."

What Causes It?

Still, many men and their partners view premature ejaculation as a problem. Most such men would really rather last longer than they do (and their lovers would likely agree). After all, who doesn't want to get more pleasure out of life?

The fundamental problem for men with premature ejaculation is that they've simply gotten into the *habit* of going directly from arousal to orgasm, without pausing to savor the sensations in between, explains Helen Singer Kaplan, M.D., Ph.D., founder of the Human Sexuality Program at New York Hospital–Cornell Medical Center, in her excellent little book *How to Overcome Premature Ejaculation.* If sex were a ten-course meal, he goes straight for dessert, missing most of the feast in the process.

"For any number of reasons, premature ejaculators never develop a normal sense of what their genitals feel like when they are highly excited and about to come," Dr. Kaplan explains. "It is this sensory deficit that is the key to the cause and also to the cure of inadequate ejaculatory control."

Often this pattern gets started early, when he learns to masturbate in the bathroom in 30 seconds flat for fear of getting caught. Or he learns to make love in the back seat of the old Chevy, or on the sofa at his girlfriend's parents' house. Because he's frightened or feels guilty or ashamed, he rushes through the experience and never really becomes familiar with full-blown, extended, erotic feelings. Rapid ejaculation becomes a *learned* behavior, a habit, which simply has to be unlearned.

By contrast, a man who's learned to control his responses can linger over the feast of sex, enjoying the sensations of full-blown arousal without having to ejaculate before he (or she) is ready. He can dally at the plateau stage of sexual arousal until his lover is satisfied, or he can push on through to orgasm and ejaculate. It's pretty much up to him.

What Doesn't Cause Premature Ejaculation

So that's all premature ejaculation is: a bad habit. It's not a dread disease or a Freudian complex. (Studies have shown that long-term psychotherapy has a dismal record of success in treating the problem.) Rapid ejaculation has nothing to do with whether or not you're circumcised, either.

Among a study group of 312 men, Masters and Johnson reported, virtually all of them accepted as "biological fact" the notion that uncircumcised men are better able to control their ejaculations because the highly sensitive glans (head of the penis) is swaddled in foreskin. But it's not true. When they tested the sensitivity of the glans in both circumcised and uncircumcised men, Masters and Johnson could find no significant difference. Besides, they point out, even if a man is uncircumcised, his foreskin will usually pull back and expose the glans to direct stimulation during intercourse.

It's also extremely unlikely that premature ejaculation is caused by a physical problem, but if you're worried about this, you shouldn't hesitate to see a urologist. A few conditions (like a hormonal imbalance, prostate infection, urethritis or some nervous system disorder) might affect ejaculation. One clue that a physical ailment might be involved, according to Dr. Kaplan, is if the problem turned up recently, after years of normal ejaculation.

Learning Ejaculatory Control

Back in 1955, a urologist at Duke University Medical School named James Semans, M.D., announced a simple little technique for treating premature ejaculation (which he'd learned from a prostitute who later became a sexual surrogate). His findings were pretty much ignored at the time, but today they're the basis of successful treatments used by sex therapists all over the country. Basically, Dr. Semans's *stop/start* technique involved stimulating the penis almost to the point of ejaculation, then stopping; stimulating it again, then stopping; and repeating this until the man learned to control his ejaculations. Later, Masters and Johnson developed a variation called the *squeeze* technique: Instead of simply stopping, the area just below the head of the penis is squeezed just before the moment of ejaculation. Today, most therapists tend to favor the stop/start method because it's simpler and seems to work just as well, says Dr. Birch.

Whether you're learning the stop/start technique as a couple or alone, the first thing you need to do is relax. The underlying idea, after all, is to get comfortable with your sexual sensations, and you can't do that if you're tense. That's why trying *too hard* not to come—such as forcing yourself to think about car wrecks, or biting your tongue—often backfires. Not only does that make you even tenser, it's also just a way of *reducing* your sexual awareness; what you're trying to do is *expand* your sexual awareness.

When couples learn the stop/start technique, they begin by getting undressed and in bed, free from distractions. They kiss and caress until he's aroused. Then she takes his penis in her hand and begins stroking it. He is to concentrate on his arousal only, selfishly, and when he gets very close to "the point of no return" just moments before ejaculation, he asks her to stop. Then they wait a little while (perhaps 10 or 20 seconds, not too long) and start again. This whole process is repeated until the man has been brought almost to the point of ejaculation three or four times. A man trying the technique himself does basically the same thing during masturbation.

When they're first learning, therapists say, men will often go a little too far and ejaculate, or they'll lose their erection when they stop and be unable to get it back. Well, just relax. It's all right if that happens. Forgive yourself. Try again tomorrow, again attempting to work up to three or four near-ejaculations before you let yourself go.

In stage two, you work up to three or four near-ejaculations again, but this time using a wet hand or a lubricant. Wetness heightens the sensations, makes ejaculation harder to control and more closely resembles a vagina. Once this exquisite drill has been mastered, the man actually enters his lover's vagina when she's mounted on top of him. (Most men don't ejaculate as rapidly with the woman on top.) When he has a firm erection, she slips down on top of him. Then, holding her hips, he gently guides her body up and down, stopping when he nears ejaculation. Once he can last 5 minutes or so, he begins moving his own hips as well. Some couples also like to use the side-by-side position, which also tends to delay ejaculation.

In the final phase of learning ejaculatory control, instead of stopping just at the point of ejaculation, the man simply slows down. Or he may deeply penetrate his lover and rock from side to side or roll his hips, churning his erection about with a circular motion rather than thrusting in and out. This helps to sustain the pleasure before both partners are ready for the climax.

A couple of things to remember: Most therapists recommend that while you're learning these exercises, you abstain from any other kind of masturbation or intercourse. You're trying to learn a new way to make love, and doing it the old way will erase your newfound gains. Also, if you're going to try learning these techniques, you should do them for several weeks, three to five times a week, just as described here. Doing them haphazardly won't do you much good at all. And finally, you need to enlist the help of your lover.

"Our extensive clinical experience has taught us that it is virtually impossible to cure a premature ejaculator if his wife or girlfriend is uncooperative," observes Dr. Kaplan.

PRIAPISM

To some men, it might sound like a dream come true: a robust and throbbing erection that doesn't go away. In reality, though, prolonged erections are a medical emergency—and unless they're treated within 4 hours, they can result in permanent impotence.

Priapism, as this painfully embarrassing condition is called, was named after the Greek fertility god Priapus, who is often pictured as a grotesque little man with an enormous, erect phallus. Medically, the condition is defined as persistent, abnormal erections, accompanied by pain and tenderness (although the erection may or may not be painful at first; sometimes it only begins to hurt later).

Priapism occurs because of a drainage problem. For one reason or another, after the erectile chambers of the penis (corpora cavernosa) become engorged with blood during arousal, they fail to drain off and go limp. The veins, which act as penile drainpipes, fail to open, so blood stagnates in the cavernosa, and the erection stays rigid. This in turn leads to inflammation, swelling, fluid retention and eventually permanent damage to circulation in the penis.

A Multitude of Causes

A whole slew of things can cause priapism, but perhaps the most common one nowadays is self-injection therapy for impotence. In this new treatment, one or more drugs are injected directly into the penis, producing long-lasting erections within minutes. But in an estimated 3 to 7 percent of cases, the erections don't go away, requiring a midnight trip to a hospital emergency room or a urologist's office. (See "Erection Problems.")

Some other things that can cause prolonged erections include:

- Drug reactions caused by substances like testosterone, the antidepressant trazodone (Desyrel), the high blood pressure medicine hydralazine (Unipres), or the aphrodisiacs yohimbine or Spanish fly (cantharis).
- Physical injury to the penis or scrotum or ruptures of pelvic blood vessels or the urethra.
- Blood disorders such as sickle cell anemia or certain types of leukemia.
- Anesthesia during surgery. Sometimes men develop rigid erections to the point where it's impossible to continue unless the erection is deflated with drugs.
- Damage to the brain or spinal cord caused by diseases like multiple sclerosis, encephalitis, meningitis or epilepsy.

Don't Wait!

The most important thing to remember, if this ever happens to you: Stifle your pride and go get medical help within 4 hours. Because most men *don't* do this—waiting instead until the erection goes away—an estimated 50 percent of them become permanently impotent.

Once you find a doctor, he or she will probably put you to bed and apply ice packs to your erection to constrict blood vessels and reduce swelling. Then you'll probably get a shot of some erection-deflating drug. A variety of medications are now being used, including steroids, sedatives, female hormones and epinephrine or dopamine. A team of researchers from Georgia Baptist Medical Center in Atlanta recently reported that the safest, most effective drug for priapism they've found is an asthma medication called terbutaline. It can even be taken in pill form, as a preventive measure, for men who are prone to too much of a good thing, they report.

P ROPHYLACTIC.

See Condom

Prostate

Most men are so completely unaware of their prostate gland that they don't even know how to say its name. (It's often mispronounced "prostrate.") Generally, this obscure wad of tissue doesn't even enter male consciousness until it starts causing trouble sometime in late middle age.

The fact is, though, that most men are probably intimately familiar with sensations produced by their prostate—feelings about as far from pain and misery as you can get. In fact, there's an inexpressibly sweet moment 2 or 3 seconds before ejaculation in which the prostate plays a starring role.

In their studies of male sexual arousal, William Masters, M.D., and Virginia Johnson, of the Masters and Johnson Institute in St. Louis, reported that ejaculation actually consists of two stages. In the first, sometimes called *emission,* the prostate and several other related glands begin heaving with rhythmic contractions. Since the main function of the prostate is to manufacture some of the fluid in semen, the purpose of these contractions is to expel the juice into the base of the urethra in preparation for ejaculation—almost like loading a bullet into the chamber of a gun. It's these rhythmic contractions that produce the sensation of *ejaculatory inevitability* (the feeling that you're about to ejaculate and can't stop). A couple of seconds later, in the second stage of ejaculation, the gun is fired, and semen explodes out of the body.

Trouble Spot

So not everything about the prostate is bad. Even so, for most men, the doggone thing means nothing but trouble. Prostatitis (an infection of the prostate) can cause fever, painful urination, scrotal pain, even low back pain, and is one of the most common reasons men visit urologists. (If it's caused by bacteria, infection can generally be blasted out with antibiotics, but if it's chronic nonbacterial prostatitis—caused by God knows what—you'll just have to suffer until it goes away.)

Another problem with the prostate is that as a man ages, it tends to gradually swell in size. Nobody knows why. Normally, it's about the size of a walnut, but it can bulge up to the size of an orange. This condition, known as benign prostatic hypertrophy, or BPH, is such a widespread male experience that it may simply be a normal part of aging. By some estimates, three-quarters of all men over 50 have some of the symptoms of prostate enlargement.

Generally, BPH is more of a nuisance than a genuine health risk (the *benign* in BPH means that it's not cancerous). The main problem derives from the prostate's location. It's wrapped around the urethra (urinary exit pipe), right at the base of the bladder, like a fat little doughnut. When it swells, it begins gradually squeezing off the flow of urine, which is why the symptoms of an enlarged prostate usually involve urination. Typically, symptoms of BPH include having to urinate more frequently; weak, hesitant, interrupted or urgent urination; getting up in the night to urinate; or a feeling that you've not completely emptied your bladder when you're through.

Surgical Treatments

In about 10 percent of cases, the prostate swells so much that medical treatment is called for. One of the most common options is a surgical procedure called a transurethral resection of the prostate, or TUR, in which a tiny tube is slipped up through the penis to remove excess tissue. (In another variation, the prostate is reached through the abdomen.) The surgery is relatively painless, relatively simple and usually very effective at relieving symptoms. It's also incredibly common: TUR is one of the most often performed surgeries in men over 65, according to Michael Barry, M.D., a prostate researcher in the General Medicine Unit at Massachusetts General Hospital in Boston.

Even so, huge numbers of men suffering from BPH avoid going to a doctor, at least partly because they fear what the surgery might do to their sexual potency. What does it do? It's usually said that the risk of developing erection problems from TUR is relatively small.

In one study, most of the practicing urologists in the state of Maine allowed all their TUR patients to be interviewed 3, 6 and 12 months after the operation. Of the 318 patients involved, almost 80 percent said their symptoms were completely gone, or nearly so, after the surgery. But 5 percent of the men who'd had no trouble getting erections before the operation reported that they couldn't get one during the year afterward. Four percent of the men reported they now had trouble with urinary incontinence (uncontrolled release of urine). And most also reported retrograde ejaculation—meaning that semen, instead of being expelled from the body during ejaculation, backs up into the bladder, where it's harmlessly passed off in urine. (This minor sexual aberration isn't serious; it just takes a little getting used to, according to men who've had the operation.)

So the operation is not without a small degree of sexual risk. Still, don't forget that 70 percent of the men in this study were over 65, a time when potency is naturally declining. And the mind, as ever, plays a powerful role in sexual potency—if you *think* you're going to have trouble, there's a good chance you may.

The future may hold safer alternatives. One new drug called Proscar, developed by Merck Sharp and Dohme, improved urinary flow in more than half the 1,600 men with BPH who tried it—and caused impotence in only 3.5 percent of them, according to reports from clinical trials. The drug became available in 1992; ask your doctor if interested.

When It's Cancer

If men fear the sexual aftermath of surgery for BPH, they're terrified of what might happen after surgery for prostate cancer—the second most common kind of cancer in men, according to the American Cancer Society.

The problem is that the growth of these tumors is fueled by testosterone, almost as if male hormones were a nutrient for such cancers. Therefore, the basic goal of treatment is to eliminate or neutralize the action of male hormones. Since 90 percent of the body's testosterone is manufactured by the testicles, one treatment is castration. Usually this dramatically slows the growth of the tumor, but it may interfere with a man's sex drive or his ability to get an erection, according to Dr. Barry. (Not always, though: A small amount of testosterone is still supplied by the adrenal glands.) Other treatments involve a sort of chemical castration, in which synthetic female hormones are given in drug form.

If the cancer hasn't spread beyond the prostate itself, doctors may choose to surgically remove the gland in an operation called a prostatectomy. In the old days, this operation nearly always resulted in impotence, because it involved severing the nerves that control erection. Today, new surgical techniques leave men sexually potent 50 to 75 percent of the time, according to studies.

Another common treatment for localized prostate cancer is radiation therapy—blasting the whole prostate region (the groin) with radiation. In the medical literature, the incidence of impotence following radiation therapy ranges from 25 to 85 percent. One theory is that the radiation damages blood vessels in the region surrounding the prostate, causing them to gradually clog up and impede blood flow to the penis.

Part of the problem with external radiation therapy is that the whole region around the prostate, including healthy tissue, is blasted with radiation. But a different kind of radiation therapy, called brachytherapy, is both more precisely targeted and less damaging to potency in most men. Instead of exposing the whole area to radiation, several tiny pellets of radioactive iodine, smaller than grains of rice, are implanted directly into the prostate gland itself. The tumor takes almost all of the blast; little radiation escapes outside the prostate's tough shell. In one study at the University of California, Irvine, 40 of 41 patients who were sexually active prior to treatment were still able to have erections afterward.

Not every type of prostate cancer is suited to this type of treatment, experts say, but if preservation of sexual potency is high on your list of priorities, and the type and stage of the tumor is appropriate, it could prove to be a happy alternative indeed. It's certainly an option to discuss with your doctor.

Sex as a Cancer Preventive

As a final thought, consider this intriguing idea: Frequent ejaculations may help keep the prostate healthy and cancer-free. This can't be considered a *proven* idea; it's just a fascinating tidbit that turned up in the medical journal *Urology* a few years ago. A British urologist, Anjan K. Banerjee of the Manchester Royal Infirmary in Manchester, England, reported that he'd tested this hypothesis on a group of 423 men. They ranged in age from 60 to 80; 274 had prostate cancer, and 149 did not. Each of the men was asked to estimate his ejaculatory frequency per week (by intercourse or any other means) during the sexually active part of his life.

Result: The men who were disease-free reported ejaculating significantly more frequently than those who had cancer. For instance, 31 percent of the men without cancer reported ejaculating five to seven times a week, but only 13 percent of men with cancer said they were that sexually active. Reduced ejaculatory frequency appears to promote the development of this disease, Dr. Banerjee suggests, although what the connection may be, he confesses, is still unclear.

Still, if it's true, the treatment is certainly the most pleasant sort of medicine ever invented.

PUBERTY

Strictly speaking, puberty (from the Latin root *pubertas,* or "adulthood") means the age at which a person first becomes capable of sexual reproduction. For a boy, that means he can produce sperm, and for a girl, that her ovaries can produce eggs. The word also refers more generally to that turbulent time of life—usually two to four years long—when the secondary sex characteristics appear. Young girls begin to menstruate, and their breasts bud. Boys start shaving and develop the ability to ejaculate. For both, life gets a lot more complicated.

Child development specialists say that American girls usually pass through puberty sometime between the ages of 11 and 14. Boys usually go through it a little later, between about 12 and 16 or so. But kids often worry so much about whether or not their development is "normal" compared with their peers that it's important to remind them of one thing: Like almost everything else about human sexuality, the variation and range of "normal" is huge. A young girl may have full breasts and be menstruating regularly, while a classmate still has the body of a child—and both are perfectly normal. Also, there's no relationship between the age at which a youngster begins to menstruate or ejaculate and how well their sexual responses will develop later in life, according to sex educator Mary S. Calderone, M.D., a founder of the Sex Education and Information Council of the United States.

(The only real cause for worry: Girls who develop breasts before the age of 8, and boys whose testicles begin to enlarge before 9, may have a hormonal condition called *precocious puberty.* Pediatric endocrinologists have developed hormonal treatments that may help.)

What Happens to Girls

For girls, the passage through puberty begins with changes that are not visible at first: Her ovaries begin producing estrogen at rates eight to ten times higher than in childhood, touching off a host of other transformations. She begins to grow like a weed. The circles around her nipples noticeably darken, then her breasts begin to swell. Pubic hair appears, first fair and downy, then coarser, curlier and darker. Hormones rearrange the distribution of her body fat, sculpting wider hips and a narrower waist. Her voice may deepen slightly, and her sex drive begins to stir. Hair appears on her underarms. Internally, her vagina deepens, and the rest of her reproductive system awakens.

Some people think that puberty begins when a girl menstruates for the first time. In some cultures, joyous public celebrations herald this event as a young girl's entry into womanhood. Actually, though, menstruation generally comes fairly late in puberty's parade of life-changing events. Although the sequence of these changes may vary, most girls begin showing newly budded breasts 2 to 3 years before they have their first period, pubic hair appears 1½ to 2½ years before, and underarm hair appears about six months before the first period, according to Dr. Calderone.

In the United States, studies have shown, the average age of first menstruation is just under 13. But just because a girl has begun to menstruate doesn't necessarily mean she can get pregnant. It may be as much as a year or more after she begins menstruating that she begins to ovulate, an in-between period sometimes called *adolescent sterility.* (There are a few cases on record where a girl has begun ovulating *before* her first period.)

What Happens to Boys

For boys, the passage through puberty tends to come a little later and be a little rockier than the experience of girls. But even though boys' overt physical development lags about two years behind that of girls, their age at first ejaculation tends to be only about six months behind the age that girls have their first period, notes Dr. Calderone. In terms of their ability to reproduce, boys and girls are not all that far apart.

In boys, a great burst of growth is often the first sign of puberty. Then, as his testicles begin pouring out testosterone, pubic hair appears, gradually growing darker and curlier. A little while later, hair appears under his arms. Not long after the first coarse, curly pubic hair appears, boys generally have their first ejaculation. This may occur during masturbation, or it may be a wet dream, but either way, it's likely to be an astonishing and wonderful event. (Lots of small boys masturbate and reach orgasm, but it's not until now that they actually ejaculate semen.) In his survey of more than 5,000 men, the late Dr. Alfred Kinsey reported that age at first ejaculation ranged from 8 to 21. For 90 percent of boys, age at first ejaculation was between 11 and 15, he found, but most boys first ejaculated at around age 13.

As puberty continues, the boy's muscle mass and bone length increase. His shoulders broaden, his hips narrow. Facial hair appears. His larynx, or voice box, enlarges, deepening his voice. Eighty percent of boys have to suffer through the embarrassment of a temporary enlargement of the breasts, caused by a brief surge in his testicles' production of female sex hormones. (This is quite normal and goes away quickly.) His penis, testicles and scrotum grow noticeably larger, and his erections seem to develop a mind of their own, appearing spontaneously and for no apparent reason. His facial skin gets oilier, often causing acne (which tends to be worse in boys). At the same time, specialized sweat glands called the apocrine glands, located around the armpits and the groin, become more active. (Some researchers speculate that these glands produce special odors, or pheromones, that are part of a primitive sex-signaling system.)

Sex before Puberty

Puberty, in many ways, appears to be a young person's sexual awakening. Many adults feel that before the storms and transformations of adolescence, kids are almost completely innocent of sex (unless we tell them about it). But the past 40 or 50 years of sex research have demonstrated that this is simply not so. Sexuality does *not* begin at puberty. For most of us, sexuality begins not long after birth. It may even begin *before* birth. According to William Masters, M.D., the grand master of sex research, ultrasound scans have shown that boy babies in the womb sometimes have erections a few weeks before they're born. And girl babies may produce vaginal lubrication when they're only a few weeks old.

In Dr. Kinsey's sample, fully 70 percent of males reported having engaged in some sort of sex play before adolescence—typically masturbation, exhibiting the genitals or touching the genitals of another child. This sort of thing seems to be less common among girls, but even so, 14 percent of adult women recalled that sometime before adolescence, they'd experienced orgasm, through either masturbation or sex play with others.

In other words, we're sexual beings, almost from Day One. It may be comforting for parents to retreat into a soft-focus vision of childhood sexual innocence, but that's not doing anybody a favor. Kids are sexual, whether they've reached puberty or not. And honestly acknowledging that sexuality is the first step toward being a genuine help to them, once they hit the heavy seas of adolescence. (For help in learning to talk to your kids about sex, see "Birds and Bees.")

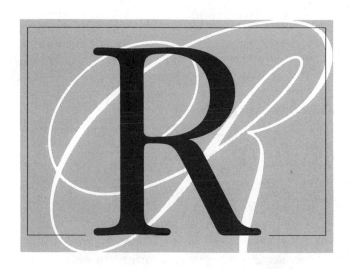

RHYTHM METHOD

The rhythm method of birth control is one of the oldest, most complicated and most unreliable methods of avoiding pregnancy. Basically, it involves figuring out the fertile days of a woman's menstrual cycle and avoiding intercourse during those times. Women can *usually* avoid getting pregnant by abstaining from unprotected vaginal intercourse for five to eight days before and three days after an egg is released from an ovary.

Actually, there's only one day or less during a woman's entire monthly cycle that the egg is properly positioned for fertilization by sperm. Usually, a woman's ovary releases an egg (an event called ovulation) about halfway between the first day of her period and the first day of her next period, give or take a couple of days. But sperm can survive in her reproductive tract for up to eight days before she ovulates. And the egg, once released, can survive for 24 hours or so. That's why you need that "safety zone" (no intercourse) for a few days before and a few days after ovulation.

Fertility Awareness Methods

The rhythm method is really one of a whole group of birth control strategies often lumped together under the general term *fertility awareness methods*. They're all ways of figuring out when a woman's fertile days occur—they just monitor different signals the woman's body gives off during those times. Many women use more than one method, because they're more reliable when used together. The body's little warning flags of fertility tend to confirm one another.

All these methods have their advantages. You don't have to buy anything, except perhaps a chart or a thermometer. They don't involve hormones or drugs. And they produce no side effects (except for the frequent mishaps and miscalculations that result in unwanted pregnancy), since they're "completely natural." In fact, since they involve such minimal intervention into the awesomely intricate process of conception, some religious groups that find other forms of contraception objectionable have no problem with fertility awareness methods. (Such methods are sometimes called *natural family planning*.) And finally, for people who are highly committed to the process, don't mind keeping careful records and have the will to abstain from sex when the woman's fertile, the method can be somewhat effective.

A Dose of Discipline

The disadvantages of fertility awareness methods are that all the methods require diligent record keeping, a rather daunting dose of self-discipline and the full cooperation of both partners. The heedless urge to make love does not always cooperate with the fertility charts, of course, and many couples sometimes just can't resist having sex during her "unsafe" days. (Experts at the World Health Organization say having unprotected sex during fertile periods probably accounts for more failures in the method than the inability to read fertility charts.) *Both* of you must agree to abstain from intercourse during the entire fertile period, or it won't work. One way to stay safe but spontaneous: Simply use condoms or some other form of birth control when she's fertile, or indulge in sex play that doesn't involve intercourse.

The bottom line, though, is that fertility awareness methods generally don't work very well, at least for most people. That's partly because the various signals a woman's body gives off during her fertile phase are not very precise and may vary considerably if she's ill, under stress or not getting enough sleep. Many women's menstrual cycles (and thus fertility) are just too irregular to predict with any degree of certainty. And of course—ah, love!—the flesh is weak.

As a result, some studies estimate that of 100 women using the rhythm method for a year, given typical patterns of use, about 20 will get pregnant. Other studies show failure rates as high as 40 percent! Even if they all used the method perfectly, with no foolishness and no mistakes, about 9 would get pregnant. By contrast, only about 3 would get pregnant if they were using the Pill or an IUD.

Finding Your Rhythm

The rhythm method is also sometimes called the calendar method, because it makes use of a calendar to track the history of a woman's periods. She begins by recording the length of her periods over six or eight months, to get a clear idea of her menstrual pattern and to determine the length of her longest and shortest cycles. Then, based on her past pattern, she predicts her future fertile days. The earliest day she's likely to be fertile is figured by subtracting 18 days from her shortest cycle. In other words, if her shortest cycle lasted 24 days, her first fertile day would be the sixth day after her period started. The last day on which she's likely to be fertile is determined by subtracting 11 days from her longest cycle. If her longest cycle is 31 days, the last day she's likely to be fertile is 20 days after her period begins.

Between these two dates, the couple needs to abstain from intercourse completely, use some other kind of birth control or get sexual in a more imaginative way than intercourse. For most couples, that means no intercourse for about ten days during the middle of the woman's cycle.

Tracking Your Temperature

The basal body temperature method is onerous in a different way: Every morning before she gets out of bed, a woman has to take her temperature and record it on a chart. That's because from the time the egg is released until she has her period, the body's temperature rises by a little less than 1°F—usually between 0.4° and 0.8°F. (The woman has to use a special thermometer that shows a range of only from 96° to 100°F, making it easier to identify such tiny temperature changes.)

This method, too, requires keeping records for about six months before actually putting it to use in order to figure out the pattern of ovulation and then predict when future ovulations will occur. By avoiding intercourse for seven days before her temperature is expected to rise and for the first three days *after* it rises, a woman can usually avoid getting pregnant. Some couples practice a stricter version of the method—no unprotected intercourse from the first day of her period until *four* days after her temperature has risen. This can dramatically increase the method's effectivness, according to Planned Parenthood.

Still, it's not terribly reliable. One study found that even when hormone tests clearly showed they'd ovulated, 6 out of 30 women had no elevation in their basal temperatures at all. The pattern can also be disrupted by illness, jet lag or interrupted sleep. The safest way to use the basal body temperature method for birth control, according to experts, is to avoid intercourse or use a backup method all through the first half of your cycle.

Monitoring Mucus

The cervical mucus method (also sometimes called the ovulation or Billings method) is a way of figuring out when a woman ovulates by studying changes in the consistency of her vaginal discharges, which are actually mucus produced by her cervix. The cervix is the doorway to the uterus, and it's through a tiny cervical opening called the os that sperm must pass in order to reach a waiting egg. (See "Cervix.") Normally, the cervical opening is blocked by a plug of mucus to protect the uterus from infection. For all of her menstrual cycle except for the few days when she's fertile, that mucus has a consistency often described as yellowish, thick, milky, white or cloudy. The vagina itself feels fairly dry.

But just before an egg is released, in response to an upsurge in estrogen, the consistency of the cervical mucus changes. It gets clear, slippery and elastic, almost like raw egg whites, so that it will stretch between your fingertips for a couple of inches or so. There's also more of it—a woman's vagina often feels wetter or more slippery when she's fertile.

By paying close attention to these changes, you can figure out your fertile days. You should avoid intercourse for a day before this clear, slippery mucus appears, all during the days your mucus has this consistency and for one day after your mucus changes, most experts say. Even so, the mucus method is probably the least reliable of all the fertility awareness methods described here. In one study, the failure rate after a year was almost 40 per 100 couples.

The preceding descriptions are all fairly brief and basic, and for a reason: If you're serious about using fertility awareness methods as your main form of birth control, you really need some professional instruction. It's best to ask your gynecologist or local family planning clinic about where you can get some help in learning how to use these methods. Clinics often offer free classes.

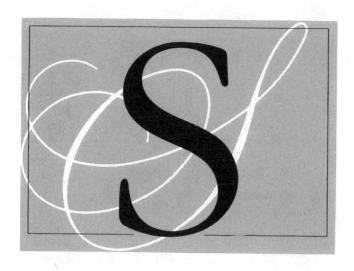

SAFER SEX

The sexual revolution of the 1960s and 1970s was nothing compared with the sexual revolution wrought by AIDS. It's changed the whole landscape of sex, perhaps forever—now "the kiss of death" is no longer a poetic metaphor but a terrifying possibility.

All is not bleak, however. Even though there's still no vaccine for the human immunodeficiency virus (HIV), which causes AIDS, and no cure for the disease itself, it's not that hard to *completely* shield yourself from the risk of becoming infected. HIV is actually quite difficult to catch. Despite its appallingly brilliant design, it's really very fragile. You can kill it instantly with a little household bleach, a bit of ordinary soap and water or vinegar. Outside the body, it dies very quickly.

You Can Block It

Almost the only way you can get AIDS is through *conscious actions* — in other words, things you can control. As former Surgeon General C. Everett Koop, M.D., Sc.D., has said: "Who you are has nothing to do with whether you are in danger of being infected with the AIDS virus. What matters is what you *do*."

Just to clarify: There are only four basic ways you can get AIDS: by using needles tainted with HIV-infected blood; through transfusions or other exposure to tainted blood or blood products; by fetal transmission, from a mother to a baby; and through unprotected sex. By far the most common mode of transmission is sex — AIDS is primarily a sexually transmitted disease (STD). And *you* are the one who controls your sexual behavior.

You simply cannot get it from casual, nonsexual contact. There's no evidence HIV has ever been transmitted by shaking hands, hugging, kissing on the cheek, crying, coughing or sneezing. You can't get it by *donating* blood. You can't get it from mosquitoes, dogs, cats, toilet seats, office furniture, pools or hot tubs. And in studies of families in which one member had AIDS, there's no evidence of transmission even though family members shared food, utensils, towels, cups, razors and toothbrushes and even kissed each other, according to the Surgeon General's Office.

A Deadly Turnabout

It's beyond the scope of this book to delve too deeply into the nature of the virus, its natural history or the available treatments for people who are HIV positive. Very briefly, though, once a person is infected, the virus enters the white blood cells, mainly those called T4 cells or T-helper cells (a part of the immune system), "rewrites" the cells' genetic blueprint and changes it to its *own* blueprint. In a deadly turnabout, the virus transforms these cells that were meant to protect the body into a factory for manufacturing more HIV. In this way, it can overwhelm the body's defenses with amazing speed.

Shortly after the initial infection, a person may experience a flulike illness (fever, swollen lymph nodes, aching joints or muscles, diarrhea). This is followed by a period in which they feel quite healthy but are probably contagious. During this period — usually from 2 to 12 weeks after infection — they will test positive for HIV antibodies in their blood. Often there's a period of latency, also during which the individual is contagious but shows no symptoms. This period sometimes lasts nine or ten years. Then the virus begins spreading like mad, and when it does, the immune system is rapidly devastated, laying the individual open to attack by conditions such as Kaposi's sarcoma (a rare skin cancer) or a certain type of pneumonia, *Pneumocystis carinii,* that has become one of the calling cards of AIDS.

Suffice it to say that everyone—especially people who are sexually active outside of stable, long-term relationships—needs to know the meaning of "safer sex."

Safer Sex Guidelines

These days doctors tend to say there *is* no safe sex, only safer sex. Here are the basics for protecting yourself from AIDS while you continue to enjoy the pleasures of a healthy sex life.

Avoid sex practices that involve sharing body fluids. Nearly all safer sex guidelines come down to this, the most important single bit of advice. That's because HIV is spread when blood, semen or vaginal secretions from somebody who's infected come into direct contact with the blood or bodily fluids of somebody who's *not* infected.

HIV concentrations are highest in semen, breast milk and blood, including menstrual blood, explains John G. Bartlett, M.D., director of the Infectious Diseases Division at Johns Hopkins Hospital in Baltimore and coauthor of *The Guide to Living with HIV Infection.* HIV has also been found, in much lower concentrations, in women's genital secretions, Dr. Barlett adds. It's sometimes found in saliva, in very low concentrations. And it has not been found at all in urine, sweat or feces.

Always use condoms. The best choice: lubricated latex condoms that are impregnated with the spermicide nonoxynol-9. Lambskin condoms may feel good, but they don't protect against HIV because they're perforated with microscopic holes large enough to allow HIV to pass through. When a condom is lubricated, it's protected against rips and tears and doesn't break as easily as an unlubricated one. And nonoxynol-9 has been shown—at least under laboratory conditions—to kill HIV on contact. Women now have another option, the female condom, marketed under the brand name Reality and available in drugstores for about $2 apiece. (For more, see "Condom.") But whatever kind of condoms you use, it's important to use them *consistently,* every time you make love, not just when you feel like it.

If you use a lubricant, make sure it's a water-based product, not an oil-based one. Oil-based lubricants cause latex to rapidly disintegrate into a gummy mess that offers no protection against AIDS (or pregnancy, for that matter). Contact with petroleum products destroys condoms. *Don't* use: Crisco, baby oil, cold cream, Vaseline or certain vaginal creams like Monistat, Premarin or Vagisil. *Do* use: K-Y Jelly, saliva, spermicidal creams or commercial lubricants like Astroglide, Lubraseptic or Lubafax.

When is it safe to *stop* using condoms in a relationship? That's the $64,000 question.

"If you've been in a mutually monogamous relationship for six months, and you've both been tested and are certain you're HIV negative, I'd say it's probably okay to stop using condoms," says Dr. Bartlett. "Of course, you still can't be *absolutely* certain you're safe."

Two possibilities why you can't be absolutely sure you're safe in such a relationship: The body develops antibodies to HIV (which is what the test measures) usually somewhere between two weeks and three months after exposure. You could have been tested *after* you were infected but before antibodies appeared (which means the test would have been negative). Or else one of you picked up the virus from somebody else after both of you were tested.

Use spermicides containing nonoxynol-9. This is the active ingredient in most spermicides sold in the United States. It's actually a mild detergent that destroys HIV by bursting its protein membrane. It also kills microbes that cause other STDs, including herpes, gonorrhea, syphilis and trichomoniasis. Generally, in fact, protecting yourself against AIDS with spermicide and condoms also protects you against a whole host of other STDs as an added bonus.

Beware of open sores. Open sores increase your risk. In order to infect a new host, the virus must somehow enter that person's bloodstream. Normally, intact, healthy skin provides a nearly insurmountable barrier against HIV, Dr. Bartlett says. Even if you get some infected blood or semen against your skin, this is "almost invariably safe." But if you have open sores on your genitals or in your mouth, the virus has a portal of entry directly into the bloodstream. Studies of homosexual men have shown that those with herpes, syphilis or chancroid (all STDs that produce open sores if untreated) are at greater risk of becoming infected with HIV than men who are free of genital ulcers. This is also why unprotected anal intercourse, which tears the lining of the rectum, is one of the riskiest of all sexual behaviors.

Can HIV penetrate the mucous lining of the vagina, rectum or mouth if there are no cuts or sores? The answer to this is not known, Dr. Bartlett says, because it's never been tested in humans (and, for ethical reasons, never will be). To protect yourself, whatever the answer: Use condoms.

Avoid high-risk practices. Being on the receiving end of unprotected anal intercourse is probably the riskiest sexual practice of all. (Don't forget, though, that *both* partners are at risk in anal intercourse.) Even using condoms is not entirely safe: With vaginal intercourse, about 1 in 100 condoms will break, but with anal intercourse, 10 in 100 will break, studies have found.

Worldwide, probably the most common mode of transmission is unprotected penis-in-vagina intercourse. Again: Don't do it without using spermicide and a condom.

Don't have unprotected sex with multiple partners, prostitutes or drug users. It's also unsafe to have sex with someone who has had sex with multiple partners, drug users or prostitutes. Unfortunately, although it's great to know the sexual history of your sex partner, the plain fact is that no area of life is more rife with secrets—and lies—than a person's sexual past. In one astounding study, 52 percent of sexually active HIV carriers admitted they had, at one time or another, concealed their illness from a sex partner. So just because a sex partner *tells* you he or she hasn't done anything risky doesn't mean you can believe it.

"When you ask people what they're doing to reduce their risk of getting AIDS, they often say, 'I'm being more careful about who I have sex with.' But this is really very little help, because you simply can't tell by looking at someone if they're infected," says Robert Kohmescher, deputy chief of mass media communication development at the Centers for Disease Control's National AIDS Information Education Program in Atlanta. "After all, how do you think people are getting infected? They're getting infected by having sex with people they think are *not* infected."

Things That Are *Possibly* Unsafe

There are a few more things to consider adding to your safer sex list.

Oral sex. There are no confirmed cases of HIV transmission solely through oral sex, but theoretically, it might be possible, experts say. The person *performing* oral sex is at greater risk, because he or she makes contact with semen or vaginal secretions. The other person is exposed only to saliva. Men should wear condoms when receiving oral sex, and women should wear dental dams over the vagina when receiving oral sex. (Dental dams are sheets of latex used by dentists, available without a prescription in drugstores and often displayed next to condoms.)

French kissing. The risk of HIV infection through kissing is "extraordinarily low," says Dr. Bartlett. For one thing, the virus has been found in saliva in only about 1 or 2 percent of people with HIV infection, and then only in very low concentrations. Also, researchers have shown that substances in saliva inhibit the growth and replication of HIV. Nevertheless, there are a number of reported cases of HIV infection through French kissing (wet kissing), according to Robert Kolodny, M.D., medical director of the Behavioral Medicine Institute in New Canaan, Connecticut.

If You're Worried, Get the Test

Are you worried that risky behavior in the past may have put you in danger?

It's easy enough to put all doubts to rest: Just get the test. Currently, the two most commonly used blood tests for antibodies to HIV (the ELISA and the Western blot test) are widely available in hospitals and clinics. At many clinics, the test is either free or very inexpensive. Since it takes weeks for HIV antibodies to appear in the blood after the initial exposure, some clinics recommend having a test three months after you think you may have been exposed and another test six months later.

For more information about transmission and prevention of AIDS and other STDs, for information about the site nearest you where you can be anonymously tested for AIDS or for treatment, support or written information, call the national AIDS hotline at 800-342-AIDS. For Spanish-speaking people, the number is 800-344-7432. For the hearing-impaired (using TTY/TDD technology), 800-243-7889.

SECOND HONEYMOON

An old German proverb makes this prophecy: "Marriage is fever in reverse—it starts with heat and ends with cold."

For some couples, the home fires just keep on burning, no matter how much time has gone by. But for others the dismal prophecy is all too true. What's the secret to keeping sex hot, even after years of marriage?

Despite all the talk about "safe sex," maybe there's something about sex that isn't always supposed to be safe. Camille Paglia, author of the book *Sexual Personae,* writes of the "dark, turbulent drama of sexual desire"—as if there's something in the very nature of our hunger for one another that's dangerous, wild, resistant to rationality. There's a certain sort of sex that's just one wild adrenal rush, with stuff getting knocked over and things busting apart at the seams—a few breathless moments stolen from death. (Remember?)

By contrast, the sort of sex we often settle for in marriage is mechanical, predictable and so safe it sometimes seems hardly worth the trouble. Boredom is death to sex.

That's why sex therapists almost invariably recommend breaking out of boring sexual routines. (Nobody's suggesting that you go seeking dangerous sex outside marriage; we're talking about keeping the sparks flying inside your *own* bedroom.) Try altering the pace, for instance. Go much faster than you usually go. Good sex doesn't always have to be lingeringly slow or even terribly considerate. Sometimes your partner may not mind if you just steal her daisy (or his) and run. (In a good relationship, your partner knows you'll come back later with a bouquet.)

"Try some sessions of nonintercourse sex, where foreplay is the main course, not just an appetizer," suggests Bernie Zilbergeld, Ph.D., a clinical psychologist in the Human Sexuality Program at the University of California, San Francisco, and author of *Male Sexuality.* "Or try some sessions where only one person gets all the goodies. Do it one time just for your partner. Then other times, she (or he) will do it all for you."

If you're always the aggressor, try letting yourself be seduced. If you're used to being seduced, try seducing. Or try *both* being aggressors, making love like lions.

Try All-Day Foreplay

"Always remember that good sex begins while your clothes are still on," say William Masters, M.D., and Virginia Johnson, of the Masters and Johnson Institute in St. Louis, and their collaborator Robert C. Kolodny, M.D. "Getting in the mood" is not just the few moments before sex; it can go on for hours, or days, beforehand. Since good sex is just one aspect of a good relationship, it's sweetest when it just grows naturally out of the time you spend together.

"The best sex times we ever have usually happen after hours and hours of talking," says one young businessman who's been married ten years. "Sometimes, usually it's Saturday, we're talking all day long. The whole day becomes a prelude to bed. If we take the time to reconnect, to really say hello again, after the madness of the work week, it just deepens the pleasure of sex."

Relocate Your Sex Play

Sleep specialists tell insomniacs never to read or watch TV or do anything else in bed except sleep. Eventually the bed becomes powerfully associated with the sensation of falling asleep. In the same way, beds can become powerfully associated with boring, predictable sex. So try getting out of the bedroom.

"I can't tell you how many people have fantasies of making love in the living room in front of a roaring fire but don't do it," says Dr. Zilbergeld. "It takes a little effort, but it's worth it. Even if you just do the same old thing, if you try it in a new location you'd be surprised how much it will add."

Think of yourself as a Hollywood location scout, looking over your whole house for promising stage sets. Kitchens are full of interesting things (remember Jack Nicholson and Jessica Lange on the kitchen table in *The Postman Always Rings Twice?*). Try the walk-in closet. Or the guest bedroom. Or the yard. Or the kids' tree house. Even the car.

Work on Newness

Address your mate from a new angle. For ideas, take a look at those classic how-to love manuals, the *Kama Sutra of Vatsyayana* or *The Perfumed Garden.* (Or just flip to "Sexual Positions" in this book.)

Most couples wind up making love at the same time, every time: after the lights are out and the kids are in bed. But that gets boring, and it probably isn't the greatest time to do it anyway, because both of you are usually exhausted. So try rescheduling the main event. Try the morning—get a babysitter to come Saturday morning at about 10, then lock the bedroom door and don't come out until you're ready. Or just skip the late news and go to bed a little earlier.

Some couples are badly in need of synchronized watches. By the time he's ready for bed, she's deep into REM sleep. By the time he's ready to face the day, she's gone. "You're going to have to agree to get up earlier, or go to bed later, in order to spend more time together between the sheets," suggests one sex therapist.

Therapists often recommend setting aside some time to be together when you're not stressed out, exhausted or trying to do two other things at once. (Yes, make a date with each other!)

Arrange to meet for a drink once a week at 8:30, after the kids are in bed, just to say hello for 15 minutes. You might be surprised how often these little scenes from a *New Yorker* cartoon turn into scenes from a different sort of magazine.

Warm Up the VCR

Generally, sex researchers say, men are more inclined to be aroused by visual stimuli (like sexy movies) than women are. But that's not to say that women don't also enjoy the occasional blue movie. In one popular magazine survey taken a couple of years ago, 85 percent of the respondents said they'd watched a sexy movie at least once, and almost half reported they watched them regularly. Watching a steamy movie at home together may lead to the most interesting sort of intermission.

It may be that one or both of you find hard-core erotica offensive. But there's softer, sweeter stuff available, if you take a bit of time to find it. (One source: The Sexuality Library, a California company that will mail you erotic films, for a variety of tastes, in a plain brown wrapper. They won't rent your name to anybody else, either. For a catalog of 300 videos and books, send $2 to The Sexuality Library, 1210 Valencia Street, San Francisco, CA 94110.)

Ask for What You Want

Communication is another key, say sex therapists. It helps to openly share sexual fantasies and intimate sexual feelings and desires with one's mate. It sounds easy, but most of us don't do it.

It's also important to keep up appearances. "One of the real keys to a satisfying, long-lasting sex life is taking pride in your appearance, keeping yourself up," says Dorothy Strauss, Ph.D., a sex therapist and associate clinical professor in the Department of Psychiatry at the Health Science Center of the State University of New York in Brooklyn. "Take your physical self seriously. Don't let yourself get sloppy." *You* notice when your mate starts getting a little seedy, putting on weight, padding around in a bathrobe all Saturday morning. Well, it works both ways.

SEMEN

The teaspoon of milky fluid that men ejaculate during orgasm is, for all the drama of its expulsion, mostly just packaging. All but a tiny dewdrop of it is a warm, sugary, protein-rich bath that's simply a transport vehicle for its most precious cargo: sperm. In a single ejaculation, the average healthy man expels anywhere from 120 million to 600 million sperm (enough, in theory, to repopulate the world in about two weeks). They're so tiny, though, that they make up only a wee fraction of semen's total volume. That's why, after a man has had a vasectomy (an operation in which the sperm ducts are severed), he won't notice any change in the amount of semen he ejaculates.

About 70 percent of the fluid in semen is produced by the seminal vesicles, a pair of saclike organs that empty into the urethra (the pipe through which urine and semen exit the body). The other 30 percent is a clear fluid manufactured by the prostate. Most men ejaculate 3 to 5 milliliters of semen each time they reach orgasm (5 milliliters being roughly a teaspoonful), but as a man gets older, the amount and the force with which it's expelled gradually diminish.

Frequent sex also diminishes semen volume, since it takes the body a few days to replenish its supply. In one Swedish study, 46 healthy, fertile men gave semen samples after one day, and then three days, of sexual abstinence. The researchers noted a "significant increase" in semen volume, as well as sperm counts, the longer these Nordic gentlemen managed to restrain themselves. (If you're having trouble getting your wife pregnant, try not trying quite so often.)

An Up-Close Look

Semen ranges in color from milky white to yellow to grayish. If it's pale red to dark brown, that's probably due to the presence of blood (a condition known as hematospermia). Usually this is not serious, and no particular cause is ever found. Still, it's important to have yourself checked by a urologist or other doctor, since blood in the semen may be a sign of infection or even prostate cancer.

Semen has an odor that's been compared to the sweet, malty smell of blossoms on a chestnut tree. When it's first expelled from the body, it's thick and sticky, but it gradually liquefies, then dries to a stiff crust. What *is* the stuff? Well, besides sperm, semen contains water, simple sugars (to provide fuel for sperm), alkalies (to buffer the acidity of the urethra and the vagina), prostaglandins (substances that cause contractions of the uterus and fallopian tubes and are thought to aid in sperm's passage to the womb), vitamin C, zinc, cholesterol and a few other things. Healthy semen, in other words, does not contain anything that's bad for your health. It's not fattening, either—an average man's ejaculate contains somewhere between 5 and 25 calories.

In the age of AIDS, it's important to remember something else about semen: Along with blood and vaginal secretions, it's one of the primary carriers of HIV, or human immunodeficiency virus, the virus that causes AIDS. (See "Safer Sex.")

Semen can also carry the organisms that cause gonorrhea, hepatitis B and chlamydia.

Semen Power

It's a tragedy of the modern age that semen has been linked to death, disease and early sorrow, because in many ancient cultures, it was venerated as a source of health, strength and long life. Among the Hindus and the Muslims of India, for instance, sexual chastity was greatly valued—not so much because it was morally virtuous but because unexpelled semen was believed to give men superhuman power, both physical and psychic. Although intercourse was justified for the purpose of having children, wasting semen was thought to be detrimental to one's health. These ideas grew out of the notion that one drop of semen was distilled from 80 drops of blood and stored in an organ in the head. To hoard this mysterious, nearly sacred "semen power," medicines were given to prevent nocturnal emissions, and masturbation was discouraged, observes anthropologist Edgar Gregersen, Ph.D., in his book *Sexual Practices.*

Among some Hindu, Jain and Buddhist sects, in fact, the devout were encouraged to practice a technique known as "nonspilling" (*askanda,* in Sanskrit) in which, even during intercourse, semen was preserved. These men learned to practice what Western medicine would consider a sexual dysfunction—retrograde ejaculation, in which semen is not expelled from the body but instead backs up into the bladder.

These ideas may seem charmingly quaint to us today, but perhaps a kind of primitive awe is in order. Semen is not *really* distilled from blood, of course. But this milky stuff—swarming with life in unimaginable numbers, ripe with life's mystery—really *is* magic.

SEX AND THE COMMON COLD

If you or your partner has a cold, the best way to avoid sharing it is to avoid all intimate contact. Trouble is, the average American adult has about two colds a year; the average parent with young kids in school has about six. Some winters, that could mean going without sex for months—and in the dismal gray light of February, that may be just too depressing to contemplate.

If you decide to have sex in spite of a cold, how likely is it that you'll both end up with it? Well, not as likely as you might think. For one thing, researchers say, a cold is most contagious for only about three days—from the moment you realize you've got one until roughly three days later. During that critical period, your body is shedding cold-causing viruses at such a furious rate that they're likely to spread. You also shed viruses for a few days before you start feeling bad and for up to three weeks after you feel great, but in such small quantities you're not usually a hazard to either your sex partner or your co-workers, researchers say.

Tip 1: Try to avoid intimate contact during the first three days of a cold.

Concerns about Kissing

Contrary to popular belief, it's harder to catch a cold by kissing somebody with the sniffles than it is by shaking hands. In one University of Wisconsin study, only 1 of 16 student volunteers who kissed other, cold-infected volunteers got sick. Other studies have demonstrated that it takes 1,000 times as much rhinovirus (one family of cold-causing viruses) to cause a cold if it's dripped onto the tongue rather than dabbed on the nasal passages. On the tongue, rhinoviruses tend to be swallowed and die a quiet death in the stomach. But the nose is the royal road to the upper respiratory passages, the favored habitat of colds. One caution: Adenoviruses (another kind of virus that causes colds) can be spread by mouth, but it's not known how frequently this occurs.

Yet another study found that about 40 percent of spouses passed the bug on to their mates. In fact, these researchers found that when one person in a family has a cold, *any* member of the family has about a 40 percent chance of getting it, too—which seems to suggest that sexual contact is not that significant a factor.

Tip 2: Just to be safe, keep face-to-face contact and wet kissing to a minimum.

Beware the Sneeze and the Handshake

Interestingly enough, despite the billions of colds the human race has suffered through, researchers still aren't completely sure how colds are usually transmitted. But most specialists now believe that the two most common modes of transmission are by hand contact and through the air.

Some researchers tend to favor the aerosol theory of transmission—sneezing can send a blast of rhinoviruses 3 feet or more. But two cold researchers at the University of Virginia School of Medicine in Charlottesville, Jack Gwaltney, M.D., and Owen Hendley, M.D., have convincingly demonstrated a sort of nose-to-hand-to-nose theory of transmission.

In one experiment, Dr. Gwaltney and Dr. Hendley had 15 college students lather their hands with the nasal secretions of people with colds, then touch their noses or eyes. Result: 11 of the 15 got a cold. By contrast, out of 12 students who just sat at a table with cold sufferers, only 1 got sick. Hence, this general theory: People with colds, whose hands are swarming with cold viruses from blowing their noses, touch a doorknob or another person's hand and in this way spread the virus to a fresh victim's hand. That person, in turn, gets infected when their hand travels to their own nose or eyes. (The researchers secretly observed doctors at conferences and noted that they touched their noses or eyes on average about once every 1½ hours.)

How to break this chain of transmission? In another experiment, Dr. Gwaltney and Dr. Hendley had mothers dip their hands in a dilute iodine solution—which kills rhinoviruses for up to 2 hours—when any family member got a cold. Result: They got sick less than half as often as mothers who didn't sterilize their hands. These research findings translate into a couple of simple ways for you and your sex partner to protect each other. When your partner has a cold, wash your hands frequently and try to keep your hands away from your nose and eyes. Remember to wash your hands (or, preferably, shower) after sex or other close contact.

To protect your mate when *you've* got a cold, always cover your mouth when you sneeze, and use *disposable* tissues rather than cloth handkerchiefs, which are rather like swaddling clothes for cold viruses (they can live for hours in there).

Chilling Out the Libido

About the only good news in all of this is that nature is on your side. When you've got a cold or the flu, you usually don't feel like having sex anyway, thus solving the whole problem. That's because part of the immune system's response to infection is a complex cascade of hormones that block appetite, sex drive and reproductive processes, according to Stanford University neuroendocrinologist Robert M. Sapolsky, Ph.D. It only stands to reason: When your body is doing battle with a viral invader, it needs to marshal all its resources for the fight, not waste them on trivialities like sensual pleasure. The body throttles back desire by reducing levels of circulating sex hormones, Dr. Sapolsky says, and if the illness lasts long enough, it even curtails sperm production and ovulation. (No sense making babies when you feel about as sexy as an old shoe.)

SEX THERAPY

One of the best things about sex therapy is that it's relatively short-term—it's not going to go on forever. Sex therapy is a form of relatively brief psychotherapy that's focused specifically on the sexual problem you and your mate are having—it's not about dredging up every childhood trauma you ever had, as might be the case with, say, Freudian psychoanalysis.

"If I'm treating a sexual problem that's occurring within a relatively intact marriage, treatment might take anywhere from 8 to 20 sessions," says Sallie Schumacher, Ph.D., a sex therapist in private practice in Winston-Salem, North Carolina. "Those sessions might be spaced out differently, and the total length of treatment varies depending on the problem, of course, but generally, it shouldn't last too terribly long. Most patients will see some noticeable progress after 3 or 4 sessions."

Other therapists say it's likely to take longer than that. Sex therapist Shirley Zussman, Ed.D., a director of the Association for Male Sexual Dysfunction in New York City and former president of the American Association of Sex Educators, Counselors and Therapists, says in her experience it generally takes a couple of months to a year to make significant progress. But compared with psychoanalysis, which may take one to three years or sometimes longer, even that is brief.

One other thing it's important to know: Sex therapy doesn't involve any actual sexual activity (at least not in the office). Generally, it usually involves an in-office talking session with a therapist every week or so, plus homework assignments. In some cases, the homework involves purely mental exercises, such as clarifying ideals and goals or reading a book. It may involve learning sexual techniques at home, such as sensate focus exercises—to help couples relearn how to enjoy leisurely, unpressured sex—or the stop/start technique—to deal with premature ejaculation. But all this is done in privacy, at home, so you don't have to worry about doing anything embarrassing in front of the therapist.

Short-Term, Long-Term

Couples or individuals come into sex therapy for a diverse array of sexual complaints, says Dr. Zussman, including erection problems (probably the most common problem), lack of orgasm, lack of desire, premature ejaculation, performance anxiety and marital conflict. But generally, she says, all sexual dysfunctions are thought to be caused by two general sorts of trouble: either immediate, short-term problems or more deep-seated, more intractable psychological difficulties. It's the shallower, more immediate problems that sex therapy is especially good at treating.

"In these cases, the therapist's job is to remove the inhibitions that are close to the surface and in the way, so the person's underlying sexual functioning can come through," says Dr. Zussman.

For instance, it's not uncommon to uncover a good deal of repressed rage in couples who are having trouble sexually. "When it's the man who's angry, his penis becomes an instrument of rage toward his partner, although he may be quite unaware of this," Dr. Zussman explains. In order for him to begin functioning sexually, the anger needs to be acknowledged and dealt with—and that's the role of sex therapy.

Sometimes, though, the trouble turns out to have a more deeply buried source, and these problems are more difficult to treat. The therapist may uncover a great fear of intimacy, for instance, or terrible guilt about sex, a strong inhibition against any kind of pleasure at all or a fear of abandonment. In some cases like this, she says, patients will be referred to another therapist for longer-term psychoanalysis. A man may have little interest in sex because he's deeply depressed, for instance, so he'll be treated for the underlying depression *first,* then come back for sex therapy focused on his erection problems (or whatever it may be).

Beyond Masters and Johnson

William Masters, M.D., and his former wife and collaborator, Virginia Johnson, were the earliest, and are still the most famous, pioneers of sex therapy. Beginning in 1959, they developed a therapeutic model in which couples would come to their clinic in St. Louis for two weeks of intensive therapy involving 14 separate sessions. Each couple would be treated by a pair of cotherapists, a man and a woman. Masters and Johnson reported very high success rates using this technique—but it's not without its drawbacks. For one thing, as a practical matter, it's much more expensive to hire two therapists than one. For another, Dr. Zussman points out, comparative studies have shown that working with a cotherapy team is not significantly more effective than working with a single therapist. Which is why, if you do decide to seek a therapist's help, it's likely only one will come to the door.

Setting Some Ground Rules

Most therapists say it's really best if you and your sex partner come to therapy *together.* (Masters and Johnson worked only with couples.) But sometimes that's just not possible, and there are many therapists who are willing to work with a single client.

"If it's possible, I like to see both partners, but I don't make that a requirement," says Dr. Schumacher. "I've found that once someone makes a change, it's almost as if other changes occur automatically. For instance, if two people are anxious and upset, and just one of them can learn not to be that way, it has a profound effect on the other."

Are there any other ground rules for successful sex therapy? That depends on the therapist. Dr. Zussman, for instance, will not treat a couple if either of them has an ongoing affair in progress. She won't see the girlfriend or boyfriend of a married client. And other therapists refuse to treat people if one is keeping a secret (an affair, bisexuality) from the other. The main ground rules, therapists say, are that you have the willingness to confront your problems, be honest about revealing them and be willing to change.

Helping Couples "Do Better"

Very early in the process—sometimes even before anything else is done—sex therapy patients will often be screened by a medical doctor to rule out any physical problems. This is particularly important if the man is having erection problems, which very often involve physical complications such as heart disease or diabetes. Some clinics have adopted a multidisciplinary approach to sex problems and may have urologists, gynecologists or other medical specialists on staff. (However, this is the exception rather than the rule.)

What sort of problems is sex therapy best able to treat successfully?

"Well, I've had 100 percent success in changing an unconsummated marriage, sometimes of long duration," reports Dr. Schumacher. "It's very rare that therapy can't help a woman reach orgasm. And premature ejaculation is not difficult to treat." But no matter what the problem, whether it's marital conflict, performance anxiety, stress or erection problems, therapy will probably help. "Overall, we can help almost all couples to do better sexually," says Dr. Schumacher. "Simply learning to talk about their problem, helping them to feel closer and learning about basic human sexuality can be therapeutic."

Finding a Good Therapist

Unfortunately, almost anybody can call themselves a sex therapist, because there's no single university degree, and no license, required to use that title. A sex therapist may turn out to be a psychiatrist or a psychologist, a medical doctor, a nurse, a counselor, a social worker or (sometimes) a fraud. That's why it's important to take care in locating a competent therapist who is qualified to help you.

One of the best ways: Get a referral from somebody you trust, preferably a physician or a psychologist. You might try contacting your local hospital; some hospitals have sex therapy clinics. A nearby university may have a sex clinic or a program for training therapists or may be able to refer you to a sex therapist near you. Or you can contact the American Association of Sex Educators, Counselors and Therapists, the only professional organization that certifies sex therapists. The association will also refer you to a certified therapist in your area. (Certification by the association means that the therapist has met certain educational and training requirements.) Contact them at 435 North Michigan Avenue, Suite 17171, Chicago, IL 60611-4067.

Once you do locate a therapist, advises Dr. Zussman, "you should ask very directly about their training and qualifications in sex therapy." Also, she adds, don't be afraid to ask how long it's going to take. Naturally, the therapist can't tell you *exactly* but should have a general idea about how long similar cases have taken in the past. Some skeptical patients may want to give sex therapy a limited trial—just attend a few sessions and see how it goes. There's nothing wrong with that, and in fact some therapists may even suggest it.

How much should it cost? Dr. Zussman says it's hard to find an experienced therapist in New York City who charges less than $125 an hour (which is also her rate). Dr. Schumacher, in North Carolina, charges $110, which is typical for her area. Fees at some sex clinics are on a sliding scale based on income, so that could take some of the sting out of the bill. And most health insurance policies that include mental health coverage do reimburse for sex therapy, Dr. Zussman adds. However, not all policies include mental health coverage—so check your policy to be sure.

SEXUAL AIDS

For sexual purists, sex toys and playthings may seem gimmicky, even a bit unfair. After all, isn't your lover's body (and your own) enough? Well, usually. Then again, you never know what you're missing until you try some of the many sexual aids currently available. Scented massage oils, or feathers, or a delicious little vibrator can expand your sexual repertoire in ways you might never have imagined.

Among sexual aids, vibrators are the old standby because they're so much fun. Some models (usually marketed as massage aids) can be strapped to the back of the hand and thereby transmit good vibrations via the fingertips to virtually any part of the body. This kind of vibrator is widely available in drugstores (and the cashier probably won't even raise an eyebrow when you buy one). More explicitly sexual vibrators, shaped like penises, torpedoes or even a pink plastic figurine with a long-eared rabbit on its back, may be battery powered or have an electric cord and sometimes come with a genuinely amazing assortment of attachments. They can be used for direct stimulation of the clitoris, penis or nipples (or wherever else you choose) or for vaginal penetration. These and other sex toys are available through these reasonably tasteful and discreet catalogs.

Good Vibrations. This is one division of a small California company owned and operated by women. It grew out of the experiences of sex therapist Joani Blank, who found that hundreds of her clients longed for a "clean, well-lighted place" in which to shop for sex toys and books. The company sells vibrators and other sexual playthings, which are mailed in the famous brown paper wrapper with Open Enterprises (the corporate name) as the return address. The company promises not to resell your name if you order something. For a catalog, send $4 to Good Vibrations, 1210 Valencia Street, San Francisco, CA 94110.

Eve's Garden. The proprietors of Eve's Garden describe their catalog as "a women's sexuality boutique." It lists sex toys, vibrators, massage oils, feathers, videos and other erotic playthings of special interest to women. For a copy, send $3 to Eve's Garden, 119 West 57th Street, Suite 420, New York, NY 10019.

The Xandria Collection. The Xandria catalog offers vibrators, stimulators, exotic lotions and lubricants, massage products, books and videos. Send $4 and a signed statement that you're over 21 to The Xandria Collection, 874 Dubuque Avenue, Department UTC, South San Francisco, CA 94080.

SEXUAL ETIQUETTE

Miss Manners can tell you which fork to use at a garden party or explain the elaborate protocol of weddings. But who's to explain the etiquette of sex? Pardon the presumption, but here's a rough sketch of an ethic of sexual decency—guidelines to ensure that we treat our lovers with kindness, decency, playfulness and pleasuring.

Remember the Golden Rule. "Do unto others as you would have them do unto you" works as well between the sheets as it does anywhere else.

Take the time to make yourself desirable. In longtime marriages, and even in longish relationships, lovers tend to let themselves go to seed without really sensing how unfair that it is to their partner. *You* notice when your partner comes to bed with face or legs covered with stubble, or without having showered, or with unbrushed teeth. Why shouldn't your partner notice when you do the same? You may *feel* desire, but if you don't take the trouble to make yourself desirable, is it really fair to ask for sex?

Ask for what you want. It's not fair or right to present yourself to a lover and say, in effect, "Here's my body—see if you can figure out what to do with it." For one thing, if you don't know how to ask for what you want, you're virtually guaranteed not to get it. For another, by not helping your partner satisfy you, you're setting him (or her) up for failure, touching off the tumble toward blame, anger and recrimination. If you have the strength and self-respect to ask, it will help your partner do the same.

Make sure that was a yes. You need to be sure that your partner has given full consent to sex. Sexual etiquette means nothing if it doesn't honor this basic sexual right. And consent is not something that's required only of college kids on a date. It's a question of propriety that applies to *any* sexual relationship, even a married one.

Take no for an answer. If your partner can't or won't give you what you want (oral sex, say), then it's unfair to bully or browbeat them into giving it anyway. To pressure a lover by withholding love, threatening them or making them feel unworthy constitutes a kind of sexual blackmail. Of course, a no may not always last forever. It's acceptable to ask again later, if you do so in a kind, undemanding way.

Take responsibility. You need to take responsibility for your own sexual needs and desires, accept them with reverence and gratitude—and let your partner know what they are.

Respect your partner's nakedness. "Where else are we as vulnerable as we are during sex?" asks Jude Cotter, Ph.D., psychologist and sex therapist in private practice in Farmington Hills, Michigan. "We are naked, physically and spiritually, and there's an obligation to be sensitive to that vulnerability."

During extended foreplay, air taken up into the vagina will sometimes escape in little farts the French call "love butterflies." A woman should feel comfortable letting fly a few butterflies in front of her lover, or saying or doing whatever else she wishes, without fear that such intimacies will later be violated. To violate the privacies that are shared during sex should be a crime. (It's not just spies who traffic in pillow talk.)

Remember to say thank you. If you thank the bagboy at the grocery store for helping you load the car, shouldn't you also always thank your lover for more important favors? (There are plenty of ways to say thank you, of course, and some of the nicest ones don't require words.)

Keep some things secret. What people say during orgasm, more lyrically known as "birdsong at morning," is private and should be kept secret. The Indians didn't keep parrots or mynah birds in their bedrooms because of how readily the birds picked up and repeated such privacies—so don't you do it, either.

SEXUAL POSITIONS

I have in this book shown how the husband, by varying the enjoyment of his wife, may live with her as with thirty-two different women, ever varying the enjoyment of her, and rendering satiety impossible.

— Twelfth-century sage Kalyana Malla
in *Ananga-Ranga,* an Indian love manual

The 32 different sexual positions described by Malla (which he calls, rather charmingly, "internal enjoyments") don't come close to covering all the possibilities. In fact, there's a long tradition—in sources as varied as old Sanskrit erotic literature, Ovid and the sex sages of ancient Arabia—of attempting to determine the total number of possible positions for human sexual intercourse. The potential is mind-boggling. One Indian sexologist counted an astounding 529, but that was mainly because he considered every tiny difference (like the angle of arms or legs) to be a completely new position.

Not that it really matters. The whole business of counting positions, sometimes called the "Kama Sutra fallacy," is about as useful a pastime as counting the dancing angels on the head of a pin. All that really matters is that we all tend to fall into boring sexual routines, and breaking out of them is nearly always a good idea.

The Missionary Position

There are probably a few stuffy people left who still believe that the missionary position (face-to-face, man on top) is the *only* right and true position for sexual intercourse, even though it's almost never practiced by animals and only rarely depicted in ancient erotic art. (The oldest known painting of human sexual intercourse, dating back to 3200 B.C. and found in the Ur excavations of Mesopotamia, shows a woman on top.) In some cultures, this position is considered positively outlandish. The Polish anthropologist Bronislaw Malinowski, Ph.D., once described how Trobriand Islanders, around the campfire, would mimic the position used by missionaries and thereby reduce their friends to tears of helpless laughter. (The islanders thought the Oceanic position, described later, was the only right and true one.)

On the other hand, the missionary position is certainly the most *common* one, at least in our culture, as the late Dr. Alfred Kinsey found in his great sex surveys of the 1940s and 1950s. He even estimated that as much as 70 percent of the U.S. population may never have tried intercourse any other way. And this position does have its advantages.

"There are some times when a man likes to dominate a woman; there are some times when a woman likes to be 'taken' by a man," says Jude Cotter, Ph.D., a psychologist and sex therapist in private practice in Farmington Hills, Michigan.

And if the goal is pregnancy, in this position the vagina is like an upright cup and thus tends to retain semen.

But the position also has major drawbacks.

"It's the worst position for the male, because he is supporting his weight with his smallest, weakest muscles (back and shoulders) and tends to tire fairly quickly," says Dr. Cotter. "If he's a lot heavier than she is, he tends to squash her. And because he's using his hands to support himself, he can't touch her clitoris directly."

The biggest disadvantage of the missionary position, though, is that her clitoris is only indirectly stimulated (if at all) by his penis, making it difficult for her to reach orgasm. In fact, in *The Hite Report,* researcher Shere Hite reported that of 1,844 women surveyed, only 30 percent reported regularly reaching orgasm during intercourse—in large part, almost certainly, because of the popularity of the missionary position.

The Coital Alignment Technique

For most women, the key to orgasm is clitoral stimulation. One way of overcoming the lack of clitoral stimulation is to use the *coital alignment* technique.

Instead of entering her straight on when using the missionary position, the man "rides high," so that his pubic bone (the hard surface just above the shaft of his penis) is applying pressure directly to her mons (the rounded protuberance above her vagina, beneath which lies the clitoris). By settling into a gentle, mutual rhythm in which he rocks his pubic bone back and forth over her clitoris, rather than focusing so much on thrusting in and out, she gets stimulated just where she needs it.

Women who've learned the coital alignment technique are able to reach orgasm more often and more pleasurably and are more likely to climax simultaneously with their partner, researchers say.

It's important to keep *continuous, steady* pressure on the clitoris, say researchers who have studied the benefits of this position. As the man bears down, the woman should apply counterpressure by pushing up with her pelvis. Also, both partners should establish a sexual rhythm that's identical in pattern and pace. Get a slow, steady, even rhythm going, each in sync with the other, and try to keep it up. There's a natural tendency for the man, as he approaches orgasm, to speed up at the same time the woman slows down or even stops. But you need to overcome this tendency and keep moving and thrusting at the same pace as your partner, the researchers say.

The man should rest the full weight of his body on the woman and not prop himself up on his elbows. The woman's legs should be wrapped around the man's thighs, with her ankles resting on his calves (bending her knees any more than that is uncomfortable and tends to immobilize her pelvis, they say).

Woman on Top

On the other hand, you could always skip the missionary position completely and let the woman get on top. Some people feel it's "just not right" for the woman to be in the "superior" position, that it is an affront to a man's authority or suggests latent homosexuality, or some other nonsense. Actually, though, it's *pleasure* that should be in the superior position. You may find the woman-on-top position to be mutually satisfying. As a rule, when the woman is on top she's much better able to fine-tune the stimulation of her clitoris and thus reach orgasm (although sometimes it may be a little more difficult for the man to keep his penis from falling out).

"Only the female-superior and lateral [side-by-side] coital positions allow direct or primary stimulation of the clitoris to be achieved with ease," report William Masters, M.D., and Virginia Johnson, of the Masters and Johnson Institute in St. Louis, in *Human Sexual Response.* "Clitoral response may develop more rapidly and with greater intensity in female-superior coition than in any other female coital position."

Which is a rather stiff way of saying it helps her get where she wants to go.

"Undoubtedly," says Dr. Cotter, "the position of choice is the female on top. When a woman is kneeling astride his erect penis, they can both last longer. He's not getting tired, she's not getting tired, since her strongest muscles are supporting her. Both his hands are free to stimulate her clitoris. He can also see her body, and this is important, because men are turned on by the visuals, which is why there should be some light source in the room."

Also, Dr. Cotter adds, in this position it's possible to deal with some erectile difficulties. If he's having trouble getting an erection, she can use the "stuff technique" and simply stuff his semierect penis into her vagina when she's ready. If he has trouble with premature ejaculation, he can usually last longer when she's on top.

Side by Side

Making love while the man and woman are lying face-to-face and side by side is sometimes called the African position, because it's widely practiced there. It has its advantages: It's restful for both parties. It's particularly nice when either partner is sick, tired or old. It's useful during the last months of pregnancy. And like the woman-on-top position, it helps men last longer than the man-on-top position.

Also, adds Dr. Cotter, "for many women, this is the preferred position, because when the man is cradling his partner with one arm, they can fall asleep in each other's arms after intercourse. Some women think this is the nicest part of making love."

Rear Entry

In the ancient love manual *The Perfumed Garden,* Tunisian poet Sheikh Nefzawi describes several variations of the rear-entry position as "after the fashion of a ram" or "coitus of the sheep." The Marquesan Islanders refer to it as "horse intercourse." All the imagery of animals is appropriate, because rear-entry intercourse is practically universal among other mammals, reptiles and birds.

In most primates, a female in heat presents herself sexually to a male by exposing her buttocks, not her breasts. In fact, the zoologist-author Desmond Morris, Ph.D., in his book *The Naked Ape,* points out that human females are the only primates with permanently enlarged breasts. It could be, he suggests, that breasts are there to evoke some primal memory of those inflamed, inviting buttocks.

Rear-entry intercourse does seem a little raunchy and animalistic, which is part of its appeal. But it has other practical benefits, such as the fact that it can be done late in pregnancy. It's the position in which the man can have probably the deepest penetration. And many women who have an erotically sensitive "G-spot" on the front, top wall of their vaginas say that it's most easily reached when the man enters from behind. (See "G–Spot.")

The disadvantage is that it's sometimes difficult for the man to keep his penis inside the vagina in this position. Sometimes men worry that their partners might think they're homosexual and thus feel threatened by this position, Dr. Cotter says. But as a practical matter, the biggest disadvantage is the lack of clitoral stimulation in the rear-entry position (although she can help with her own hands).

A Few Exotic Variations

Actually, Dr. Cotter says, the best position of all is one we don't use in our culture, because we can't. The woman lies on her back with her knees raised, and the man enters her while squatting between her legs "like a catcher on a baseball team." In certain cultures people who are accustomed to squatting can greatly prolong intercourse in this position, but we civilized chair-sitters would probably find it terribly uncomfortable, Dr. Cotter says. It's this position, sometimes called the Oceanic position, that's favored by many Pacific Islanders (including those who found the missionary position so hilarious).

In the Truk Islands of Micronesia, another variation is sometimes practiced, writes anthropologist Edgar Gregersen, Ph.D., of the City University of New York, in his book *Sexual Practices:* "The man sits on the ground with his legs wide open and stretched out in front of him. The woman faces him, kneeling. The man places the head of his penis just inside the opening of her vagina. He does not really insert it but moves his penis up and down with his hand in order to stimulate her clitoris. As the couple approach climax, the man draws the woman toward him and finally completes the insertion of his penis."

Sitting Positions

Art or literature depicting seated lovemaking is fairly rare in other cultures, although the Chinese are particularly fond of depicting intercourse involving a man sitting in a chair, according to Dr. Gregersen. Although they may be somewhat uncomfortable, seated positions have the advantage of being not too strenuous on the man and may help him delay ejaculation.

Standing Up

In almost all cultures, standing positions are associated with brief, illicit encounters, according to Dr. Gregersen. Sheikh Nefzawi describes one variation called "driving the peg home" in which the woman wraps her legs around the man's waist, wraps her arms around his neck and leans her back against a wall to steady them both. The *Kama Sutra* describes another variation, called *avalambitaka,* or "suspended congress." The man stands up, leaning back against a wall. The woman sits on his clasped hands, facing him and holding onto his waist with her thighs, with her arms around his neck. She moves by pushing her feet against the wall that's supporting the man.

Obviously, these positions (despite their erotic potential) should be attempted only with care, because they require strength, flexibility and a great lower back.

SMELLS, SEXUAL

In bed her heavy resilient hair
— a living censer, like a sachet —
released its animal perfume,
and from discarded underclothes
still fervent with her sacred body's
form, there rose a scent of fur.

Those steamy lines from Baudelaire, poet of the sensuous, suggest the erotic power of aroma better than anything modern science has to offer. Sex and sexuality are bathed in the faint mist of erotic musk, and —even though sex researchers have had a hard time proving it—almost everybody knows odors have the power to arouse. In fact, erotic literature from many ancient cultures (ranging from classical Greece to the Orient) often refers to the aphrodisiac power of sexual smells.

(The British writer Somerset Maugham is supposed to have asked one of H. G. Wells's girlfriends why such a fat, homely fellow had so much luck with women. "He smells of honey," she replied.)

Of course, not all body odors qualify as sensual.

In the modern world, people are probably inclined to associate body odors more with repulsiveness than with sexiness. And of course, it's unfair to expect your partner to be aroused if you haven't bathed since last Tuesday. (Sex therapists report that this is a fairly common complaint, especially from women.)

Still, by going to such extraordinary lengths to mask our own smells, we've certainly lost something, and perhaps something important.

Search for the Pheromone

It's well known that many other animals—including bees, wasps, moths and mammals—use special odors known as pheromones as a kind of sexual signaling mechanism, to let the males know when the females are ready to mate. Female rhesus monkeys, when they're in heat, release chemical compounds in their vaginal secretions called copulins, which seem to attract males. And female codling moths entice their mates by exuding an amorous pheromone that males detect with their antennae.

Do humans also give off come-hither aromas when they're ready for sex? It's a question that has intrigued scientists for decades—and the answer is no and yes, according to David M. Quadagno, Ph.D., a professor in the Medical Science Program at Florida State University in Tallahassee. There are actually two different kinds of pheromones, he explains. *Signaling pheromones,* of the type favored by moths, have an immediate, sexually enticing effect, almost like the mythic Love Potion Number Nine. There's no evidence (so far) that humans exude this kind of pheromone. The second type, *releaser pheromones,* has a much slower effect and only works after prolonged exposure. It's this second type that's been shown to exist in humans.

In 1986, scientists at the Monell Chemical Sciences Center and the University of Pennsylvania Medical School announced findings that showed, for the first time, that releaser pheromones do play a role in human sexuality. There is, these researchers concluded, some chemical pheromone exuded by a man in his natural body odor that women either smell or absorb through their skin during intimate sexual contact and that tends to make women sexually healthy. Women who have sex with a man at least once a week have normal-length menstrual cycles and milder menopause and are more fertile, compared with women who are celibate or have sex irregularly, they found. Their prime suspect: an odiferous pheromone secreted by special sweat glands (the apocrine glands) in men's armpits and around their genitals.

In one test of this theory, a group of women who had periods longer than 33 days or shorter than 26 days (compared with a national average of 29½ days) came to the Philadelphia clinic three times a week. There they partook of an exceedingly odd sort of medicine: Pads that male volunteers had worn under their armpits were rubbed under the women's noses. After 12 to 14 weeks of this, the women's cycles gradually shifted, slowing down or speeding up until they approached a normal 29½ day cycle. In some mysterious way, the "male essence" in the pads seemed to have calmed and steadied their reproductive systems.

The researchers also found a "female essence" in the secretions of women—an aromatic pheromone that has a profound effect on the sexual physiology of other women. It's this smell, researchers believe, that's behind the odd but well-known phenomenon called *menstrual synchrony.* When college-age women share a dorm room, their menstrual periods gradually shift until they're all having their periods within a few days of one another (and they shift apart when the women go home for the summer). The researchers rubbed pads on the underarms of women who were having their periods, then rubbed this odiferous stuff on the upper lips of women who were not having periods—and in a matter of a few months, their periods had shifted into sync with one another.

(One intriguing difference between "male essence" and "female essence": Women's pheromones can disperse across a room, the researchers found, but men's pheromones require direct, intimate contact to have an impact.)

This sort of research has touched off a frenzy of research in the labs of perfume companies, who smell money in the idea of a bona fide sexual attractant. A few companies have even marketed fragrances with such alleged powers (usually containing a substance called androstenol, secreted by both men and women). There's never been any convincing evidence that the stuff works, however, despite all sorts of ingenious scientific attempts to prove it.

On the other hand—who knows?—maybe tomorrow researchers will discover that just beneath the threshold of consciousness, we've been signaling each other by smell all along. Interestingly enough, it's known that the apocrine glands are largest during the reproductive years, so that the body odors of young, sexually active adults differ from those of older people or children. With his talk of "animal perfume," Baudelaire may have been more right than he knew.

SMOKING

The after-sex smoke may be a cherished romantic ritual (at least in the movies), but the truth is that smoking is about as unsexy as you can get.

Smoking can be harmful to the reproductive systems of both men and women. Women who smoke during pregnancy are considerably more likely to give birth before their babies have reached full term. And in men, smoking has been shown to significantly decrease the number and liveliness of sperm cells. In one study researchers found that semen samples from smokers were twice as likely to have the lower end of normal sperm densities (40 million per milliliter) as those from nonsmokers.

And women who are trying to *avoid* making babies by taking the Pill are at greater risk for complications if they smoke. The most serious complications associated with oral contraceptives are circulatory problems like heart attack, stroke and thromboembolitis (blockage of an artery by a blood clot), and the risk of all these things is increased by smoking, especially among women who are over 35. (See "The Pill.")

Smoking and Impotence

There's also evidence suggesting that smoking may interfere with a man's ability to get or maintain an erection. A team of urologists at Queen's University in Kingston, Ontario, examined 178 impotent men and found that 80 percent were either current or former smokers—a much higher percentage than would be found in the general population. Heavy cigarette smoking (25 or more cigarettes a day) was more than twice as prevalent among these men as among the general population.

Measurements of the men's penile blood pressure (blood flow to the penis) was also revealing, since robust blood flow is critical for producing a rigid erection. Twenty percent of the impotent men who had a history of smoking had abnormally low penile blood pressure, compared with only 9 percent of the impotent men who were nonsmokers. This suggests, say the researchers, that "smoking may be an important risk factor in impotence."

This evidence is not totally conclusive, but it's highly suggestive. It's known that one of the most common causes of erection problems is inadequate blood flow. Way back in 1979, the U.S. Surgeon General's report on smoking and health concluded that smoking is one of the most important causes of peripheral vascular disease—that is, damage to small arteries like the ones that supply the penis. It seems reasonable to conclude that when it comes to sex—especially in older men already inclined to have vascular problems—smoking could mean nothing but trouble.

Sexual Cancer

Research also suggests that smoking can increase the risk of cancer of the cervix in women and cancer of the penis in men. Swedish researchers compared

247 Swedish men with penile cancer with a group of similar men who were cancer-free. The men with cancer, they found, were much more likely to be smokers than the healthy men. They also found a "dose-response relation" between smoking and penile cancer — meaning that men who smoked more than ten cigarettes a day had a "significantly higher risk" than men who smoked fewer than that.

The researchers also point out that in women who smoke, high concentrations of nicotine and other tobacco by-products have been found in the cervix. (One theory holds that substances in cigarette smoke not only cause cancer in parts of the body in direct contact with smoke, like the lungs or the larynx, but also travel to places far afield from the original site of injury via the circulatory system.)

In uncircumcised men, tobacco by-products become concentrated in smegma — the cheesy secretions that build up beneath the foreskin of the penis. This is especially true in men who have a condition called phimosis — a tightening-up of the foreskin, which prevents it from being drawn back over the head of the penis. Phimosis, which is a known risk factor for penile cancer, encourages smegma to accumulate beneath the skin, and when smoking makes these secretions toxic, you've got double trouble.

These findings seem to provide at least one reasonable argument in favor of circumcision. If you're an adult, of course, penis surgery is a bit drastic. But it's never too late to give up the smokes.

SNORING

Everybody snores a little from time to time, but some people — usually overweight, middle-aged men — snore so heavily that their mates, in desperation, send them off to sleep in the guest room. Snoring can put enormous stress on an otherwise contented marriage, which is perhaps partly why there are over 300 antisnoring gadgets listed in the gazettes of the U.S. Government Office of Patents. Not only is it extraordinarily unsexy, but it can actually have a profound effect on sexual functioning. Researchers have found that a significant number of heavy snorers suffer from reduced sex drive, and a good number of log-sawing men are also impotent, according to Derek S. Lipman, M.D., author of *Stop Your Husband from Snoring,* who is an ear, nose and throat specialist in private practice in Portland, Oregon.

That's because heavy snoring is the classic symptom of a more serious syndrome known as obstructive sleep apnea (OSA). While sleeping, people with OSA momentarily stop breathing—typically, hundreds of times a night—because their upper airways become blocked by tongue, tonsils, soft palate or some other part of their respiratory anatomy. Because sleep is repeatedly interrupted during the night, OSA can have profound effects on the body. It inhibits sexuality, doctors believe, because of the combined effects of oxygen deprivation, fatigue and depression. It can also lead to other serious complications, including high blood pressure, increased risk of heart attack or stroke, excessive daytime sleepiness—even, in rare cases, death.

People with OSA should be under a doctor's care. There are a number of treatments, including surgery, for the disorder. In fact, anyone who snores on a regular basis should see a doctor to rule out the possibility of OSA.

Other Things to Try

Once you're sure that honking and wheezing is nothing more than plain old snoring, consider taking these more moderate steps.

Lose some weight. Doctors invariably counsel people who snore to drop a few pounds, because this reduces the symptoms. Weight loss of 10 to 25 percent can sometimes take care of the problem completely, or at least can greatly reduce the number of episodes.

Lay off the booze. Drinking alcohol within a few hours of going to bed increases snoring episodes. In one study, middle-aged men who seldom snored began snoring like crazy after heavy drinking just before bed; those who already snored did so much more heavily.

Sleep on a firm mattress with a low pillow. This ensures that your neck is straight and your airway is not obstructed, suggests Dr. Lipman.

Don't take sleeping pills, sedatives or narcotics before going to bed. These are central nervous system depressants, and they increase the severity of snoring spells. Some cold remedies will do the same thing.

Quit smoking. Doctors also invariably counsel people who snore to quit smoking, because smoking worsens snoring by irritating and swelling mucous membranes in the throat and reducing oxygen uptake in the lungs.

Try a "snore ball." It may sound crazy, but some people have found that sewing a pocket into the back of their pajama top and slipping in a golf or tennis ball keeps them from snoring so much. The reason: It helps you avoid sleeping on your back, which has long been known as the most snore-prone position. Some people find that after using a snore ball for a couple of months, they can get rid of the ball—and still not snore.

SPERMICIDES

Sperm-killing concoctions that are tucked into the vagina just before intercourse are among the oldest and simplest of all birth control devices. Egyptian papyri dating back to as early as 1850 B.C. give recipes for primitive spermicides made of honey, carbonate of soda, acacia tree tips and the dung of crocodiles and elephants. Horrific as this may sound, it turns out that the Egyptian physicians may have known more than they knew they knew. Twentieth-century researchers have learned that oily, gummy or gluey things (like honey) tend to slow a sperm's mobility; that lactic acid (produced by acacia trees) is deadly to sperm; and that acidic things (like elephant dung) discourage fertilization. These odiferous ancient recipes must have worked reasonably well, because they're repeatedly mentioned by writers in the Mediterranean region for over 3,000 years, according to Reay Tannahill, author of the wonderful book *Sex in History.*

The Modern Alternatives

Today, highly effective spermicidal products are available without a prescription in almost any drugstore (and they're completely dung-free!). Although they come in a variety of forms, all spermicides consist of two parts: a base material that disperses the active ingredient throughout the vagina, especially over the cervix, and the active ingredient itself. There are only two such sperm-killing chemicals available in the United States: nonoxynol-9 (the active ingredient in the great majority of spermicidal products) and octoxynol. Both of these substances are surfactants, meaning that they work by destroying the surface membrane of sperm cells. Soaps and detergents are also surfactants; spermicides, in effect, are a specialized form of soap.

In stores, you'll find several different types of spermicides.

Foams. These come in an aerosol can. After being shaken (it's important to shake the can at least 20 times before use), the foam is sprayed into an applicator, which is inserted into the vagina. The foam rapidly disperses, covering the cervix and giving good protection for half an hour (when the foam starts going flat, requiring a new application). Some foams come in prefilled applicators that can be conveniently slipped into a purse.

Gels and creams. By use of an applicator, these spermicides are also inserted into the vagina as deep as is comfortable. They tend to be a little less messy than foams, but they, too, begin losing their effectiveness after about 30 minutes and should be reapplied if sex play continues longer than that. According to lab studies, foams and creams disperse better than gels and suppositories.

Vaginal suppositories. These are capsules, tablets or thin sheets of film that are melted by body heat after being slipped deep into the vagina, with either a freshly washed finger or an applicator. Some of these tablets foam or effervesce, creating a physical barrier to sperm as well as a chemical one. One disadvantage of foaming tablets, suppositories and film is that you have to wait a while (usually 10 to 15 minutes) after insertion before you can make love. It takes that amount of time for the product to dissolve adequately. With foams, gels and creams, on the other hand, you can make love immediately after insertion (which, under certain circumstances, can be the difference between heaven and purgatory).

Some foaming tablets generate heat as they dissolve, which both partners are likely to feel (and some people find strangely pleasurable). In fact, when marketers of a foaming tablet called Neo Sampoon discovered that men in the Philippines found the heat highly erotic, the company kicked off a campaign with the slogan "Neo Sampoon—for that warm sensation!"

Spermicides should be left in place for 6 to 8 hours after intercourse. It's not necessary to douche afterward, but if a woman wants to douche, she should wait 6 to 8 hours before doing so.

How Effective Are They?

Probably the biggest drawback to spermicides is that they have a fairly high failure rate. Numerous studies have shown that this is a failure not so much of the products themselves (which are quite effective if used correctly) but of the way they're actually used. It's important to use spermicides *every time* you make love, and carefully follow the product instructions, but lots of people do so only haphazardly.

As a result, typical-use failure rates, for 100 women using spermicides for a year, would result in about 20 pregnancies, according to a report from the Population Information Program at Johns Hopkins University in Baltimore. (Theoretically, if you used spermicides perfectly, every time, only about 3 pregnancies would occur.) By comparison, typical-use failure rates for sterilization are considerably less than 1 pregnancy per 100 women per year, about 3 for the Pill and the IUD and around 12 for condoms, according to Planned Parenthood.

It's really much better to use spermicides *in combination* with some other barrier method, like condoms, a diaphragm or a cervical cap. Even though some spermicidal products are marketed for use without any other form of backup birth control and can be used this way, you greatly reduce your chances of getting pregnant by "doubling up" your protection.

Minor Problems

One of the biggest selling points for spermicides is their safety. Unlike other forms of birth control, there have never been any reports of serious side effects from spermicidal creams, foams or jellies—the most dangerous potential side effect of spermicides, in fact, is pregnancy. Other than that, though, about the worst side effect you're likely to encounter is a little local irritation of the penis or vagina. It's possible the irritation is caused by the active ingredient, which (being a form of detergent) can irritate the skin just as detergents do. Or it's possible it's caused by something else in the product. If you experience irritation from a spermicide, try switching products.

It's also possible you may be having a mild allergic reaction. About 5 percent of people who use nonoxynol-9 experience some localized allergic reaction to it, says Philip Darney, M.D., associate professor of obstetrics and gynecology at San Francisco General Hospital. Generally, such reactions are not very serious, though, and can be overcome by switching to a product that contains octoxynol instead of nonoxynol-9. A man can try using condoms to avoid direct contact with the stuff. (For more, see "Allergies.")

There have been lingering safety concerns about whether a sperm cell that was damaged by a spermicide before it fertilized an egg might be more inclined to result in a malformed fetus. This is a serious question, and it's been extensively investigated, but a huge number of these studies have failed to show that there's any connection between spermicide use and fetal defects.

On a lighter note, some people complain that spermicides have an unpleasant taste and so interfere with oral sex. This may present a problem of timing, but there's no reason to worry that spermicides might be harmful to your health. Spermicides are safe enough to eat.

STD Protection and Other Advantages

Spermicides are readily available in almost any drugstore, and they don't require a prescription. They're also convenient to use. They don't require any assistance from your partner. For some women (especially those who have intercourse fairly infrequently) there's another special advantage: You have to use spermicide only when you want to make love. You can avoid the risk, effort and expense of some other method (like an IUD) that must be used all the time, no matter how frequently you have sex.

Spermicides also have the added benefit of providing some protection against sexually transmitted diseases. Clinical studies have shown that nonoxynol-9 offers women significant protection against both chlamydia and gonorrhea.

In laboratory tests, nonoxynol-9 has been shown to be lethal to the organisms that cause gonorrhea, genital herpes, trichomoniasis, syphilis and AIDS. It's important to remember, though, that these findings came from tidy little experiments done in glass dishes, not from real sex, and there's a difference. For one thing, all these organisms penetrate human cells, and when they're hiding inside a cell, they've got some protection against spermicides. For another, these organisms can rapidly penetrate the body through open sores and may escape the spermicide this way. Also, given the haphazard patterns of human behavior (especially sexual behavior), there's no assurance that the spermicide will be properly dispersed throughout the vagina or even that you'll remember to use it at all. That's why you can't count on spermicides to offer you perfect, fail-safe protection from sexually transmitted diseases. They help, but you still need to be careful.

STRESS

At the heart of sex is an odd, almost Zen-like irony: In order to perform your best, you mustn't try *too hard*. You've got to relax, get out of your body's way and just let it happen by itself. But when your body is wracked with stress, tension and anxiety, and your mind is wracked with worry and distractions, sweet sex is nearly impossible. You wind up having sex as a way of releasing stress: lovemaking as aerobics class.

And that's just not the way it's supposed to be.

"Stress and fatigue are probably the most common barriers to good sex in a world of two-paycheck families, tough economic times and our own expectation that we can still 'have it all,' " says Allan Elkin, Ph.D., a sex therapist, clinical psychologist and director of the Stress Management and Counseling Center in New York City. "These days I see a tremendous number of people suffering from what I call 'disarousal'—disorders of arousal, or low sexual desire, caused by the exhaustion, worry and distractions of a stressful life."

How Stress Interferes with Sex

Stress is deadly to sex because it makes trouble on three different levels, Dr. Elkin explains: physiologically, emotionally and on the mundane level of day-to-day life.

On the physical level, when the body is under chronic stress, it is continuously readying itself for combat or escape (the famous "fight or flight" response). The muscles tense, heart rate and respiration speed up, and blood vessels constrict, squeezing off the blood flow to the extremities. That's why your palms feel cold and clammy when you're anxious—and why many stressed-out men have trouble getting erections.

Stress also touches off a complex cascade of hormones that can have a negative effect on sex, Dr. Elkin says. In studies of military recruits subjected to a variety of stresses (a parachute jump, boot camp, combat training), testosterone levels in these nervous young men dropped significantly, thus wilting their sex drive. It only stands to reason: When you're preparing to face imminent danger, or at least some sort of action, the last thing your body needs to waste energy on is sex.

On a fundamental level, in other words, preparing the body for war is almost precisely the opposite of preparing it for love.

Mental Stress Takes a Toll

There's also an emotional aspect to stress: Psychiatrists say that in the depths of the psyche, chronic stress can be transformed into anxiety, depression, anger, guilt or some dispiriting combination of those four emotions.

And "anxiety, anger, depression and guilt have long been seen as crucial in sexual dysfunctions in general and in the loss of sexual desire in particular," reports a team of psychiatrists from the University of Manitoba, in Winnipeg.

Something else happens to the mind under stress: You can't seem to concentrate on anything. Like a fidgety gunfighter anticipating an onslaught of lead, the mind starts jumping all over the place but never rests in any one place for very long. An endless parade of worries and distractions begins racing through your mind—about money and work, about your health and your kids, about your relationships, about yesterday and tomorrow. In several studies, the stress-induced presence of distracting thoughts has been shown to impair sexual responses—and the more a person's thoughts wander, the more difficult it is to become aroused.

"If you're distracted and worried because you're overstressed, and you don't perform well sexually, there may also be a kind of 'rebound effect' that makes things even worse," Dr. Elkin says. "The next time you have sex, you begin to worry that you'll perform poorly again, which compounds the stress, which may lead to a secondary sexual dysfunction."

Then of course, there's the unprofound, day-to-day aspect of stress: You're overscheduled, underpaid and exhausted, and by the end of the day there's just not enough energy left for love.

What to Do

It's easy to describe the effects of stress, but it's harder to say what to do about them. Modern life is rife with tension and anxiety and perhaps always will be. We're *all* stressed out to one degree or another (how would *you* like to have a 140,000-word book due in six weeks?). Still, sometimes simple things can make an enormous difference.

Make a date. "Lots of people say, 'Sex is supposed to be spontaneous'—but in order to nourish a relationship, sexually and in every other way, a couple really needs to schedule time to be together and honor the commitment to protecting that time," says Georgianna S. Hoffmann, R.N., a certified sex therapist in Iowa City, Iowa. Your special time together doesn't have to involve intercourse, or even getting sexual at all—it just has to be calm, uninterrupted time, and it has to be regular. At a minimum, she ways, couples should schedule one weeknight and one weekend night to be together. "That time together should be as important as any other part of your life, including a meeting with the chairman of the board," she says. You say you just don't have time? "If we consider something a high priority, we can always find time to do it," she responds.

Don't leave sex 'til last. "We tend to leave sex to the dregs of the day, when we're too tired to perform—even though our desire and interest in sex may be perfectly healthy," says Dr. Elkin. So if you're going to make a commitment to spending more time with your mate, also commit to rescheduling your life a little. Turn off the TV before you're completely exhausted. Try having sex on Saturday morning or another morning. Try nooners. Again: If you give your sexual relationship a higher priority in your life, there will always be enough time for it.

Try massage. "Relaxed, sensuous touch is one of the best relievers of stress," says Hoffmann. Trading short massages with your mate (whether or not it leads to sex) can be something close to magic. Hoffmann, who instructs her sex therapy patients in the gentle arts of touch, distinguishes between *caressing* and *massage.* A caress, she says, is "a very light, very, very slow touching of the surface of the skin, so lightly and so slowly that the skin ahead of the touch begins to anticipate the touch." Men, she says, tend to touch women too firmly, with too much muscle. "If men can learn to caress," she says, "it makes a world of difference."

Massage is a deeper, firmer form of touch. There are many different kinds, of course, but in general massage is a great "sex-enhancer," because it so effectively dissipates the effects of stress, according to Gordon Inkeles, author of *The Art of Sensual Massage.* Muscles that are under continual stress, he explains, gradually accumulate nasty acidic wastes—especially if you're just sitting at your desk all day. Without exercise to burn off these lactic and carbonic acid wastes, it may take days or weeks for them to seep away naturally. But deep massage can force the gunk out of your muscles in a matter of minutes, inducing a sense of luxuriant relaxation that's a perfect prelude to sex. (For more, see "Massage.")

Get moving. It's been said a thousand times, but it's still worth repeating: One of the all-time greatest stress-reducers is exercise, preferably 30 or 40 minutes, three times a week. (See "Exercise.")

Change just one thing. Former sex counselor Michael Castleman, in his book *Sexual Solutions,* suggests that it may be helpful to try to identify the biggest stress factors in your life and then to try to change *just one.* If you try to change them all, you'll probably give up in despair. And of course, some stressful things you can't or don't want to change (like a baby in the house). But if you feel like overwork is destroying your sex life, for example, try delegating one job responsibility at work. If you don't seem to have enough time for sex, you may have to cut something else out (but just one thing).

Get the kids to bed. When both husband and wife work, what tends to happen is that the kids are allowed to stay up late because Mom and Dad want to share a little time with them at the end of the day, Hoffmann says. But the upshot of it all is that there's no time left for Mom and Dad, and that's not good for anybody. "You've got to set a reasonable bedtime and stick to it," she says.

Follow your bliss. It's important to have something in your life that truly, deeply relaxes you and to give that to yourself regularly. It could be yoga, could be gardening, could be drinking tea and talking with a friend. But whatever it is, Castleman says, you'll know it's the right thing because all true follow-your-bliss activities have three things in common: When you're doing them, you have a sensation that time is suspended, a sense that you're really alive in the present moment and a sense that you've "lost yourself" in what you're doing.

Sounds a little like good sex, and a little like Zen, doesn't it?

Syphilis

The good news about syphilis is that if it's diagnosed early, it's not all that difficult to cure. One course of antibiotics (typically penicillin, tetracycline and/or doxycycline) can usually knock it right out of your system.

The bad news is that undiagnosed syphilis is an extremely dangerous sexually transmitted disease that can lead to degeneration of the heart, brain or spinal cord, blindness, paralysis and even death. To make things worse, its symptoms can be so variable that doctors often fail to diagnose it correctly, researchers say. This may be part of the reason syphilis has begun making a comeback in recent years. It's now at its highest level since 1950, with roughly 40,000 new cases (and probably many more) turning up in the United States each year, according to researchers.

Dubious Cures

Not so very long ago, syphilis was a sexual scourge of epidemic proportions. In sixteenth- and seventeenth-century Europe, it was widespread, and in desperation sufferers were subjected to a variety of dangerous (and mostly useless) treatments. In the early 1900s, syphilis patients (including Danish writer Isak Dinesen, author of *Out of Africa)* were given bismuth and arsenic, which was sometimes more deadly than the disease. And in the late 1920s, a new treatment was introduced: Patients were deliberately infected with malaria, which induced a 106°F fever for several days and "burned out" the syphilis—or else killed you.

In the 1940s, the first really effective drug for syphilis was introduced— penicillin. Even today, penicillin remains "the drug of first choice" for all stages of syphilis, according to Connie Whiteside, M.D., of the Division of General Medicine at the University of California, Davis, Medical Center. Penicillin was so effective at reducing infection rates, in fact, that during the 1950s some doctors optimistically described syphilis as a "vanishing disease." But in the late 1980s, syphilis began rearing its ugly head again, especially in the inner cities and among prostitutes and drug abusers. Reckless behavior like the exchange of sexual favors for drugs is one reason syphilis has taken hold and seems to be spreading again in the 1990s, public health officials say.

What Causes It

Syphilis is caused by a spiral-shaped bacterium, or spirochete, called *Treponema pallidum.* Almost always transmitted to a new host through sexual intercourse or oral sex, this microscopic creature drills its way through the skin and from there spreads like crazy. Hours after they've penetrated the skin, the spirochetes generally make it into the bloodstream, and within a week they've spread throughout the body.

If untreated, the infection generally progresses through three stages over a period of many years. During the first stage (primary syphilis), a single painless sore appears at the spot the spirochete entered the body. This sore, or chancre, usually shows up anywhere from 10 to 90 days after infection, almost always on the genitals. Typically, syphilitic chancres have a smooth center and a raised, firm border and are sometimes filled with yellow pus like a blister or pimple, according to Dr. Whiteside. In men, these sores usually show up on or near the head of the penis. In women, they're usually on the labia (lips of the vagina)—but sometimes they're down inside the vagina where they can't be seen or felt. Occasionally, they appear on the mouth, breast, fingers, tongue or face.

Then the disease gets tricky. In a month or two, the sores heal and disappear— leading many infected people to conclude that the infection has gone away, too. Wrong. It has simply disappeared inside the body and continues to do damage in places it can't be seen. (This is why *any* genital sore should be checked by a doctor. Don't just wait until it goes away, because with syphilis, it will. You're still infected, though—and you're probably contagious.)

Later Stages

Phase two (secondary syphilis) generally shows up two to six months after the sores go away and may last up to two years. By then, the spirochetes have spread so widely they may have invaded almost any part of the body. The resulting symptoms can vary so much syphilis is sometimes called the Great Imitator.

The most common sign of secondary syphilis is a nonitchy, often measlelike rash that typically appears on the palms of the hands and soles of the feet, often accompanied by what feels like the flu, according to Ted Rosen, M.D., associate professor of dermatology at Baylor College of Medicine in Houston. You may also feel headachy, have swollen glands, lose weight and feel generally lousy. About a third of patients have whitish sores in their mouth or throat and may begin to lose their hair in patches, according to Dr. Whiteside. The disease is highly contagious at this stage and (if there are sores in the mouth) can be spread through kissing.

The last act of the disease (tertiary syphilis) generally comes after a dormant period, which may last for up to 20 or even 30 years. During this time, there may be few if any outward signs of the infection. Although it's much less contagious in this last stage (syphilis is usually only contagious during the first few years you have it), it can do devastating damage to the carrier, invading the bones, heart, spinal cord and even the brain.

Although syphilis is almost always sexually transmitted, it can also be spread from a mother to a baby, which is why it's crucial to have a blood test for the disease early in a pregnancy. Treatment before the fifth month can prevent infection, but an infected mother who is *not* treated has only a one in six chance of delivering a healthy baby.

Imperfect Testing

Syphilis, in short, can be the worst sort of news.

If your doctor suspects you may have it, he or she will undoubtedly order tests to verify the presence of the spirochetes or of antibodies to them in your blood. Unfortunately, there's no perfect test for syphilis, only a series of imperfect tests, the accuracy of which varies depending on the stage of the disease.

The most accurate test for primary syphilis is examination of scrapings from lesions under a special kind of microscope. Since the lesions are generally swarming with these noxious organisms, they can actually be seen. Unfortunately, this test takes special expertise, and the equipment is not widely available.

Two of the most accurate blood tests for secondary syphilis are one developed by the Venereal Disease Research Laboratory (VDRL) and the rapid plasma reagin tests. Both tests, which detect antibodies to *T. pallidum* in the blood, are inexpensive and easy to perform. However, these tests also produce a fairly high number of false positives. Other infections (like herpes, mononucleosis and hepatitis), vaccinations, pregnancy or drug abuse can incorrectly suggest that you've got syphilis. That's why a more expensive, more precise test may be used to confirm an initial positive result from the VDRL test.

What You Should Do

In the battle against syphilis, here are a couple of things to keep in mind.

Syphilis is stubborn, and there's no real assurance the disease has been completely eliminated even after you've taken the antibiotics. That's why it's important to return to the doctor for all the follow-up blood tests. Doctors also recommend a return visit two years after the initial treatment.

If you're diagnosed as having syphilis, you need to inform your sexual partner(s) and convince them to go to a doctor for evaluation and possible treatment. Until you're cured, you should avoid sex, or at least use condoms to prevent the spread of the disease.

Researchers have recently found that syphilis and AIDS often go hand in hand, partly because the genital sores of syphilis provide a ready pathway for the AIDS virus to enter the body. If you're diagnosed with syphilis, you probably should also be tested for AIDS.

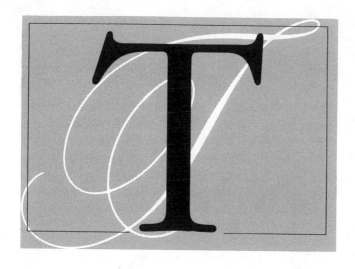

TERMS

Here are some brief definitions of a few useful though often misunderstood sexual terms.

Bestiality. Sex with animals. This practice is not as uncommon as you might think—the late Dr. Alfred Kinsey found that about 8 percent of the men he surveyed had had sexual contact with animals, although usually only once or twice in their lifetimes.

Exhibitionism. A sexual behavior in which a person (usually male) is aroused by exposing his or her genitals to strangers. It's the shock, dismay and panic that's the real turn-on, according to renowned sex expert John Money, Ph.D., professor of medical psychology and pediatrics at Johns Hopkins University and Hospital in Baltimore. If you don't act shocked by a flasher, you'll at least deprive him of the sexual pleasure he gets out of the experience. Exhibitionists are rarely dangerous and don't usually move on to more violent behavior like rape.

Fetishism. A fetish is an inanimate object endowed with magical or supernatural power. A sexual fetish is an object endowed with sexual power. Sexual fetishes can be objects or body parts such as panties, bras, hair, breasts, feet or even pictures of feet. The objects might provide tactile sensations (leather, latex, fur) or emit smells (soiled underwear) that stimulate the fetishist. (A fetishist is a person who gets aroused by a fetish.) Some fetishists have sex *only* with fetish objects and may actually derive greater pleasure from that than from intercourse. For others, fetishes are only an accessory to lovemaking with another person. Sex experts theorize that because they are so terrified or revolted by their own feelings of "sinful," "wicked" lust, fetishists transfer their sexual feelings to objects. The fetish itself becomes sinful, arousing and a substitute for a lover, according to Dr. Money. Fetishism is thought to be much more common in men than in women, perhaps because men seem to be more easily aroused by sights and smells than women are.

Frotteurism. A sexual behavior in which someone gets sexual pleasure, and may even reach orgasm, from rubbing up against strangers in a crowd.

Hermaphroditism. Having the attributes of both sexes (from *Hermes* and *Aphrodite,* god and goddess of love). Human hermaphrodites suffer from a birth defect called intersexuality, in which their reproductive systems and/or chromosomes are not quite male or female. A true hermaphrodite (very rare) may have both female fallopian tubes and a male vas deferens, for instance. A pseudohermaphrodite (more common) has the chromosomes and interior reproductive system of a woman but the genitals of a man, or vice versa.

Hermaphroditism is not uncommon among animals—some oysters, snails and worms function as both males and females during reproduction (simultaneous hermaphrodites), and hermaphroditic fish actually change from one sex to another during their lives (sequential hermaphrodites).

Incubus. A mythological evil spirit that assumes the form of a man and has intercourse with someone, usually a woman, at night in bed.

Nymphomania. Insatiable sexual desire in a woman, nowadays sometimes referred to as a *sexual addiction.* Typically, such women have a compulsion to lure a series of casual sex partners for one-night stands, then reject them, because the thrill of newness and conquest is the only thing that enables them to reach orgasm—although even then orgasm is not very satisfying.

Paraphilia. A general term for sexual behavior that is outside the realm of what's usually considered normal (what used to be called "perversions.") In a way, all paraphilias are a way of separating oneself from the "wickedness" of sexuality—such as transferring it to some inanimate object (fetishism) or having to be punished for feeling lust (sadomasochism). The key thing about a paraphilia is that it *must* be there in order for a person to become sexually aroused.

Sadomasochism. A sexual behavior in which sexual pleasure results from the giving (sadism) or receiving (masochism) of pain and humiliation. Partners may always play the same role or may reverse roles. More men than women are thought to enjoy these practices.

Satyriasis. The male version of nymphomania, sometimes also called *Don Juanism* or *sexual addiction.* After *satyr,* the mythological attendants of Bacchus who were half-goat, half-man and famous for their merriment and lechery.

Sodomy. This term usually refers to anal intercourse. However, it may also refer to mouth/genital contact or sex with animals. It's also sometimes used euphemistically (and vaguely) to refer to any "unnatural" sexual behavior.

Succubus. A mythological evil spirit that assumes the form of a woman and has intercourse with someone, usually a man, at night in bed.

Transsexualism. Transsexuals are those whose sexual self-image or gender identity does not match the sex of their physical body. They may undergo sex-change surgery and hormone treatment to become (as nearly as medically possible) their "true selves"—someone of the opposite sex. Transsexuals do not view themselves as homosexuals but as heterosexuals who at birth were "trapped in the wrong body." This unhappiness with one's own sex is also sometimes called *gender dysphoria.*

Transvestitism. A sexual behavior (also called *cross-dressing*) in which a person is sexually aroused by dressing up in the clothes, especially the underwear, of the opposite sex. Studies have shown that transvestites are almost always male and usually heterosexual. That is, even though they dress up like women, they still think of themselves as male and are attracted to women. They don't want to become a woman (unlike a transsexual, who does); they're simply aroused by the experience of wearing women's clothes.

Voyeurism. A sexual behavior in which a person becomes aroused from the risk of being discovered while secretly watching a stranger undressing or having sex. Peeping Toms are rarely rapists; they spy, and then later they "re-view" these secret mental movies during sex, either alone or with a partner.

Zoophilia. Sex with animals (same as bestiality).

TESTICLES

Why did God put the testicles—those exquisitely delicate, jumbo-jelly-bean-shaped glands upon which the whole human race depends— *outside* the body? They hang there in their pendulous sac of flesh, the scrotum, just begging to be kicked (and probably no man has escaped experiencing the agonizing pain of that occurrence at least once). Well, strictly speaking, it's because the testicles can't manufacture sperm at the body's core temperature. They must be kept mildly refrigerated, at a constant 94°F, in order to be optimally productive. That's why they're suspended a few inches outside the body—and why the cremaster muscles lower the elevation of the testicles to cool them off when it's hot outside and hoist them up when they get chilly.

Their Role in Arousal

Most people know that a man's testicles have two basic jobs: to manufacture sperm (in order to impregnate a woman) and to manufacture testosterone (the male hormone that fires up the *desire* to impregnate a woman). But it's less well known that the testicles also have a role to play in the drama of sexual arousal. In the 1960s, during their real-life observations of human sexual activity, the research team of William Masters, M.D., and Virginia Johnson, of the Masters and Johnson Institute in St. Louis, made the rather extraordinary discovery that the testicles are dramatically elevated just before ejaculation. As sexual excitement mounts, they found, the cremaster muscles reel in the testicles so tightly that just before orgasm they actually make direct contact with the body. (In about 85 percent of men, they add, the left testicle dangles a little lower than the right, and during arousal, the right one rises first, followed by the left.)

This discovery is of "extreme physiologic importance," Masters and Johnson reported, because if the testes don't undergo at least partial elevation during arousal, a man will not fully ejaculate. Some men, especially men older than 50, ejaculate when their testicles are only partially elevated. But when this happens, they found, there's a "marked reduction in ejaculatory pressure." With few exceptions, younger men simply cannot ejaculate fully until testicular elevation has occurred.

Something else rather odd happens to the testicles during arousal: They vastly increase in size. It's well known that *vasocongestion* (the temporary damming-up of blood) is one of the key characteristics of sexual arousal. That's what causes erections, "sex flush" and the swelling of the nipples, vulva and earlobes. It also causes the skin of the scrotum to swell and thicken during arousal and the testicles to swell. Typically, Masters and Johnson reported, a man's testicles swell by about 50 percent at the height of arousal, and if sexual excitement is sustained for long enough, they actually may almost *double* in size. This amazing, little-known sexual side effect tends to taper off as a man gets older, though. Men beyond their late fifties often show little if any increase in testicular size during arousal, they found.

A 60-Second Anatomy Lesson

The testicle is rather like a spacewalking astronaut, floating freely at the end of a tether called the spermatic cord, a bundle of blood vessels, nerves and ducts that connect it to the rest of the body. It doesn't really float in space, of course, but inside a lubricated, fluid-filled sac called the scrotum. The testicle itself is divided into about 250 tiny compartments, each containing a bewildering maze of seminiferous tubules, tiny tubes in which sperm are manufactured. Once the sperm cells mature, these frantically lashing cells, loaded with their genetic instructions, enter the seminal vesicles and the epididymis, a small mass of coiled ducts that can be felt on the back side of each testicle. The sperm dally there until they're ejaculated through the vas deferens—a duct leading up through the spermatic cord to the penis—during orgasm. (It's the vas deferens that's cut in a vasectomy, the male sterilization operation.)

Elsewhere in the depths of testicles, the Leydig cells are busy manufacturing testosterone, which (besides inflaming the libido) also orchestrates the development during puberty of secondary sexual characteristics like beard growth, increased muscle mass and deeper voice. Interestingly enough, one testicle has the capacity to manufacture all the testosterone a man needs to fuel his libido and grow a male body, although under normal conditions both testicles actively produce this hormone. The other one is really just a "backup," according to Richard E. Berger, M.D., professor of urology at the University of Washington and coauthor of *BioPotency: A Guide to Sexual Success.*

Actually, Dr. Berger explains, the testicles' testosterone-producing machinery is quite separate from their sperm-producing machinery and far more resistant to damage. That's why the great majority of infertile men have a perfectly robust sex drive and no trouble getting erections. But that doesn't mean that things can't go wrong. For instance, infections of the epididymis (called epididymitis) are painfully common. Often they occur when bacteria back up in the urinary tract and invade this dark maze of ducts. But although there are tiny valves that allow sperm made in the testicles free passage *up* into the epididymis, the valves are also designed to prevent bacteria from flowing *down* into the testicle, where they might damage the testosterone factories. It's not uncommon for a man to have a terrific infection of the epididymis, complete with pain and swelling, while the testicle itself remains serenely unaffected.

What Can Go Wrong

Occasionally, baby boys are born with a condition called cryptorchidism, or undescended testicles. Their tiny scrotums are empty, as if they'd had their pockets picked. That's because normally, during embryonic development, the testes begin to grow up near the kidneys, and late in the pregnancy they gradually descend through the abdominal wall into the waiting scrotum. But sometimes they get stuck on the way down. It's easy enough to fix this problem with a simple operation, but it's important to do so, because undescended testicles are likely to become infertile (partly because they're too hot). They're also 40 to 50 times more likely to become cancerous than a normal testicle, according to urologist and microsurgeon Sherman J. Silber, M.D., author of *The Male*.

An amazingly high percentage of men (1 out of every 400 to 700, by some estimates) is born with a condition called Klinefelter's syndrome, in which the testicles are extremely tiny, don't produce adequate testosterone and often produce no sperm at all. The problem: Rather than being born with an XY pattern of chromosomes (like a normal male) or an XX pattern (like a female), they're born with an XXY pattern. Such men are often treated with testosterone injections, which returns their sex drive to normal.

Despite their exposed location, it's amazing how seldom the testicles are seriously injured, Dr. Silber notes. Sometimes, though, a powerful blow to the groin causes the spermatic cord to get kinked or twisted around. When *torsion* of the testicle occurs, arterial blood flow continues to pour in under pressure, but venous outflow is blocked, so the testicle becomes massively swollen. If something isn't done within 4 to 8 hours, Dr. Silber warns, the testicle will die "a slow and agonizing death." In a couple of days it can grow to the size of a grapefruit, then over a period of three months shrink down to the size of a pea—a lifeless cinder. Severe swelling, bleeding or bruising of the testicles should be checked by a urologist or other doctor *immediately*, he warns.

Testicular Cancer

One other misfortune that may befall the innocent testicle: cancer. Testicular cancer is actually quite rare, but among men aged 20 to 40, it's the most common type, according to Neil H. Baum, M.D., clinical professor of urology at Tulane Medical School in New Orleans. The good news: If detected early, it's one of the easiest kinds of cancer to cure.

As a first line of defense, many urologists recommend that men learn the testicular self-exam and do it regularly (ideally, once a month). The procedure works best if you do it just after you get out of the shower, when the scrotal skin is smooth and soft. Just roll each testicle gently between the thumb and fingers of both hands (using both hands on each testicle, and doing them one at a time). If the testicle feels soft and spongy, rather like a peeled hard-boiled egg, that's the way it's supposed to feel.

But if you detect a lump (usually about the size of a pea), a hard spot or any other irregularity on the front or side of the testicle, have it checked by a urologist or other doctor. (Remember that on the back side of the testicle, you'll feel the soft, irregular swelling of the epididymis.) A lump is probably nothing—but if it's cancer, the sooner you have it treated, the better your chances of living a long, ardent life.

Testosterone

Testosterone is often referred to as a male hormone, and in many ways it is. Testosterone transforms a young boy's body into that of a man. During puberty, when his testicles start manufacturing the stuff like mad, it deepens his voice, gives him pubic hair and a beard, broadens his shoulders and packs on muscle mass. Testosterone inflames his sex drive. It's testosterone that also helps fuel aggression, the thirst for competition and the "typically male" drive for dominance.

"In males of all animal species studied, the development and maintenance of aggressive and sexual behavior require testosterone," observes Walter A. Brown, M.D., of the Providence Veterans Administration Medical Center in Rhode Island. If a normal adult male human is castrated, his sex drive will gradually taper off to nearly nothing (although this happens rather slowly and unevenly, researchers say). Male sex offenders, who seem to be abnormally sensitive to testosterone, are sometimes given a synthetic female hormone called Depo-Provera, which shuts down testosterone production and lays a calming hand on their out-of-control sex drive.

Testosterone in Women

Even so, it's really not accurate to say that testosterone is the sole property of the male. Because in humans—unlike nearly every other animal species—testosterone fuels sex drive in both males and females. In almost every other species, sex drive in females is orchestrated by female hormones, and females are interested in sex only for the few days or weeks when they're ovulating.

"The human sex drive, from a hormonal point of view, is neither male nor female but rather an undifferentiated basic urge created by a single hormone, testosterone," writes urologist and microsurgeon Sherman J. Silber, M.D., in his great little book *The Male.*

It's true that men's bodies contain about ten times as much circulating testosterone as women's bodies do. But women have a heightened sensitivity to its seductions, so their smaller supply goes a lot farther.

Some of the testosterone produced by a woman's body comes from her ovaries, but most of it comes from the adrenals, a pair of peanut-sized glands perched atop her kidneys. That's why, when a woman's ovaries gradually cease to function after menopause, her sex drive does not go away completely—the adrenals just keep quietly pumping out sex juice. Still, after menopause women often complain of a loss of interest in sex. And in many cases, doctors have discovered, their sexual fires can be stoked up again by giving them replacement testosterone.

Today, many older women on hormone replacement therapy have testosterone added to the hormonal mix as a way of boosting their libido and overall sense of well-being. "In something better than half the women given an estrogen/testosterone combination, there will be a self-reported increase in sexual interest and sexual activity," says Judith H. Seifer, Ph.D., R.N., clinical professor of psychiatry and obstetrics/gynecology at Wright State University School of Medicine in Dayton, Ohio. On the other hand, testosterone sometimes lives up to its reputation as a male hormone when given to women, Dr. Seifer adds. In a small number of cases, it can produce masculinizing side effects, such as facial hair, weight gain, a deepening of the voice, acne and some disturbances in blood cholesterol levels (one of the most unpleasant legacies of maleness).

"If a woman is already hairy or has problems with acne, she's going to want to hesitate before taking testosterone," Dr. Seifer says. (See also "Hormone Replacement Therapy.")

What Testosterone Can't Do

Testosterone is amazing stuff, but there are limits to what it can do. Not so long ago, for instance, many doctors and researchers believed that erectile problems and loss of libido in aging men had a lot to do with a gradual, age-related decline in testosterone levels. As a result, many older men whose fires were burning low were given replacement testosterone, either in pill form or by injection. But the hormonal story is not quite that simple, and it turns out that this treatment is usually a lousy idea.

For one thing, it's now known that testosterone has little to do with the ability to get an erection. It seems to stimulate *desire* but doesn't affect performance. (Little boys, who have very low testosterone levels, get erections quite regularly.)

In a man with normal testosterone levels, testosterone pills or shots may arouse his sexual appetite or heat up his sexual fantasy life, but he'll be no more able to get an erection than he ever was.

"I think the practice of giving testosterone injections to men having erectile difficulties is still fairly widespread; it's certainly not uncommon," says Richard E. Berger, M.D., professor of urology at the University of Washington and coauthor of *BioPotency: A Guide to Sexual Success*. "But in the absence of low testosterone, you're doing the person a disservice, because this causes the body to shut off its own production. Therefore, if you give testosterone injections long enough, it's hard for the body to recover and start producing its own supply again. Given in very large doses, testosterone can increase libido briefly, but this is short-lived. Unless there's a genuine shortage of testosterone, it's not a good treatment."

This is the same sort of thing that happens in male athletes who take anabolic steroids to boost muscle mass and sports performance. Because the steroids suppress their natural production of testosterone, taking them can eventually result in sterility, shrinkage of the testicles and liver damage. For women, taking steroids can interfere with menstrual cycles and ovulation.

There's another danger in giving testosterone to men with erection problems, Dr. Berger adds. Older men—the very sort of chaps who are inclined to have erectile troubles—are also prone to prostate cancer. And it's well known that testosterone stimulates the growth of prostate tumors, almost as if it were a nutrient for cancer. So by dumping additional testosterone into the body, it's possible that a small, undetected tumor may be "fertilized" and begin growing like a weed. (Testosterone doesn't *cause* prostate cancer, but if the tumor is already there, it stimulates its growth. That's why treatment for prostate cancer involves shutting off testosterone production, either by castration or with female hormones.)

About the only time testosterone injections really work is in the comparatively rare cases where a man's testosterone levels are genuinely low, Dr. Berger says. This is often caused by a condition called hypogonadism, or underfunctioning testes, which is thought to be the cause of erectile problems in perhaps 5 percent of cases. (It can be diagnosed only by a blood test.) If that's your problem, testosterone really can make a dramatic difference, he says. (See also "Erection Problems.")

What about Homosexuals?

If you think of testosterone as a hairy-chested, howling-in-the-woods sort of hormone, it's easy to understand something else that was once widely believed:

that homosexuals have lower levels of male hormones than heterosexuals. Some early, widely reported research supported this notion, but it's now been pretty thoroughly discredited. Homosexuals and heterosexuals do not seem to have significantly different testosterone levels. When homosexuals are given massive doses of testosterone, it doesn't turn them into heterosexuals, either, Dr. Silber says. It may temporarily boost a gay man's libido somewhat, but it will not change his sexual preference. Sexual preference is far more complex than mere hormones can explain (so complex, in fact, that nobody fully understands it).

Which brings us to the bottom line on testosterone: It's amazing, but it's not magic. It's not a panacea or a love potion. Its role is to stimulate our desire to seek a sexual partner, but whether we act on those urges, whom we seek if we do act on them and whatever else we do with our sexuality—well, that's up to us.

TUBAL STERILIZATION

At a certain point in life, many women run out of patience with temporary birth control methods and begin considering a one-stop solution: permanent sterilization. After all, a married woman is likely to decide she doesn't want any more kids by the time she's 30 or 35, but she can still get pregnant until she's 50 or so, when menopause signals the end of her childbearing days. That means as much as two decades of nagging worry about pregnancy whenever she has sex.

In fact, about 31 percent of all married women in America have had the operation, making it the most popular method of birth control among married women in the United States, according to the National Center for Health Statistics. By comparison, about 20 percent of married women use the Pill, and 17 percent rely on their husband's vasectomy for protection from surprise motherhood.

"The typical woman who gets the operation is married, thirtyish, with a couple of kids, someone who's decided her family is completed," says Pam Harper, public information officer at the New York City–based Association for Voluntary Surgical Contraception.

Why don't more women convince their husbands to be sterilized—since, after all, vasectomy (the male sterilization operation) is cheaper, safer and even more effective than female sterilization? (See "Vasectomy.")

"That's a complex question, and there are lots of theories—but the most obvious explanation is that it's women who get pregnant and have babies," says Harper. "It's usually the partner who wants to end childbearing the most, the one who's most highly motivated, who is the one who gets the surgery."

If you decide that sterilization is appropriate for you, what's involved?

Variations on a Theme

There are a number of variations on the operation, but they all have one goal: to block off the fallopian tubes so egg and sperm cannot meet. Eggs, manufactured in the ovaries, voyage down the fallopian tubes toward the uterus, hoping to make contact with sperm. But if the fallopian tubes are blocked, the eggs can't go anywhere. Although the ovaries continue to produce them, they're harmlessly reabsorbed into the body. "Having your tubes tied" or even "tubal ligation" is not a strictly accurate description—sometimes the fallopian tubes are ligated (tied off), but sometimes they're sealed off (electrocautery) or pinched off by means of clips, clamps or rings.

Here is a brief description of the most common techniques.

Laparoscopy. First a woman's abdomen is slightly inflated with ordinary air or another harmless gas so her reproductive organs can be seen clearly. Then a small incision is made in the abdominal wall, and a rodlike viewing device (called a laparoscope) is inserted through the opening. Once the tubes are located, additional instruments are slipped through the same incision, the tubes are tied off, the instruments are withdrawn, and the incision is closed. In the double-puncture technique, two incisions (one for the viewing device, the other for surgical tools) are made. Laparoscopies leave only a tiny scar, and the woman is free to resume sex as soon as she feels comfortable. Complications (usually bleeding or infection) occur in about 0.5 percent of cases.

However, medical experts say, laparoscopies are highly dependent on surgical skill. Surgeons who do fewer than 100 operations a year have a four times higher complication rate than those who do them more often. Make sure you have the operation done by a surgeon who's done plenty of them.

Minilaparotomy. A small incision is made in the lower abdomen, just above the pubic hairline. Through the incision, the surgeon locates the tubes, seals them off and closes the incision. This involves only local anesthesia, and recovery takes only a few days. Unlike laparoscopy, no visualizing instrument is used. This operation is generally done four or more weeks after delivery of a baby. A variation, called a subumbilical minilaparotomy, in which the incision is made closer to the navel, is generally performed within 48 hours after delivery.

Laparotomy. This is the old-fashioned "tubal ligation"—once the most common method of female sterilization. It's still considered major surgery. A laparotomy involves making a 2- to 5-inch incision in the abdomen. If it's done after delivery, it takes only 20 minutes. However, it may add one or two days to a woman's hospital stay, followed by several weeks of recovery at home.

Vaginal methods. Rather than making an incision in the abdominal wall, other techniques involve reaching the fallopian tubes through an incision on the roof of the vagina. In culdoscopy, a viewing instrument with a light on the end is inserted through the incision; a similar procedure, called colpotomy, involves no viewing instrument. Neither operation leaves a visible scar. However, in studies from around the world, vaginal procedures have been found to have higher infection rates and higher failure rates than either laparoscopies or laparotomies, so these operations are becoming increasingly less common.

The Big Pluses

Provided a woman is really ready for it, female sterilization, no matter how it's done, certainly has its advantages: no more fumbling in the dark with condoms or a diaphragm, and no more worries about pregnancy, because the operation is practically foolproof. Most studies show that failure rates are well below 1 percent—somewhere between 0.2 and 0.4 percent in the first year. This means that out of 1,000 women using the method for a year, 2 to 4 would get pregnant. (By comparison, about 30 would get pregnant using an IUD or the Pill.) In fact, except for vasectomy or a nunnery, female sterilization is the most effective birth control method available.

Does It Affect Sex?

Because so little about a woman's reproductive system is altered in the operation, tubal sterilization has few side effects. A large number of studies have shown that sterilization has little or no effect on a woman's enjoyment of sex, for instance. In one study of 200 American women, 97 percent said they were pleased with the operation, and many reported that complete freedom from the risk of pregnancy actually *increased* their sexual pleasure. (Other studies have not painted quite so rosy a picture; one British study suggested that up to 10 percent of women express some regret over having the operation, and a few request reversals.)

Since no gland is removed or altered in the operation, a woman's hormones (and her femininity) should not be affected at all. The operation does not bring on menopause. (In a hysterectomy, the hormone-producing ovaries are sometimes removed, which *does* trigger an artificial menopause—but sterilization doesn't touch the ovaries.) And tubal sterilization doesn't affect a woman's menstrual cycles, which continue in their usual pattern.

Consider It Permanent

Even so, it's crucial to remember the most important thing about sterilization: It's permanent. (Or at least, it should be *considered* permanent.) Before a woman and her partner decide this is the route they wish to take, they should be *absolutely* certain that they don't want any more children and never will. A woman shouldn't have the operation because she wants to delay having kids until later in life, shouldn't let herself be swayed by a sexual partner, friends or family if *she* doesn't want it and shouldn't do it because of temporary troubles like marital, sexual or financial problems. All those things are likely to change, but your operation will not—once it's done.

"It's important for women considering the operation to look ahead over their lives and ask themselves, if things were to change—if they remarried, if a husband died, if a child died—would they feel differently?" says Harper.

Studies have shown that the women most likely to regret the decision are those under 30 and those who are in unstable marriages when they're sterilized. Typically, such women regret the decision when they remarry and want to start a new family. Because of the importance of making the decision in a conscious, informed way, it's standard practice for doctors who do the operation to have patients sign an informed consent form beforehand.

Strictly speaking, it *is* possible to reverse the operation and restore a woman's fertility in many cases. However, because reversal is not possible in every case, you should never have a sterilization operation with the thought in mind that it "can always be reversed later." The success rates of reversal operations have dramatically increased in recent years—according to one report, among women considered suitable for operation, the chances of reversing a sterilization and having a successful pregnancy have increased from 22 percent in 1975 to over 80 percent in some circumstances today. Most other studies put a woman's chances of success at reversing the operation closer to 60 percent. The reversal operation is expensive, though, and the rate of ectopic or tubal pregnancy, a potentially serious complication, remains at about 3 percent.

How Safe Is It?

Years ago, having your tubes tied involved major abdominal surgery—several days in the hospital followed by a couple of weeks of recovery. Today, though, there's a strong national trend toward procedures that don't involve major surgery or an overnight stay in the hospital. You come into a clinic in the morning, have a 20- to 30-minute procedure, recover for a few hours and go home the same day, Harper explains. In about half of all cases, the surgery is performed shortly after delivery of a baby.

Overall, female sterilization is quite safe. Complications (usually bleeding or infection) develop in 1 to 4 percent of operations performed through the abdomen and 2 to 13 percent of procedures done through the vagina. In one survey of thousands of operations, researchers reported 2.29 deaths per 100,000 laparotomies and 4.72 per 100,000 laparoscopies. Don't forget, though, that childbirth is much more dangerous than that: In the United States, the mortality rate for delivery is about 14 for every 100,000 live births.

In 1992, the cost of an outpatient sterilization was running about $1,200 to $2,500, depending on the location, the surgeon and the technique used, according to Planned Parenthood. If you have to stay overnight in the hospital, it's more, of course, although many health insurance polices cover all or most of the cost.

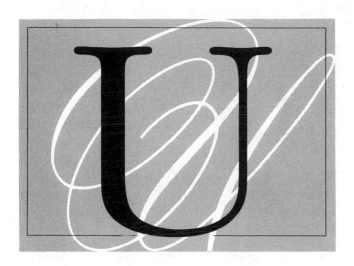

URINARY TRACT INFECTIONS

Gynecologists have often observed that young women are more likely to begin developing infections of the urinary tract and bladder (UTIs) after they become sexually active. It seems to go with the territory: There's something about sexual intercourse itself that increases the risk of infection.

One study conducted by researchers at the Infectious Diseases Clinic of the Health Sciences Centre in Winnipeg found that among young women with a history of recurrent UTIs, 75 percent of the episodes occurred within 24 hours after they'd had intercourse.

What's the Explanation?

UTIs occur when bacteria that normally inhabit the intestines and rectum (usually *Escherichia coli*) spread up into the vagina and from there infect the urinary tract, or urethra. UTIs include bladder infections (cystitis) and infections of the urethra (urethritis). Untreated UTIs can ascend to the kidneys, resulting in potentially serious infection.

UTIs are much more common in women for two simple reasons: Women's genital. anatomy puts the rectum unfortunately close to the opening of the urethra, and their urethra is shorter than a man's, making it easier for bacteria to make the trip up into the bladder. (A woman's urethra is about 2 inches long, a man's about 8 inches long, since it has to stretch all the way to the tip of the penis.)

But there are other reasons, less well understood, why sex and UTIs seem to go together. The Canadian researchers, in a particularly indelicate turn of phrase, suggest that intercourse may have a "mechanical milking" effect, pumping bacteria and other organisms from the vagina up into the urethra, where they may then spread to the bladder. Other researchers feel that intercourse (especially the rear-entry position) may help transfer bacteria directly from the rectal region into the vagina. Then there's what's sometimes called *honeymoon cystitis*—a condition in which intercourse (especially prolonged, enthusiastic intercourse) irritates the urethra and helps bacteria make their way up the urethra to the bladder.

The Danger of Diaphragms

In recent years, researchers have discovered another UTI/sex connection: Both the diaphragm and spermicides seem to significantly increase the risk of UTIs. In one study comparing 182 users of birth control pills with 192 women using diaphragms, UTIs were found to be about twice as common among women using diaphragms.

These researchers offered a couple of explanations for this. Diaphragms can slightly obstruct the urethra, they say, blocking urine flow and thus increasing the risk of infection. (Warm, stagnant urine is a prime breeding ground for bacteria.) Diaphragm use might also predispose women to UTIs by disturbing the complex flora of a normal, healthy vagina. Most of the time, the researchers note, just before a woman develops a UTI, "good" vaginal bacteria (mostly lactobacilli) are replaced by "bad" bacteria (usually *E. coli*). And that's precisely what happens among diaphragm users: Organisms like *E. coli* are recovered from vaginal cultures in those using diaphragms two to three times as often as from women using other contraceptive methods, researchers observe.

Spermicides also seem to increase the risk of UTIs by altering vaginal flora, since they kill beneficial bacteria (including lactobacilli) along with sperm.

Symptoms and Treatment

The classic symptoms of a UTI include painful urination, pain during intercourse, increased frequency and urgency of urination, having to urinate at night, itching and sometimes nausea. Sometimes there may also be a little blood in the urine or a feeling of fullness that's not relieved by urination. If the infection has spread up into the kidneys, doctors say, the symptoms may include low back pain or pain in the genitals.

Fortunately, UTIs are normally not too difficult to treat. Bacterial cystitis is generally treated with antimicrobial drugs like Bactrim or Septra (sometimes in a single, massive dose). Urethritis is usually treated with one to two weeks of antibiotics.

One thing to remember: Quite a few other kinds of genital infections can produce the very same or similar symptoms as a UTI, especially in young, sexually active women with multiple or new sex partners. According to one study, what you think is a UTI may actually turn out to be a vaginal yeast infection caused by *Candida albicans*. (See "Yeast Infections.") Or it could be a sexually transmitted organism like those that cause chlamydia, trichomoniasis, herpes or even gonorrhea. That's why it's important to have your doctor take a culture to make sure the actual culprit is correctly identified.

Banishing UTIs

If you are plagued by recurring UTIs, there are a number of things you can do to protect yourself.

Drink up. Doctors say that women who experience frequent UTIs should drink plenty of fluids to continuously flush microorganisms out of the urethra. Urinate when you first have the urge; don't wait until your bladder is full. It also helps to urinate, even if only a few drops, just after you have intercourse.

Wipe from front to back. It's important to wipe from the vagina toward the rectum, rather than the other way around, to avoid spreading rectal bacteria into the vagina. Also, if fingers or sex toys make contact with the rectum during lovemaking, be sure to wash them before touching the vagina with them. And if UTIs are a recurrent problem, avoid rear-entry vaginal intercourse.

Have your diaphragm refitted. If you use a diaphragm and are troubled by recurrent UTIs, you might ask your doctor to refit you with a smaller one or one with a different rim style. If that doesn't help, you might ask your doctor about trying a different form of birth control. (You might try a cervical cap, which is basically just a very small diaphragm. Caps do not affect urine flow the way diaphragms do.)

Try cranberry juice. Some women troubled by recurrent infections swear by cranberry juice, which acidifies the urine and may help kill bacteria.

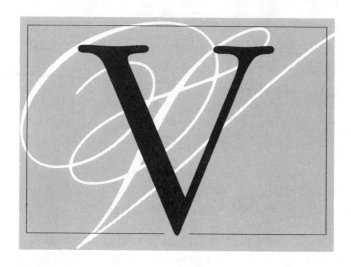

VAGINA

Despite its pivotal role in human history, until quite recently the interior of the vagina was nearly as mysterious as the dark side of the moon. But during the late 1950s and early 1960s, in a series of breathtaking explorations, William Masters, M.D., and Virginia Johnson, of the Masters and Johnson Institute in St. Louis, were able to directly observe something that had never been seen before: what happens deep inside the vagina during sexual arousal and intercourse. They performed this amazing feat by having women masturbate to orgasm using an ingenious camera–equipped plastic penis, complete with a special cold light to illuminate the mysterious, lightless interior.

In its normal, unstimulated state, they reported, the vagina is "a potential rather than an actual space"—its soft walls are collapsed together, touching each other. But during the first stage of the sexual response cycle, shortly after sexual stimulation begins, two things happen: The vagina begins to lubricate and to expand. Lubrication is the first physiological sign of arousal in women: Within 10 to 30 seconds after stimulation begins, Masters and Johnson found, little beads of fluid begin forming all over the vaginal walls, making them look almost like a sweat-beaded forehead. The little beads rapidly spread to form a smooth, glistening covering.

As a woman becomes increasingly aroused, the deepest two-thirds of her vagina begin blowing up, almost like a balloon—lengthening and expanding in what Masters and Johnson described as a "tenting" effect. The uterus and the cervix pull slowly up and back, out of harm's way. (If a woman has a retroverted, or tipped, uterus, the cervix stays where it is, suspended into this ever-widening vaginal cavity—where the man's penis may batter it, sometimes painfully, during intercourse.)

Meanwhile, the vaginal walls dramatically change in color. From their usual purplish red cast, they darken into a distinctly purplish hue as a result of vasocongestion—the damming-up of blood that's the central event of sexual arousal.

As sexual excitement reaches the plateau stage (the second stage of the sexual response cycle), the outer third of the vagina swells with blood, to the point where it actually narrows the vaginal entrance by up to 50 percent. (The deeper part of the vagina is expanding; the outer part is narrowing.) They called this outer third, swollen by vasocongestion, the "orgasmic platform," and it was this area, they discovered, that reacted most dramatically during orgasm. At the moment of climax, this whole outer ring begins spasmodically contracting at 0.8-second intervals, anywhere from 3 to 15 times. At the very highest levels of sexual excitement, Masters and Johnson found, some women experience a sort of superorgasm: The orgasmic platform explodes into a spastic contraction lasting 2 to 4 seconds, then downshifts into the 0.8-second contractions of normal orgasm.

Afterward (during the third, or resolution, phase of the sexual response cycle), the orgasmic platform rapidly drains of blood, the vaginal opening expands, and the inner, distended part of the vagina shrinks back to its original state. Its usual color returns within 10 to 15 minutes, and life returns to normal. Whew!

Masters and Johnson's spectacular findings point to one rather distressing conclusion—most men labor under some pretty odd notions about what actually turns women on.

Debunking the Deep Penetration Myth

The greatest misconception most men have about the vagina is that deep, pounding penetration drives women wild. Male-oriented erotic literature endlessly conjures up the imagery of deep penetration: spikes, spears, swords, lances, scimitars, all of them plunging hungrily down to the hilt.

But the truth is that for most women, the deepest two-thirds of the vagina are practically numb to the touch. Researchers have found that deep inside, the vaginal walls have so few nerve endings that they're similar to an internal organ (and if somebody touched your kidney, you'd hardly know it). By contrast, the outer third of the vagina and the introitus, or vaginal opening (including the labia and clitoris), are exceedingly sensitive to touch.

These regions of sensitivity were demonstrated long ago in a series of famous experiments conducted by the late Dr. Alfred Kinsey and his colleagues, who had five gynecologists explore the sensitivity of the whole genital region in 879 women. Using a glass, metal or cotton-tipped probe, the gynecologists touched or gently stroked each different area, including the clitoris, labia, the vestibule (opening) of the vagina, the deep walls of the vagina and the cervix. When the probe made contact with the women's deep vaginal walls, the gynecologists reported, less than 14 percent of the women could even feel it. By contrast, when the probe stroked the clitoris, labia or virtually anywhere else around the vaginal opening, 97 percent of the women were "distinctly conscious" of the touch.

Dr. Kinsey also noted something else, which he considered an indirect confirmation of this finding: Only a very few of the women who masturbated said they usually did so by inserting something deep into the vagina. Eighty-four percent of the women said they masturbated mostly by stimulating the clitoris and labia; a few others said they inserted things, but only occasionally.

On the other hand, sex researchers since Dr. Kinsey's day have established that some women do find deep vaginal penetration incredibly pleasurable, reporting that this triggers a "deep" orgasm that's different from an orgasm touched off by clitoral stimulation. Since the vaginal walls have so little feeling, other sources have been suggested to account for these sensations. Some women, sex researchers now believe, particularly enjoy the deep muscular contractions of the uterus and muscles of the pelvic floor, which occur during orgasm (and miss these sensations terribly when the uterus is removed in a hysterectomy). Other women seem to be especially responsive to firm pressure on the top front wall of the vagina, the so-called G-spot. (See "G-Spot.")

Basically, what we're saying here is that when it comes to sexual enjoyment—and sexual equipment—we're all alike . . . but we're also different.

Dancing Woman Meets Coyote Man

Almost anybody who's frequented a locker room has noticed the great and wonderful variety of human body types, including the genitalia. Vaginas and penises are as different as faces, hair and hands. In fact, there have been repeated attempts down through the ages—from the Hindu sages of the Indian Middle Ages to Cherokee Nation medicine men—to classify men and women according to the appearance of their genitals.

For instance, among the Cherokees, the vagina is given the lovely name *tupuli,* or "feathered flying serpent," and its depth and nature are thought to be related to a woman's entire sexual temperament, according to Harley Swiftdeer, author of the *Quodoushka Manual.* The Cherokees describe five different female genital anatomy types and five male types. Dancing Woman, for instance, has a vagina of average depth, small labial lips, a clitoris that is tiny and very high (three to four fingers above the vaginal opening) and that pops out easily from beneath its hood. Such a woman, the Cherokees say, prefers a Coyote Man, whose penis (otherwise known as a *tipili,* or "sacred snake") tends to be quite short and thin. Sheep Woman, by contrast, has a deeper vagina, larger, thicker lips and a lower, more hooded clitoris; she tends to lubricate copiously and cannot seem to reach orgasm unless she has some heart connection to her partner. She, too, prefers Coyote Man (that lucky dog).

Such teachings, fanciful as they may seem, simply underscore a great truth about human sexuality: Our bodies, and our sexuality, are an expression of our uniqueness, and there's no "right" or "wrong" about it.

Vaginismus

Vaginismus is a condition in which the ring of muscles that surrounds the vagina goes into spasm, clamping down the vaginal opening so tightly that penetration (by a penis, a tampon or anything else) is extremely painful or even impossible. Women suffering from vaginismus have sometimes never consummated their marriages, or even had a pelvic exam or inserted a tampon, because it hurts too much.

It may sound like a sexual oddity, but it's not. Vaginismus is the third most common female sexual dysfunction, after lack of orgasm (anorgasmia) and painful intercourse (dyspareunia), according to Emanual Fliegelman, D.O., professor of obstetrics and gynecology and director of Human Sexuality Programs at the Osteopathic Medical Center of Philadelphia.

A Sad Little Dance

At bottom, say experts, vaginismus is nearly always a psychosomatic disorder (meaning that it's caused by the mind).

Sometimes the whole thing gets started as a sort of sad little dance between body and mind. First, some underlying *physical* problem makes penetration painful. (The underlying disorder could be any number of things, from an unperforated hymen or a dry, atrophied vagina to endometriosis.) Then, anticipating pain the next time intercourse is attempted, the mind signals the muscles to slam the vagina shut. Because the vagina is so tightly closed, attempted penetration becomes even more painful. Which causes the muscles to squeeze even more tightly. In the end, the whole process seems to get beyond the woman's conscious control, and normally voluntary muscles behave like involuntary ones.

In a case like this, even after the physical cause is found and treated, it's likely the vaginismus will persist. Then it will take some gentle counseling or even psychotherapy before a woman finally learns to relax those muscles enough for intercourse.

Inhibitions Become Physical

In other cases, vaginismus develops as a result of some purely psychological problem or traumatic event. Rape, incest or childhood molestation or a sexual phobia of one sort or another may cause it. More commonly though, women with vaginismus are the product of a severely repressive, sex-negative, often highly religious kind of upbringing. Their vaginas slam shut because sex is sin. Robert Birch, Ph.D., director of the Arlington Center for Marital and Sexual Concerns in Columbus, Ohio, tells the story of a woman who used to be known as "old iron-pants" in Catholic school, because none of the boys could ever get into her pants. "She wore this nickname as a badge of honor—but after she got married, she couldn't get the badge off," Dr. Birch says. "She came in for therapy after 13 years of marriage, which had never been consummated." Often, he says, such couples never show up for therapy at all until they want to have a baby.

Opening Closed Doors

The good news is that treatment for vaginismus has one of the highest success rates of any sexual dysfunction—nearly 100 percent, according to various studies. Generally, the treatment begins with a little training in deep muscle relation. Often the woman is taught to do Kegel exercises, tightening and loosening the pelvic muscles in order to relax them and to develop a better sense of control over the muscles that have gone into spasm. (See "Kegel Exercises.")

After she's learned to relax, she's shown how to insert the smallest of a series of vaginal dilators into her vagina. (Vaginal dilators, generally made of hard plastic, are shaped rather like the bishop in a chest set and come in a graduated series, from smaller than a little finger to penis-size.) The first dilator is left in place for 10 minutes or so, then removed. Some doctors give patients a set of dilators that they can use at home a couple of times a day, keeping them in place for 15 to 30 minutes at a time and sometimes even sleeping with them in. With daily practice, over a period of weeks or months, the woman gradually progresses to the largest dilator in the series. Eventually, she should be ready for intercourse. (Therapists generally discourage intercourse before she's ready, because a bad experience could set the whole vicious cycle in motion again.)

Some doctors suggest that instead of using dilators, a woman use one lubricated finger, then two fingers, then her husband's fingers. Once he's able to get both fingers in, he can gently attempt intercourse (without thrusting at first). Other therapists suggest starting out with a lubricated little finger or a lubricated cotton swab, then moving up to peeled, penis-size vegetables like zucchini or carrots.

Overcoming vaginismus is not something that involves only a woman—her sex partner is deeply affected by it all, too. Not surprisingly, some husbands develop erection problems because they fear hurting their wives by attempting intercourse or because repeated attempts at entry have failed. That's why many therapists like to involve both members of the couple in therapy—and why patience, kindness and gentleness (from both parties) is so important.

VASECTOMY

The bottom line on vasectomy, the male sterilization operation, is this: It should not affect your sex drive or performance in any way. The operation is safe, simple, inexpensive and nearly painless. And it's the most effective form of birth control that there is, short of never having sex at all.

How's that for a sales pitch?

There's just one major drawback: It's permanent. Although it *is* possible to restore a man's fertility after he's had a vasectomy—sometimes many years afterward—it's not something you should count on. The vasectomy reversal operation (which involves astoundingly delicate microsurgery) is very difficult, may cost $3,000 to $7,000 and has only slightly better than a 50 percent chance of success. No microsurgeon can *guarantee* success, even if you're a good candidate. So for all practical purposes, you should never have a vasectomy unless you're *completely* at peace with the idea of never making any more babies.

What It Doesn't Do

Just for the record, here's what a vasectomy *doesn't* do.

The operation does not affect a man's ability to ejaculate or make any noticeable difference in the appearance or volume of his semen. All the operation does is cut off the supply of sperm—but sperm are so tiny they make up less than 1 percent of the total volume of ejaculate. (The rest is a warm protein stew manufactured by the seminal vesicles and the prostate.)

A vasectomy doesn't affect a man's sex drive or his ability to have erections. Vasectomy is *not* castration, so it has no effect on hormones. Castration, the surgical removal of the testicles, does affect a man's state of mind, because testosterone—the hormone that triggers libido—is produced by the testes. But vasectomy doesn't even touch the testes.

According to William Masters, M.D., and Virginia Johnson, of the Masters and Johnson Institute in St. Louis, fewer than 1 man in 20 reports decreased sexual pleasure after a vasectomy, close to half say their pleasure increased after the operation, and a quarter say they have intercourse more frequently now that they're "sperm-free."

Surgery 101

The operation itself is so simple it generally takes only 15 or 20 minutes and is usually performed in a doctor's office under local anesthesia. Once the scrotum is shaved, sterilized and numbed, a tiny incision is made in the scrotal skin. The physician reaches through this opening and locates the pair of tubes (the vas deferens) that transport sperm from the testes, where sperm is manufactured, to the urethra, where it exits the body. Each vas, in turn, is snipped in two, and the ends are stitched shut, clipped shut or cauterized. Sometimes only one of the two ends is tied off. Sometimes a little section of the vas is removed, just for good measure. Then the scrotal incision is stitched back up—and that, more or less, is that.

The ultimate result: Sperm cells are unable to escape from the body, although the testicles continue to produce them. Instead of being ejaculated, they're harmlessly broken down and reabsorbed by scavenger cells called phagocytes.

The operation usually costs less than $1,000 and is covered by many medical insurance plans. Afterward, the man is free to go home, although he's usually advised to avoid strenuous activity for up to a week. Some doctors recommend that patients rest for about two days afterward and stay on intimate terms with an ice pack.

You can resume sexual intercourse after two or three days—but it's important to remember that you're not sterile the moment the operation is through. Even after the vas has been severed, it generally takes up to 20 ejaculations before all the sperm-loaded semen that's stored up in a man's reproductive duct work is cleared out. For this reason, most urologists require two sperm-free semen samples before a man can officially be recognized as shooting blanks.

Generally, the failure rate for vasectomy is given as around 0.1 percent. This number means that in the first year after their partners had a vasectomy, about 1 in 1,000 women will get pregnant. But some of these pregnancies occur because couples had sex before all the sperm was cleared out of the man's system—so the real numbers may be even lower.

The No-Scalpel Vasectomy

In this relatively new procedure, the doctor makes a tiny puncture hole in the scrotum instead of the traditional incision. It's faster, safer and virtually bloodless, and it produces considerably less discomfort than other techniques. After the injection of a local anesthetic, one of two specially designed surgical tools gently holds one of the vas deferens while the other tool makes the puncture. Then each vas deferens is lifted out, cut and tied and pushed back into the scrotum.

While still relatively rare in this country, this technique is now standard practice in China—so far eight million Chinese men have undergone this procedure.

Minor Complications

Out of every 100 men who have a vasectomy, something like 4 or 5 develop minor complications—but most are easily treated with ice packs or wearing a jockstrap (to support the scrotum) for a few days. The most common problems are pain, swelling and discoloration due to bleeding beneath the skin. Sometimes the occluded end of the cut vas leaks a little sperm, which forms a tiny lump, or granuloma. Although they generally go away in a few days, sperm granulomas can be painful. Sometimes minor infections occur. And sometimes the fragile duct work called the epididymis, under pressure from all that backed-up sperm, blows out, causing a sometimes painful condition called epididymitis. All these problems generally go away within a week, though.

Are there any really serious, long-term health problems associated with vasectomy? This, of course, has been a continuing concern to medical researchers— but so far, nobody has convincingly shown that there are any. In the late 1970s, a couple of studies on monkeys suggested that vasectomy might increase the risk of heart disease—but since that time, a whole raft of follow-up studies in humans failed to support this. A team of researchers at Boston University School of Medicine, after studying over 2,000 men who'd had a vasectomy, concluded that "there is little cause for concern" that vasectomy increases the risk of heart attack, even in men already predisposed to them. And a more recent Scottish study, which suggested that vasectomy might slightly increase the risk of testicular cancer, has so far not been confirmed by other researchers.

Safer Than a Tubal

It's usually married couples over 30 who've had quite enough kids, thank you, who choose sterilization as a form of permanent birth control. For them, the question usually comes down to this: Should he do it, or should she? And from that point of view, vasectomy wins hands down. Medical experts agree that the male sterilization operation is quicker, simpler, safer and less expensive than the female version—the tubal ligation.

A tubal, after all, involves abdominal surgery; a vasectomy involves a couple of snips in a doctor's office.

Female sterilization is also roughly twice as expensive as a vasectomy. And in the event that you want to have the surgery reversed, the male reversal process is much cheaper and safer (although neither has a very high rate of success).

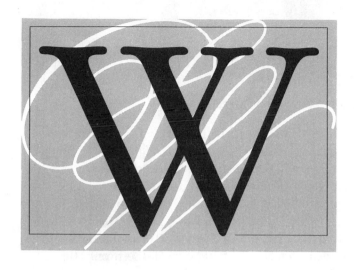

WARTS, GENITAL

If you think that sexually transmitted diseases are limited to gonorrhea, syphilis and AIDS, guess again. One of the real biggies is warts—genital warts, caused by the human papillomavirus (HPV). "In the college-age population, it's one of the most common sexually transmitted diseases we see. And even though HPV used to be thought of as little more than a nuisance, we now know that these infections need to be taken seriously," says Sandra Samuels, M.D., director of Student Health Services at Rutgers University in New Brunswick, New Jersey.

Some researchers estimate that the incidence of genital warts has doubled in the past decade—something like three million new cases of these infections are diagnosed annually in the United States, according to the U.S. Department of Health and Human Services. Their favorite target: young, sexually active people in their teens and twenties, especially women. The main danger, researchers now believe, is that several kinds of HPV play an important role in the development of certain kinds of cancer, especially cervical cancer.

You Can't Always See Them

Genital warts, also sometimes called venereal warts, are known to doctors as *condylomata acuminata* ("pointed knob"). Actually, though, all those names are something of a misnomer, because very often there's no wart (or any other visible evidence) to indicate that you're infected. In one study sponsored by the National Institute of Allergy and Infectious Diseases, almost half of women with HPV infections had no visible symptoms at all. Other researchers say there's no visible evidence (at least visible to the naked eye) in closer to *90 percent* of cases. In most cases, they say, the evidence of HPV infection can be seen only through a microscope, or the warts are tucked away out of view (such as up inside the vagina, inside the rectum or on the cervix).

If you're a man and unlucky enough to discover visible evidence of genital warts, though, they're likely to show up on or around the head of the penis or (in uncircumcised men) under the foreskin. They can also turn up on the shaft of the penis, on the scrotum, inside the urethra (often making urination painful) or around the anus. In women, warts usually show up on the lips of the vagina, inside the vagina, around the anus or on the cervix. Occasionally, they may even appear inside the mouth of someone who has been having oral sex with a partner who's infected.

Genital warts can vary quite a bit in appearance, doctors say—sometimes they don't bulge at all but appear as low bumps or hard, flat spots. Or sometimes they're bulging, fleshy warts that may be pink, red or whitish and grow fairly rapidly. If left untreated, they take on a cauliflower-like appearance, or there may be so many of them, so close together, that they look like a carpet or mosaic of warts, according to Alan N. Gordon, M.D., a gynecologist in Austin, Texas.

The Biggest Worry

One thing to remember about HPV infection, says Dr. Samuels, is that it's highly contagious. Even if you don't have any visible signs of infection, you still can unwittingly transmit the virus to your partner. In fact, HPV is so tirelessly contagious that researchers estimate about 70 percent of the sexual partners of HPV-infected people are also infected. Which is why, if you're diagnosed as being a carrier, you should drag your partner down to the clinic for treatment, too, or at least inform him or her that you're infected. (Since the incubation period may vary from a few weeks to a couple of years, it may sometimes be difficult to know which past sexual partner is to blame.)

If it were only the fact that warts are unsightly, HPV might be easier to ignore. But researchers have now learned that HPV infection is also strongly associated with precancerous changes of the cervix, vulva, penis and anus. Many genital cancers, it's now believed, progress through a multistep process before they actually become malignant tumors. And certain strains of HPV, under certain conditions, may transform a benign wart into a precancerous growth called *dysplasia*. In women, the cervix is a particularly favored location for these precancerous dysplasias. In fact, according to Dr. Gordon, HPV is the most common Pap test abnormality of the cervix.

That's why sexually active women (all women, in fact) should have Pap tests done religiously to monitor the cellular health of their cervix. One thing to remember, though: Since the Pap test detects only abnormal cell growth and not HPV infection itself, some doctors now recommend getting one additional test at the same time you get your Pap test. The Virapap test, recently approved by the Food and Drug Administration, is a more accurate screening test because it can detect five strains of HPV that have been most closely linked to cervical cancer. If you're sexually active or have reason to be especially worried about genital warts, ask your doctor about this test.

Declaring War on Warts

The basic treatment for genital warts is to destroy the wart and the surrounding infected tissue—crude, true, but reasonably effective. Small warts can be removed by freezing them with liquid nitrogen or nitrous oxide gas (cryotherapy), burning them off (electrocautery) or vaporizing them with lasers. Unfortunately, doctors say, even when surrounding tissue is removed, in about 20 percent of cases the warts come back because the HPV virus has penetrated what looks like normal, healthy skin. That's one characteristic of genital warts: The buggers often come back.

Sometimes a topical ointment that eats away the wart when applied directly to the skin is prescribed. One common medication is a solution containing podophyllin, a toxic substance extracted from the rhizomes of a plant that grows in the Himalayas. The solution is applied to the warts once or twice a week for a month or so, or until the warts go away. Podophyllin is powerful stuff, though, and it can be applied only by a doctor. It's also not recommended for pregnant women, because it can be absorbed through the skin and damage the fetus. It doesn't work terribly well, either: In one study, it got rid of warts in only 40 percent of cases.

Other, less potent solutions (such as trichloroacetic acid) can be prescribed for at-home use. For especially stubborn infections, a relatively new treatment is interferon (a natural substance that can kill certain viruses like HPV), which is given either orally or by injection.

What Can You Do?

There are a couple of things you need to remember to protect yourself.

Some researchers say there's no convincing evidence that using condoms helps to protect against the spread of genital warts. Others say condoms do offer some protection, although it may be imperfect. The bottom line is that if you're sexually active in this day and age, you should be using condoms anyway.

If you discover a suspicious-looking wart, sore or any kind of lesion on or around your genitals, you should not hesitate to have your doctor take a look at it. With HPV infections, especially, the sooner it's treated, the safer you'll be.

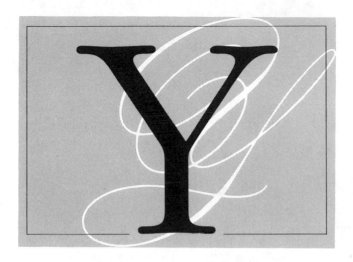

YEAST INFECTIONS

Nothing takes the joy out of sex like a vaginal yeast infection. The most common symptom, present in 90 percent of cases, is intense itching of the vaginal opening and vulva (which is about as sexy as an old shoe). There may also be burning during urination and intercourse, redness and inflammation of vaginal tissues and a curdlike discharge that resembles cottage cheese. Some women say it smells like baking bread.

Unfortunately, this dismal litany of complaints is not at all uncommon. Yeast infections are one of the most frequently diagnosed diseases in gynecology, paying an unwelcome visit to three out of every four women at some point during their childbearing years. A quarter of these women have multiple, recurrent infections, doctors say.

Usually, the culprit turns out to be a globe-trotting fungus called *Candida albicans,* in which case the infection is called vulvovaginal candidiasis. Like most fungi, candida thrives in warm, dark, wet places, and the vagina is perfect (although the fungus can also thrive in the throat or in the intestines).

What Causes It?

"All women have yeast in their vaginas, along with a whole host of other microorganisms. What we call 'yeast infections' occur when, for one reason or another, the natural ecology of the vaginal flora gets disrupted," explains micro-biologist Marjorie Crandall, Ph.D., founder of Yeast Consulting Services in Torrance, California.

Normally, this self-contained ecosystem keeps the vagina slightly acidic, which in turn keeps any one microorganism (including candida) from multiplying out of control, Dr. Crandall explains. But a number of things are known to disrupt this vaginal balance and can lead to yeast infections.

Antibiotics. Because they kill the bacteria needed to maintain the normal acidity of the vagina, antibiotics are one of the most common causes of yeast infections, according to Terry Kriedman, M.D., of the Department of Obstetrics and Gynecology at the Medical College of Pennsylvania in Philadelphia. Some antibiotics, especially tetracycline, may also directly stimulate yeast cells.

Female hormones. Women taking estrogen in birth control pills, or older women on hormone replacement therapy, are more inclined to develop yeast infections. Estrogen causes a host of metabolic changes, and it may (in some as yet unknown way) stimulate yeast cells directly. It's also known that estrogen increases the vagina's glycogen content by 50 percent or more—and since glyco-gen breaks down to sugar, it may also be that yeast cells are simply feeding on sugar (as they do in a brewer's vat). However, the yeast infection/sugar link has never been proven, Dr. Crandall points out.

Corticosteroids. These drugs, used to treat asthma and autoimmune diseases like lupus, can have a "devastating" effect on the body's immune system and increase the risk of yeast infection, Dr. Crandall says. They're also precisely the same substances the body produces under stress—which may explain why stress can also contribute to yeast infections.

Pregnancy. Fourteen percent of women develop yeast infections during pregnancy because of hormonal changes that alter the vaginal environment. Half these women have to be treated for yeast infections more than once during their pregnancies.

Menstruation. Some women are more susceptible to infections before or during their periods because menstrual blood makes the vagina less acid. (Acidity inhibits yeast growth.)

Diabetes. High blood sugar levels increase susceptibility to infection.

Infections That Keep On Coming

Usually, gynecologists treat a yeast infection with one of three medications, for three days to a week: miconazole (Monistat), clotrimazole (Gyne-Lotrimin) or nystatin (Mycostatin or Nilstat). In about three-quarters of cases, the medication takes care of the problem. But for millions of women, nothing seems to work, and recurrent yeast infections become a recurrent nightmare. To find any real, permanent relief, they may have to alter their lifestyle significantly.

Is it possible for a yeast infection to be passed back and forth, from partner to partner, in a sort of infernal sexual Ping-Pong? Well, studies have shown that sex partners usually harbor the very same strain of yeast organism, which strongly suggests the answer is yes. It is also known that men can harbor candida on the skin of their genitals, underneath the foreskin or in the prostate, where it infects the semen, Dr. Crandall says. Sometimes an infected man will develop a rash on the skin of his genitals, or (if his prostate is infected) he'll feel a bit of pain in the urethra during ejaculation. Usually, though, yeast-infected men are completely without symptoms. (No, life is not fair.)

On the other hand, women can develop yeast infections without any sexual contact at all. (One popular theory: Candida is also present in the intestine, which serves as a "reservoir" of organisms that repeatedly reinfect the vagina.)

Doctors who cultured the semen of sex partners of women with recurrent yeast infections found most of the men were carriers (probably because of a prostate infection). When both partners were treated for two weeks with 200 milligrams a day of the antifungal drug ketoconazole, 31 of 33 women were cured and remained infection-free for a year. Some doctors suggest that women plagued by recurrent infections have their partners get their semen cultured for yeast and use an antifungal cream (such as Mycostatin) on their genitals.

Look-Alike Infections

Sometimes what appears to be a yeast infection may be caused not by yeast at all but by some other equally unpleasant organism. That's why, when women go to the doctor with a vaginal infection, they should insist on a pelvic exam and a smear, or microscopic examination of vaginal fluids, Dr. Crandall says. (A gynecologist is more likely to be properly equipped for such testing than a family doctor, she adds.)

Sometimes the offending organism turns out to be a bacterium called *Gardnerella vaginalis* (the infection is called *bacterial vaginosis*). The most common symptom is a foul-smelling vaginal discharge that's milky, frothy, white or gray. Some infected women notice that just after intercourse, they have a fishy smell. (One classic test, widely used in clinics, is the "sniff test": If you mix vaginal discharge with potassium hydroxide and it produces a fishy odor, you know *G. vaginalis* has found a new home.)

Another common offender: *Trichomonas vaginalis,* a nasty protozoan with a characteristic whiplike tail. Usually the chief complaint is a profuse yellow or green discharge with a particularly offensive odor. In severe cases, there may also be itching, redness and swelling of vaginal tissue. Strictly speaking, trichomoniasis (sometimes called "trick") is a sexually transmitted disease, because it's almost never found in women who aren't sexually active. It's also more common in women with multiple sex partners.

For both trichomoniasis and gardnerella, the antibiotic Flagyl is usually prescribed, and *both* partners should be treated, specialists in sexually transmitted diseases say.

How to Prevent Infection

All this may sound like a certain number of vaginal infections are every woman's lot. Not so. You *can* fight back. Here's how.

Try changing your contraceptive. Studies have shown that oral contraceptives, the IUD, vaginal spermicides and the contraceptive sponge may increase a woman's likelihood of developing a yeast infection. The IUD seems to increase vaginal secretions that are favorable to yeast growth. The sponge increases risk because it contains spermicides that kill bacteria as well as sperm. In one study of prostitutes in Bangkok, Thailand, sponge users were more than twice as likely as nonusers to develop yeast infections. Consider switching to a barrier method, like condoms or the cervical cap, which are not associated with increased risk.

Avoid tight underwear. Moisture and heat are the perfect combination for yeast growth. Sunbathing in a wet swimsuit or wearing nylon underwear, panty hose, leotards or tight jeans is just asking for trouble. It's best to wear loose-fitting clothes and white cotton underwear, or at least panty hose with a cotton crotch, doctors say. (White is best because some dyes can be irritating.)

Avoid sugary foods. "There's very little scientific evidence, but a great deal of anecdotal evidence, that by avoiding sugary foods women can reduce the likelihood that they'll get yeast infections," Dr. Crandall says. The reason, apparently: less glucose in the vagina.

Be gentle. Anything that irritates vaginal tissue can predispose a woman to yeast infections. So avoid feminine deodorant hygiene sprays, perfumed toilet paper or too-frequent douching. Dr. Crandall recommends douching only with water, if at all, and avoiding vinegar, bicarbonate, Betadine or other harsh chemicals. Some women who are hypersensitive and have a history of yeast infections should avoid *all* chemicals, including soaps, bath oils, bubble baths, lubricating jellies or deodorized tampons, she says. Some women also say tampons seem to increase susceptibility to infection, so try using sanitary pads instead.

Try yogurt. Although conclusive scientific evidence is lacking, many women swear that eating yogurt helps (perhaps by restoring bacteria that fight candida). In one small study at Long Island Jewish Medical Center in New York, 11 women with recurrent candidal infections were monitored for six months, then they ate 1 cup of yogurt containing *Lactobacillus acidophilus* daily for six months. Result: An average of three infections fell to less than one during the six months the women ate yogurt. The researchers note that you've got to find yogurt containing active *L. acidophilus,* which may not be easy. (*Don't* apply yogurt directly to the vagina; it can add a bacterial infection to your existing problems.)

Some doctors even recommend taking three or four *L. acidophilus* capsules (available at health food stores and some pharmacies) every time you take a dose of antibiotics, in order to restore vaginal flora.

YOHIMBINE

Yohimbine is a chemical derived from the African yohimbe tree. Tea made from the tree's bark has a long, exotic folk history as a "love potion." The modern-day chemical derivative is a newly respectable prescription drug used in the treatment of male impotence.

Clinical studies done at reputable scientific institutions have shown that yohimbine restores erections—either fully or partially—in up to a third of the impotent men who try it. Although that's a success rate considerably lower than other, more drastic impotence treatments (like self-injection or implants), it also has advantages they don't have: It is noninvasive and fairly inexpensive and has very few side effects. (There is a possibility that it affects blood pressure—we'll get to that shortly.)

Skeptics say that yohimbine is really nothing more than a placebo—a worthless pill that works only because men believe it will. Still, some studies have shown that yohimbine works as well for organic impotence (caused by physical ills such as diabetes or vascular disease) as it does for erection problems caused by psychogenic (psychological) troubles. In fact, yohimbine is now the most commonly used nonhormonal drug for the treatment of impotence. Many urologists feel that the most rational use of the drug is as a sort of "first try" screening tool: If it works, fine. If not, then it's easy enough to move on to treatments that are more invasive, expensive and complicated.

Exaggerated Early Reports

Part of the skepticism many doctors still feel about yohimbine may stem from studies published in the late 1960s and early 1970s that claimed amazing success rates in treating impotent men with yohimbine. One research team reported that in a study of 10,000 men with erection problems, up to 80 percent reported "good to excellent" results while taking the drug. Another study reported that, measured in terms of erections and/or orgasms, yohimbine was up to five times as effective as a placebo.

The trouble was, it turned out that the "miracle cure" used in the studies was a drug called Afrodex. This drug was not pure yohimbine but a whole witch's brew of stuff—yohimbine, plus methyl testosterone, plus nux vomica, the plant source of the powerful poison strychnine. More careful review of these studies revealed some dubious statistics—and some suggestion that the drug itself might be toxic. The Food and Drug Administration removed Afrodex from the market in 1973. (Impotence, after all, is better than death.)

Encouraging New Research

But a new generation of researchers, using careful study designs and pure pharmaceutical yohimbine—nothing else—have shown that the drug really does seem to work for a small but consistent portion of the male population. It doesn't work as well as those fevered early reports claimed, but it does seem to work.

In one study, a team of researchers from Kingston General Hospital and Queen's University, in Ontario, tested the drug on 48 men who'd met strict criteria showing that their erection problems were psychogenic in origin, rather than being caused by any physical problem. For ten weeks, the men were given either yohimbine (18 milligrams daily, in the form of a 6-milligram tablet three times a day) or an identical-looking but totally inactive placebo.

Overall, the researchers found, 46 percent of the men taking yohimbine noticed either complete or partial improvement in the rigidity of their erections. (Only 16 percent of the placebo group noticed any improvement.) Interestingly enough, these same researchers also tested yohimbine on a group of men with organic impotence and found it was almost equally effective—43 percent of these men also reported some improvement, including 20 percent who claimed *complete* recovery. (Just to confound matters, 27 percent also responded to the placebo, however.)

"Until other pharmacological substances have been tested in controlled trials, yohimbine should be considered among the first treatment options for psychogenically impotent patients," the researchers concluded.

Harder Case, Higher Dose

Sixteen or 18 milligrams a day is the typical dosage used in most yohimbine studies. But in an older, sicker population of men, higher doses have also been used—with rather striking success.

In one study, researchers tested the drug on 82 impotent men who came into a Veterans Administration hospital in Rhode Island. These men were older (mean age 61) and sicker (many had diabetes, heart disease, nutritional deficiencies or a history of alcoholism) than the men in most other studies. So the researchers tried this plan: They started them off on four tablets a day and gradually raised the dosage to eight (42 milligrams) or until they found what seemed an optimum minimal dose.

After one month, the researchers found, 34 percent of the men were responding to the drug—ten of the men (14 percent) having experienced the joyful restoration of "full and sustained erections," and 20 percent experiencing a partial response (stronger erections, occasionally rigid enough for penetration). For the remaining 65 percent of the men, the drug trial was a complete washout. A few patients experienced mild side effects— anxiety, nausea, dizziness, increased urination, chills, headache—but these went away within two days of stopping the drug.

Yohimbine was most effective, these researchers found, in younger men with mild sexual problems of recent duration—80 percent of the patients who said they'd been impotent less than two years got better on yohimbine. Also, it worked better on patients with normal blood flow into the penile arteries and normal testosterone levels.

These researchers suggest that in men with performance anxiety—perhaps the most common cause of psychogenic impotence—the drug could be used to restore a man's sexual confidence, then gradually withdrawn. In fact, one man needed only a month of treatment before he was back to his old tricks.

How Does It Work?

It's still unclear exactly how the stuff works, when it does work. Some investigators think it acts directly on the central nervous system, and others, through complex hormonal pathways. One mystery: It's known that yohimbine clears out of the blood 35 minutes after it's taken, yet most studies have shown that men usually don't notice any improvement until they've taken the drug for two to three weeks. Some researchers feel this suggests it's not yohimbine itself that's doing the trick—it's some metabolite, or breakdown product, that forms in the blood while yohimbine is being digested.

Just to clarify here: *Yohimbe* is the name of a mild-mannered over-the-counter product made from the bark of the yohimbe tree. It's sold in health food stores and elsewhere, often in pill or capsule form, in potencies ranging from 500 to 750 milligrams. But pharmaceutical yohimbine (yohimbine hydrochloride, or yohimbine HCl) is the active ingredient in the bark—extracted and refined to a purity greater than 99 percent. The research studies described here all used pharmaceutical yohimbine, generally available in 5.4-milligram tablets and sold under the brand names Yocon, Yohimex, Aphrodyne or others. The drug ranges in price up to $40 for 100 tablets.

According to a survey conducted by *Men's Health Newsletter,* the potencies— and the prices—of various mail-order yohimbe concoctions are likely to vary wildly. Even the potency of pills in the same bottle may vary. So if you're seriously interested in giving yohimbine a try, it's best to have a doctor prescribe it for you. A physician can adjust the dosage, monitor your progress and—if it doesn't work—recommend the next treatment to try.

There is one precautionary note, however: Some researchers have found that yohimbine can boost blood pressure, at least a little, in some men. In one study at Wayne State University in Detroit, for instance, researchers found that yohimbine tended to increase systolic blood pressure (that's the higher number in the blood pressure reading), although not significantly, in the men under study. It *did* significantly increase the men's heart rate, though, as well as boost blood flow in their forearms—leading the researchers to suggest that it might be useful as a treatment for *low* blood pressure in some patients. On the other hand, in another study in which 33 men were treated with the drug, researchers reported that there was no effect on blood pressure, nor were there any other side effects associated with yohimbine.

The bottom line in all this? If you're going to try yohimbine, and you're prone to high blood pressure, you need to keep an eye on your pressure—and quit taking the drug if it goes up.

INDEX

Stefan Bechtel is the former executive editor of *Men's Health* magazine and a former senior editor of *Prevention*. His articles on health, sexuality and psychology have appeared in *Esquire, Reader's Digest* and other national magazines.